+RC569.5 .F3 C35 1984

Nursing Care of Victims of Family Violence

RC 569.5 F3 C35 1984

Campbell, Jacquelyn.

Nursing care of victims of family violence

Nursing Care
of Victims of Family Violence

Jacquelyn Campbell, *M.S., R.N.*
Janice Humphreys, *M.S., R.N., C.*

RESTON PUBLISHING COMPANY, INC.
A Prentice-Hall Company
Reston, Virginia

Library of Congress Cataloging in Publication Data

Nursing care of victims of family violence.

   Includes index.
   1. Family violence. 2. Nursing. I. Campbell, Jacquelyn. II. Humphreys, Janice. [DNLM: 1. Nursing care. 2. Child abuse—Nursing texts. 3. Spouse abuse—Nursing texts. 4. Violence—Nursing texts. 5. Family—Nursing texts. WY 150 C188n]
RC569.5.F3N87   1984   362.8′283   83-13979
ISBN 0-8359-5042-5

Copyright 1984 by
Reston Publishing Company, Inc.
A Prentice-Hall Company
11480 Sunset Hills Road
Reston, Virginia   22090

All rights reserved. No part of this book may be reproduced in any way, or by any means, without permission in writing from the publisher.

10   9   8   7   6   5   4   3   2   1

Printed in the United States of America

To Lewis, Christy, Brad and my parents for their support
and love   J.C.

To my mother, my father and Bill for their unwavering
love and belief in me   J.H.

To Mary Denyes
for her generous sharing of self, scholarly guidance
and friendship   J.C. & J.H.

About the Authors

Jacquelyn Campbell, MS, RN is a full time doctoral student at the University of Rochester School of Nursing. She will build upon former research on violence against women by investigating the strengths of battered women in her dissertation research. For three years she provided nursing interventions to battered women in shelters and as a member of the board of directors of an inner city shelter and a tri-county domestic violence coalition. Formerly an assistant professor at Wayne State University College of Nursing, she also has extensive experience and involvement in community health nursing and nursing education.

Janice C. Humphreys, MS, RN, C is presently a full time Ph.D. student in nursing at Wayne State University. She is an American Nurses' Association certified pediatric nurse practitioner with nursing experience in hospital inpatient, health maintenance organization, and public health settings. She is also first vice chairperson of the board of management of Interim House, the largest battered women's shelter in the United States, and has provided nursing care to its residents since its opening. As a former faculty member of Wayne State University, she and Ms. Campbell developed and taught the first undergraduate course in the College of Nursing on violence in families.

James D. Bannon, Ph.D. is currently executive deputy chief of the Detroit Police Department. He is nationally known for his research, publications, and lectures in the area of domestic violence. He presently serves as the chairperson of the State of Michigan's Domestic Violence Prevention and Treatment Board.

About the Authors

Sara Barrett, BA, RN is pursuing her Ph.D. in sociology with a minor in gerontological nursing at Wayne State University, Detroit, Michigan. She has research experience in the areas of domestic abuse and criminal victimization of the elderly as well as working with newborns who have been abused or are at high risk for being abused.

Ann Wolbert Burgess, Ph.D., RN is currently the van Ameringen professor of psychiatric nursing at the University of Pennsylvania. She is nationally known for her research and publications on the sexual victimization of children, the responses of women who have been raped, and nursing interventions with rape victims.

William O. Humphreys, JD is a graduate of the University of California, Los Angeles, Western State University College of Law, Fullerton, and currently is a practicing attorney in southern California. In addition to his experience with the Orange County American Civil Liberties Union, employment, and sex discrimination litigation, he is currently providing legal information to battered women in the nation's second largest shelter.

Isaiah McKinnon, Ph.D. is a veteran with 18 years of experience with the Detroit Police Department. He is currently the commanding officer of the Tactical Services Section and assistant professor at Mercy College of Detroit. In addition to his three years experience both as commanding officer of the Sex Crimes Unit and commanding officer of the Youth Section, he is the author of articles in the areas of rape and child abuse.

Susan Blanch Meister, Ph.D., RN is a research associate in health policy at the Division of Health Policy Research and Education, Harvard Medical School, conducting research on families and health. She received an American Nurses' Foundation Extramural Grant as an American Journal of Nursing Company Scholar in 1981 and a Distinguished Alumni Award from Loyola University in 1982.

Joyce Underwood Munro, JD has been a staff attorney with the Juvenile Defender Office in Detroit, Michigan since 1977, representing abused, neglected, and delinquent children in Wayne County Juvenile Court. Her special area of interest is failure-to-thrive infants and children suffering from psychosocial short stature.

Mary C. Sengstock, Ph.D. is a professor of sociology at Wayne State University. She is associated with the university's Institute of Gerontology, where she is conducting research on domestic abuse of the aged. Other areas of completed research include criminal victimization, spouse abuse, and social services for victims of domestic violence.

About the Authors

Bonnie Westra, MSN, RN is a founding member of the Women's Shelter, Rochester, Minnesota, and has extensive experience working in battered women's shelters providing counseling and support groups for battered women and their children. She conducted research on identifying problems encountered by children from violent homes where women were abused, and has published and presented the findings in multiple forums.

Contents

Foreword   xvii
Preface   xix

1 Introduction: Nursing and Family Violence   1
By J. Humphreys and J. Campbell

The Scope of Family Violence   3
Family Violence As a Health Problem   3
Relevance to Nursing   4
Present Economics Necessitating Increased Role for Nursing   5
The Nurse As Coordinator of Care   6
The Need for Nursing Research   7
Theoretical Frameworks   8
Unit of Focus: Family Functioning   8
Family Violence From a Nursing Perspective: Prevention   9
Review of Book Contents   10
Summary   10

2 Theories of Violence   13
By J. Campbell

Concept Analysis   14
Historical Background   16
Theoretical Frameworks Explaining Violence   17

The Biological Perspective   17
Psychological Theories of Violence   24
Sociological Forces Affecting Violence   32
Insights From Anthropology   38
Summary   41

3   Family Well-Being   53
By S. Meister

The Concept of Family Well-Being   54
Family As a Convoy of Relationships   56
Family Contributions To Aggregate and Individual Needs   60
Family Well-Being: Definitions and Issues   65
Links Between the Construct of Family Well-Being and Violence   67
Summary   69

4   Abuse of Female Partners   74
By J. Campbell

The Parameters of Abuse of Female Partners   75
Historical Perspective   81
Theoretical Frameworks   84
Summary   108

5   Child Abuse   119
By J. Humphreys

Scope   120
Definition of Child Abuse and Neglect   123
Historical Background on the Maltreatment of Children   125
Culture and Child Maltreatment   127
Child Protection in the United States   128
Theoretical Frameworks   129
Patterns of Behavior   136
Summary   138

6	**Domestic Abuse of the Elderly**	**145**
	By M. Sengstock and S. Barrett	

Characteristics and Frequency of Domestic Abuse of the Aged   147
Characteristics of Abused and Abusers   151
Proposed Causes of Elder Abuse   156
Means Used by Agencies in Identifying and Serving Abused Aged   168
Suggested Nursing Care For Elder Abuse Victims   173
Summary   183

7	**Intra-familial Sexual Abuse**	**189**
	By A. Burgess	

Forms of Intra-familial Sexual Abuse   191
Theoretical Frameworks of Causation   194
Patterns of Victim Response   201
Summary   211

8	**Nursing Care of Families Using Violence**	**216**
	By J. Campbell	

The Family As a Violence-Producing Institution   218
The Intergenerational Transmission of Violence   218
The Connections Between Wife Abuse and Child Abuse   219
Assessment   220
Planning   228
Nursing Intervention   229
Evaluation   238
Sample Nursing Process   239
Summary   239

9	**Nursing Care of Abused Women**	**246**
	By J. Campbell	

Approaching the Battered Woman   247
Assessment   249
Planning   257

Nursing Intervention 258
Evaluation 273
Sample Nursing Process 274
Summary 275

10 Nursing Care of Abused Children 281
By J. Humphreys

Self Awareness 282
Assessment 283
Planning 291
Nursing Intervention 292
Evaluation 305
Sample Nursing Process 305
Summary 306

11 Nursing Care of Children of Violent Families 315
By B. Westra

Incidence 316
Social Learning Theory 316
Children of Battered Women 317
Identification of Children of Violent Families 318
High-Risk Characteristics 318
Assessment Techniques 321
Planning 328
Nursing Intervention 328
Evaluation 335
Summary 336

12 The Nurse and the Police: Dealing With Abused Women 340
By J. Bannon

Introduction 341
Scope of the Problem 341
Historical Background 343
Interface with Nursing 354
Summary 357

13 The Nurse and the Police: Dealing With Abused Children 359
By I. McKinnon

Overview 360
Definition of Child Abuse and Neglect 361
Variations of Definitions 361
Reporting Child Abuse and Neglect 361
Protective Services 362
Law Enforcement Involvement 362
The Patrol Officer 363
Investigation 363
Sexual Abuse 365
Interface with Nursing 366
The Detection of Child Abuse 367
Gathering Evidence 367
Arrest 368
Summary 369

14 The Nurse and the Legal System: Dealing With Abused Women 370
By W. Humphreys

The Legal Concept of Wife Abuse 371
The Laws and the Abused Woman 372
The Abused Wife in the Legal System 374
New Beliefs, Better Understandings 375
The Nurse in the Legal System 378
Summary 381

15 The Nurse and the Legal System: Dealing With Abused Children 384
By J. Munro

The Legal Concept of Child Abuse 385
Infanticide and the Law 385
Corporal Punishment 387
The Modern Idea of Child Abuse 388
The Law and Violent Families 389
Interaction Between Nursing and the Legal System 393
Summary 401

16	**Implications for Nursing** 403
	By J. Humphreys

Nursing Conceptual Model of Family Violence 404
Nursing Theory and Family Violence 406
Nursing Research and Family Violence 409
Nursing Practice 411
Nursing Education and Family Violence 413
Course Description 415
Summary 417

Selected References 419

Theories of Violence and Aggression 419
Abuse of Female Partners 425
Child Abuse 430
Sexual Abuse 433
Elderly Abuse 434

Index 436

Foreword

The increased evidence of violence in our society is a serious concern for all persons. Violence within the home is seldom presented to the public until a dramatic incident such as a reported death or a seriously damaged victim is identified. Public reaction is thus apt to be directed against the accused and so remains an aberration rather than a social concern. Yet the accumulated data present a picture of a need to address the problems. Research in all areas of family violence remains a critical need as evident in the authors' summary.

Nursing Care of Victims of Family Violence is a book directed toward nurses with documentation of the scope of the problem as indicated by current statistical evidence and with direction for nurses who are in positions within the health care delivery system to address individual and family care. There is also a clear message that nurses can serve as advocates for social change. Increased consciousness raising through knowledge of the problem is a first step, but continued attention through use of nursing histories and assessment can serve to clarify family actions and behaviors that may be predictors of violence or abuse.

It is evident that nurses have many points of entry into the health care delivery system. Nurses are found throughout the community in community health programs, ambulatory clinics, emergency rooms, acute care settings, nursing homes, school health programs, community mental health centers, nurse clinics, home health care programs and physicians' offices. Nurses have noted the victims of abuse. Earlier studies of child abuse including incest are now augmented by studies of spouse abuse, most often women as victims, and of violence against the elderly. Early presentation of health problems that may be a result of suspected abuse can be identified. Nurses in all settings need more information and programs directed at assessment and planned intervention prior to the increased violence. Violence and abuse within family settings tend to escalate in intensity and in frequency. Violence within the family seldom remains directed at a single victim.

Early identification is a high priority for health care intervention. Nurses by nature of their positions may well be gatekeepers for many victims and for deeply troubled families. The holistic approach of this presentation in *Nursing Care of Victims of Family Violence* by nurse clinicians and scholars is an outstanding effort to provide direction for nurses and to the nursing profession.

The authors have sought nurses who have participated in research and in development of health care programs for victims of abuse. In addition, they have sought the assistance of a sociologist concerned with abuse of the elderly, leaders in the criminal justice system who have long had to cope with the end results of family violence and with attorneys who have experience with the prosecution of aggressors or the protection of the victims.

The topics are not easy to address. The personalized responses to the victims and to the aggressors are often barriers for health professionals and for others. The evidence of assault and violence often evokes revulsion and anger. The identified tendency of the victims to conceal the abuse and to protect the aggressor is difficult for caretakers to accept or understand. Such responses decrease the potential for rational long-term commitment to planned change. One has to find a balance between coping with situations of today while advancing programs to resolve the larger health and social issues.

Nursing Care of Victims of Family Violence is a book that addresses the needs of current families and the needs for future direction. All persons who have been involved in family abuse situations give credence to the belief that the incidence is far greater than the recorded statistical data. The need for research in all areas of family violence is clearly underscored. Nurses and other health care professionals do need to work with other personnel to address the larger health and social issues. Interdisciplinary investigations are essential to local and national programs aimed at reduction of family violence.

The book offers a challenge to the nursing profession to become accountable in health care for a special population group whose health needs are clearly holistic. One cannot simply nurse the physical evidence of abuse. One must address family or group health as well as the physical and psychological health of the victim.

Lorene R. Fischer
Professor and Dean
Wayne State University
College of Nursing
Detroit, Michigan

Preface

This book evolved out of our clinical nursing practice with victims of family violence and development of a senior undergraduate nursing course addressing the same concern. A number of people and ideas that we felt the need to attend to could no where else be discussed. We choose to deal with them now.

We jointly made the decision to refer to *the nurse* as *she*. We acknowledge that an ever enlarging percentage of nurses are males. The reality, however, continues to be that the majority of nurses are female. We refer to the nurse as she not without recognition of our male colleagues, but rather as an effort to facilitate the flow of reading.

For the existence of this text we owe a great many thanks.

To our many friends and colleagues who provided support and indulgence.

To Julie Ploshenanski for patience, interest and skillful typing of the manuscript.

To Beth Elderd and Shelley Gelbert for their advice, tolerance and editorial assistance.

To Rose Odum for constructive, knowledgeable review.

To our students who have challenged us to grow.

To the faculty and staff of the College of Nursing, Wayne State University for their high standards, encouragement of our work, and constant interest.

To Susan Venters and the women of Shelter for their evocative poetry.

To the battered women and children who freely shared their problems and concerns.

To the profession of nursing for providing an opportunity to care about the needs of other human beings.

To each other for continuing friendship, and sharing of ideas.

Introduction: Nursing and Family Violence

Janice Humphreys and *Jacquelyn Campbell*

> heartless
> is the cold empty carcass
> of a world
> once full of love
> we must go back
> to the time of the female
> eons
> and
> eons
> ago
> back to caress
> of the great mother
> nurture and care we need
> she's calling
>
>   Susan Venters

Reprinted from *Every Twelve Seconds*, compiled by Susan Venters (Hillsboro, Oregon: Shelter, 1981) by permission of the author.

A woman enters the emergency room with facial bruises and severe abdominal pain. She is asked perfunctorily how her injuries occurred, and she mumbles that she fell down a flight of stairs. Her male companion glowers in the doorway of the cubicle. The nurse firmly asks him to wait outside and gently proceeds with obtaining a detailed history from the woman, including assessment for family violence. In another part of the hospital, a newly postpartum battered mother in the obstetrical unit fears going home and does not know where to go. Her primary care nurse helps arrange her discharge directly to a wife abuse shelter. A fourteen-year-old daughter of a woman who has five other children is being seen in the outpatient clinic with her mother. The mother voices the concern, "I don't want to have to 'do time' for what I might do to her." Mother and daughter are counseled by the nurse.

These are three illustrations of the multitude of possible interfaces of nursing and family violence. Family violence is a significant health problem, widespread in American society. "A person is more likely to be hit or killed in his or her home by another family member than anywhere else or by anyone else."[1] Nursing has an important role to play in the prevention, detection, treatment, and scholarly investigation of this health concern.

A violent act is one of physical force which results in injury or abuse to the recipient.[2] Within the family, violence can be directed toward any member by another and can include sexual acts as well as other forms of physical aggression. No matter if the violent action is perpetrated by the father against the mother, the mother against the child, or the adolescent against the grandfather, violence in the family is a profound event that affects the whole family. To look at wife abuse, child abuse, or abuse of elderly family members in isolation is to see only a portion of the effects of violence in American families. The problem needs to be addressed in its totality in order to see the full picture with all its ramifications.

All the clients in the introductory examples are "victims" of family violence in that they are "subjected to oppression, deprivation or suffering" within violent families, whether or not they are the actual recipients of the aggressive acts.[3] At the same time, the philosophy of this text is that these people and their family units have significant strengths upon which appropriate nursing care will build. The other basic assumptions of the book are that nursing care of victims of family violence takes into account the whole family, is based upon a firm theoretical foundation, and can be a significant force in all levels of prevention of this problem. The major purpose of the book is to integrate nursing practice in family violence with existing theory and research. The need for increased nursing theoretical development and nursing research in this area is also a consistent theme.

THE SCOPE OF FAMILY VIOLENCE

Estimates of the amount of violence within families in the United States vary widely. Definitions of abuse and methods of reporting differ significantly from community to community, and it is generally recognized that official reports of family violence only scratch the surface and especially underestimate prevalence in middle-class homes. Probably the most reliable national figures are derived from the nationally representative sample of 2,143 individual family members responding to a self-report survey conducted by Murray Straus, Richard J. Gelles, and Suzanne K. Steinmetz in 1976.[4] The investigators reported an incidence of 3.8 percent of American children, aged three to seventeen years, as being abused each year. When projected to the 46 million children of this age group who lived with both parents during the study period, the percentage translates to 1.5 to 2 million children being abused by their parents, not including those under three years old and/or living with a single parent. The same study revealed that 3.8 percent of the wives reported violence from their husbands serious enough to be considered abuse, which results in a 1.8 million battered women figure, without incorporating women in cohabitating relationships but not married.

Sexual abuse within the family, violence toward elderly family members, and physical aggression by adolescents toward other family members were not measured by the Straus, Gelles, and Steinmetz study. Each of these forms of family violence constitute significant health problems in and of themselves, and the prevalence rates are just beginning to be estimated. To begin to conceptualize the extent of the phenomenon in everyday language, it is noteworthy that wife abuse is more prevalent than rape by a stranger and child abuse is more common than chicken pox.

There is evidence to suggest that violence in the American home has always been common.[5] Certainly women, children, and the elderly have long been subjected to maltreatment by the dominant male head of household. Whether or not the incidence is currently rising is somewhat controversial. More child and wife abuse is being reported and recognized than ever before, but this may be as much because of increased awareness of the problem as actual increase in cases. Abuse of the elderly is just beginning to be recognized as a health problem so that where almost no cases were officially recognized before, case finding is now being pursued vigorously, and the numbers will undoubtedly rise dramatically.

FAMILY VIOLENCE AS A HEALTH PROBLEM

Seventeen percent of Kentucky housewives who were battered used hospital emergency services for treatment of injuries as reported by a 1979 Harris poll.[6] Based on this figure, approximately 1 million battered women would be seen in an emergency room each year nationally.[7] Evan Stark et al. estimate that more than one in four visits by women to emergency services at an urban hospital were made by battered women.[8] R. Emerson Dobash and Russell Dobash report that in their sample of 109 abused women, 80 percent had sought medical attention for their injuries at least once.[9] As Stark and her associates state:

> Battered women comprise a significant percentage of rape victims, suicide attempts, psychiatric patients, mothers of abused children, alcoholics, and women who miscarry or abort. Finally . . . battered women make multiple visits to the medical and psychiatric service for general health problems that are as much a part of the battering syndrome as physical injury but are not recognized as related to assault.[10]

Similarly, abused children, adolescents, and elderly family members are frequently seen in health care settings. Even when the presenting problem is not directly the result of physical aggression, the family violence must be considered in a holistic assessment. In addition, the entire family should be taken into account in the health care provided, extending the problem significantly.

RELEVANCE TO NURSING

The definition of nursing given by the American Nurses Association in its Social Policy Statement is, "the diagnosis and treatment of human responses to actual or potential health problems."[11] Nursing care of victims of family violence fits well within the scope of this definition and thereby includes the prevention of family violence as well as detection and treatment.

Nursing from the time of Nightingale has been concerned with the individual, the family, and the community. Professional nurses develop a plan of care only after thorough consideration of the client's community. In turn, nursing as a profession must adapt to the ever-changing needs of the community and society. For example, if violence in the family is common and may be on the increase, then the professional nurse must alter the process by which she develops, initiates, and evaluates her care to include the likelihood of violence in families. The actual and potential alterations in individual and family health that are associated with violence are immense, complex, and in need of nursing consideration if maximum levels of wellness are to be achieved. Stress on the family is a major contributing factor to the occurrence of violence in families. The professional nurse, aware of this influence and practicing in an area of increasing unemployment, would be remiss if she failed to consider and adapt to the increased potential for family violence when conducting her assessment.

The mere awareness of the problem of family violence is not enough. Nurses need to act as client advocates. In the case of family violence, the nurse may begin by educating other professionals as to the dynamics of the problem. For instance, she may help the many other people who become involved in a case of child abuse to understand that an incident of physical harm done to a dependent child by a parent is really just an isolated act in the interactions of a complex family unit.

Nursing is furthermore in an excellent position to prevent, identify, or intervene

Introduction: Nursing and Family Violence

against family violence. In hospitals nurses may administer nursing care to patients with a wide range of needs related to potential or actual family violence (such as the teenage boy with a gunshot wound, the infant who has been abandoned, and the chronically ill elderly woman who is preparing to move in with her daughter's family.) Mental health and obstetrical inpatient units are also areas where patient needs arising out of violence can be found if nurses know how to look for them. Client advocacy, in the clinic and community as well as the hospital, involves active searching for victims and attention to prevention, as well as education and direct intervention.

The professional nurse has always had as her primary focus the client rather than "the problem." Such a focus allows the nurse to be perceived as more helping and better prepared to assist clients who experience family violence than many other professionals. Nursing's ability "to conceptualize the familial and social context of problems of violence" has recently been identified by other health professionals as well.[12]

Because of their sheer numbers, variety of practice locations, and client needs, and in particular the nature of their practice, nurses are in an ideal position to take action to decrease the likelihood of family violence and mitigate its effects. Nurses provide care to families in more settings than probably any other health care provider. Nurses see family members in the hospital clinic, school, community, and in private practice. They have traditionally provided care to whole families even though the initial request for care may have come from an individual. The nurse routinely includes information about the individual's family, culture, and health attitudes and practices when doing an assessment. She is frequently seen as help by families when they can trust no other health professional.[13]

PRESENT ECONOMICS NECESSITATING INCREASED ROLE FOR NURSING

The economic recession of the 1980s is associated with factors that contribute to the concern the nurse must have about family violence. In many areas of the country unemployment rates of well over 10 percent have been in existence for several years. Inflation further decreases the value of the little money people do have. As jobs are increasingly difficult to find, expenses rise faster than income, and stress on families builds. For many families the 1980s bring with them a first-time dependence upon social service agencies. Families who had previously functioned independently are now experiencing great difficulty. It is an ultimate irony that just when the need for social service resources is increasing many federal, state, and local service agencies are being subjected to the most severe cutbacks or complete elimination. This includes many programs directed against intrafamily abuse. Again, a discrepancy exists; numbers of families in need of social services are increasing; social services available are decreasing.

The loss of social service programs affects the potentially violent family in a variety of ways. Initially the family may experience some general difficulty in its functioning and may wish to seek counseling. Such a family therapy program could prevent family violence by assisting the family to identify alternative methods of functioning. If no family counseling programs are available or easily accessible the potentially violent family must do without. The next need for social service agency assistance may occur with a father's indefinite layoff from his job. At this point numerous social agencies become involved with the family. Limited income and assistance become available to the family through unemployment compensation, food stamps, and possibly other social service programs, but usually case workers have too many families to address general family issues. The stress on the family and its individual members, however, increases. The earlier problem of family functioning continues to grow. Violence may occur at any time in some families under severe stress. When it does occur, as in the case of child abuse, the professional must report the harmful act. Here again a discrepancy exists in that child abuse must, by law, be reported. The appropriate reporting agency is in the Department of Social Services which may have known the family much earlier, before the violence had occurred, if the resources had not been eliminated due to economic cutbacks.

The nurse has contact with families as a whole or through individual members, for a variety of reasons. She has been educated to provide nursing care in a manner that is generally perceived by the client and family as helpful rather than bureaucratic or authoritative. Clinical practice takes a nurse into the homes and lives of families in a confidential and intimate way. The nurse sees and cares for families in a manner unique to the profession at a time when they may trust no one else, when they are violent. The trust of the nurse-client or nurse-family relationship engenders an ideal opportunity for exploring these issues. The current lack of other resources has curtailed appropriate referral agencies, so the nurse must frequently take the responsibility for initiating care. The nurse then needs to be familiar with the knowledge to date on family violence, apply nursing theoretical frameworks to the problem, and be able to carry out appropriate nursing interventions and evaluation.

THE NURSE AS COORDINATOR OF CARE

The problem of family violence is multidimensional. The professional nurse cannot be expected to meet the needs of every member of a violent family in every respect without help. Rather, violent families require a broad range of interventions and teamwork. Many other professionals are likely to have contact with the members of the violent family. Social workers, physicians, lawyers, police officers, and dentists all may be involved in their own form of intervention with the violent family. According to Eli H. Newberger, a physician, the necessary involvement of professionals from different backgrounds can result in difficulties. "Each professional does what he or she can, within the ethical definition of his domain. Yet the family and its individual members can be harmed—not helped—by these well-intended, independent actions."[14] It is thus necessary that one professional serve as a coordinator of these varied interventions. The professional nurse is in a prime position in many instances to initiate, coordinate, and evaluate the multidisciplinary approach to the care of violent families. She is in a much less threatening position to elicit information from a battered woman or abusing parent and to make sure that the individual client and/or family has the paramount role in decision making beyond what the law requires. When the setting, agency, family, or situation indicates that another professional would be better suited as coordinator, the nurse, when well informed and aware, is still an integral member of the team. This book is designed to give the nurse the necessary background to understand, identify, assess, coordinate care of, and provide interventions for potential and actual victims of family violence.

THE NEED FOR NURSING RESEARCH

A major problem exists in attempting to apply the nursing process to family violence; nursing has a limited knowledge base in this area. It has been left to other disciplines to conduct the majority of analysis and study. There are recent and noteworthy exceptions to this lack, but the dearth of nursing contributions is particularly unfortunate when the potential role for nursing in decreasing family violence is reconsidered.

Law enforcement and social work are two such professions which have contributed extensively to what is known about family violence from their particular perspectives,[15] and literature from these fields describes extensive problems that exist for those who work with family violence. Executive Deputy Police Chief James Bannon reports that the individual who is most likely to be called upon in a case of "domestic violence" is himself the epitome of violence and machismo, the police officer.[16] In their training, however, police officers receive only minimal instruction in conflict intervention.[17] Surely leaving family violence completely to the police is unsatisfactory to both law enforcement and nursing professionals. Social workers, mainly because of staggering case loads and the complexities of the problems, have been severely criticized for well-publicized dramatic failures in handling child abuse cases leading to severe injuries or death of a few children.[18] The "ideology and supporting theories of the social work profession . . . are based fundamentally on the notions of the sanctity of the family and marriage" which can be obstructive in working with battered women.[19] Social work is certainly a key part of the solution to the problem of family violence as is a more self-aware, more sensitized law enforcement system, but nursing needs to make a better focused, more extensive contribution to the efforts being made.

Medicine is also becoming more aware of family violence and beginning to include both research and medical guidelines in its literature. However, the main emphasis is on physical symptomatology to alert physicians to the presence of family violence.[20] The medical model generally leads to assumptions of pathology in victims as well as perpetrators, and treatment recommendations are usually in terms of psychiatric care. A nursing perspective would appropriately emphasize the healthy aspects of the families experiencing violence, an approach well supported by actual research on victims.[21]

Law enforcement, social work, medicine, and, to date, nursing have generally based interventions with families experiencing violence on the research carried out by sociology and psychology scholars in the field. There are problematic biases in this literature as well as inadequate theory building.[22] In addition, there is the familiar problem of adapting the information to a uniquely nursing framework and finally to practice. Nursing does have literature of its own on the subject of family violence, which fortunately is increasing. Original nursing research has been included as much as possible in this book, and the Bibliography at the end of the text can be used for additional nursing references. However, a discrepancy exists between the potential magnitude of the role of nursing in the care of violent families and the amount of nursing knowledge and research available. Family violence is an appropriate area for nursing research as it involves the person (family), the environment, health, nursing, and their interrelatedness.[23] Suggested specific areas for nursing research are given in the final chapter.

Dobash and Dobash, leading theorists in the field of wife abuse, have developed "a form of analysis that established the linkages between contemporary and historical processes and interrelated interactional, institutional, and cultural aspects of the problem."[24] Jo Ann Ashley, nurse historian, has also insisted that nurses should be cognizant of history and societal influences when analyzing health problems.[25] This text will continue in this pattern, looking at the roots of the problem of violence and its cultural and structural supports as well as the more traditional physical, social, and psychological nursing approaches in developing and discussing theoretical frameworks.

UNIT OF FOCUS: FAMILY FUNCTIONING

The purpose of this book is to address the nursing care of victims of family violence, including victims of child abuse, wife abuse, and abuse of the elderly. As can be seen from this statement, violence will be examined as an indicator of family needs and issues. Often abuse of a family member is viewed as an isolated interaction involving at the most the victim and the perpetrator. As will be shown, every violent act within a family affects each of its members. The family and its functioning are the major unit of focus.

The concept of family well-being, as described by Susan Meister in Chapter 3, will be used in this text as a comprehensive and flexible construct within which current knowledge about families can be organized and applied to violent families. This conceptualization is consistent with the

THEORETICAL FRAMEWORKS

The professional nurse in practice requires a theoretical basis upon which to develop her plan of care. Nursing care of victims of family violence requires the same theoretical base. An attempt has been made to include the majority of pertinent theories in each area of abuse of a family member. Further, the current conflicts of opinion in the particular area of abuse are discussed. Whenever possible a usable nursing approach has been synthesized.

emphasis on determining and building upon the strengths of families and their members in designing nursing care which addresses family violence.

If the violent family is to be the major focus of the present work, it is necessary to examine the consequences of violence on each family member. Literature on child abuse is far more extensive than that on abuse of any other family member. The present text will include violence against children, and the facets less commonly discussed, abuse of women and the elderly, and the effects of violence in the home on all the children. The kind of abuse perpetrated against all family members is not limited to physical violence. Sexual abuse, emotional abuse, incest, and neglect are discussed where appropriate.

FAMILY VIOLENCE FROM A NURSING PERSPECTIVE: PREVENTION

The attempt is made in this book to present care of violent families in a manner heretofore not found, a nursing perspective. The nursing care of violent families will be presented from a holistic, preventive standpoint. First, holism requires that the nurse be concerned with any factor which affects the client's health. Second, prevention has long been "the heart of community health nursing."[26] It therefore seems appropriate to present the nursing care of a problem that involves families and the community in such a manner.

Some confusion exists as to what is meant by "levels of prevention." For the purpose of the present text levels of prevention are used as defined by Sherry L. Shamansky and Cherie L. Clausen.[27] Briefly, *"primary prevention* is prevention in the true sense of the word; it precedes disease or dysfunction and is applied to a generally healthy population. It does not require identification of a problem and may be a generalized enhancement of overall health approach or be specifically aimed at a particular health problem."[28] "The purpose is to decrease the vulnerability of the individual to illness or dysfunction. Health promotion encourages optimum health and personality development to strengthen the individual's capacity to withstand physical and emotional stressors."[29] Primary prevention takes place before dysfunction exists; however, it may involve interventions with individuals or families who are considered "at risk."

Secondary prevention occurs when some kind of disease or dysfunction has been identified or is suspected. "Secondary prevention emphasizes early diagnosis and prompt intervention to halt the pathological process, thereby shortening its duration and severity and enabling the individual to regain normal functioning at the earliest possible point."[30] Secondary prevention includes screening programs, problem identification, and treatment which attempts to decrease the severity of impact of a problem.

Finally, *"tertiary prevention* comes into play when a defect or disability is fixed, stabilized, or irreversible. Rehabilitation, the goal of tertiary prevention, is more than halting the disease process itself; it is restoring the individual to an optimum level of functioning within the constraints of the disability."[31]

The application of each level of prevention in the nursing care of abused women, abused children, and the abused elderly can be found in the appropriate subsequent chapters.

REVIEW OF BOOK CONTENTS

The present text attempts to provide the professional nurse with information needed so that she can more confidently and successfully provide nursing care to violent families. By virtue of the contribution of chapters by several different authors of diverse backgrounds, certain variations exist in the format of individual sections. Each chapter is relevant to the overall text theme, theory, research, and practice in nursing care of victims of family violence. The differing perspectives on violence in the family offer the reader valuable assistance in viewing the central issues from multiple stylistic as well as cognitive perspectives. The attempt has been to provide a text wherein the overall result is a unique presentation which is comprehensive, informative, and thought-provoking.

The reality of the nature of nursing practice results in nurses who are, more often than not, specialists in one or more areas. Family violence, in contrast, can occur in any family member, of any age, in any stage of development or wellness state. In an effort to provide both a generalist nursing approach and a text from which a nurse can select certain relevant sections, each chapter is designed to thoroughly address its topic and may briefly restate discussions found in other chapters.

The book has been divided into two main sections, the first presenting essentially the theory components of family violence (Chapters 2 through 7), and the second the clinical application of theory (Chapters 8 through 15). The second section has been subdivided into four chapters approaching nursing care from the perspective of professional nursing (Chapters 8 through 11) and four written by law enforcement and legal professionals (Chapters 12 through 15). Nursing is well versed in the need for collaboration with other disciplines in its approach to most health problems. However, the interface of nursing with law enforcement and the legal profession in regards to family violence is an unexplored area which these chapters address. The final chapter provides a look to the future and examination of nursing education and research implications in the area.

Summary

Violence in the American family is common and a health problem of possibly increasing magnitude. Violence occurs against all family members and is an indicator of complex family needs and issues. Nursing is in an excellent position to be actively involved with other professionals by initiating, coordinating, and evaluating the multidisciplinary approach to violent families, but has a limited knowledge base about family violence. The current text attempts to provide knowledge to nurses in a format which bases suggested nursing interventions on existing theories and research about families and violence, extends nursing care to all members of violent families and all forms of family violence, and emphasizes the strengths and health potential of victims and families so that nursing can be an important part of the prevention of this major health concern.

Introduction: Nursing and Family Violence

Chapter 1

1. Richard J. Gelles and Murray A. Straus, "Violence in the American Family," *Journal of Social Issues* 35, No. 2 (1979): 15.
2. *Webster's Third New International Dictionary*, s.v. "violence."
3. Ibid., s.v. "victim."
4. Murray A. Straus, Richard J. Gelles, and Suzanne K. Steinmetz, *Behind Closed Doors: Violence in the American Family* (Garden City, N.Y. Doubleday, 1980).
5. Richard J. Gelles and Murray A. Straus, "Violence in the American Family," p. 16.
6. Louis Harris, *A Survey of Spousal Violence Against Women in Kentucky* (Frankfort, Ky.: Kentucky Commission of Women, 1979).
7. Evan Stark et al., *Wife Abuse in the Medical Setting* (Rockvile, Md.: National Clearinghouse on Domestic Violence, 1981), p. v.
8. Ibid.
9. R. Emerson Dobash and Russell Dobash, *Violence Against Wives* (New York: The Free Press, 1979).
10. Stark et al., *Wife Abuse in the Medical Setting*, p. v.
11. American Nurses Association, *Nursing: A Social Policy Statement* (Kansas City, Mo.: American Nurses Association, 1980).
12. Eli H. Newberger and Richard Bourne, "The Medicalization and Legalization of Child Abuse," *American Journal of Orthopsychiatry* 48 (October 1978): 604.
13. Elaine Hiberman and Kit Munson, "Sixty Battered Women," *Victimology: An International Journal* 2 (1978): 469.
14. Eli H. Newberger, "A Physician's Perspective on the Interdisciplinary Management of Child Abuse," *Psychiatric Opinion*, 13 No. 2 (April 1976): 15.
15. David G. Gil, "Violence Against Children," *Journal of Marriage and the Family* 32 No. 11 (November 1971): 637-48.

James Bannon, "Law Enforcement Problems with Intra-Family Violence" (Paper presented at the Academy of Criminal Justice Sciences Annual Meeting, 14 March 1981).

16. Bannon, "Law Enforcement Problems," p. 4.
17. U.S. Civil Rights Commission, Connecticut Advisory Committee. James Bannon. "Presentation on Police Difficulties with Female Battering Cases," Hearings of 26 September 1977, p. 10.
18. Jacquie Roberts, "Social Work and Child Abuse: The Reasons for Failure and the Way to Success," in *Violence and the Family*, J. P. Martin, Ed. (Chichester: John Wiley & Sons, 1978): 255-91.
19. North West Region of the National Women's Aid Federation, "Battered Women and Social Work," in *Violence and the Family*, J. P. Martin, Ed. (Chichester: John Wiley & Sons, 1978): 322.
20. Richard O'Toole, Patrick Turbett, and Claire Nalepka, "Theories, Professional Knowledge, and Diagnosis of Child Abuse," in *The Dark Side of Families*, David Finkelhor et al., eds. (Beverly Hills, Calif: Sage Publications, 1983): 360.
21. Ibid., pp. 351, 357; Laurie Wardell, Dair L. Gillespie, and Ann Leffler, "Science and Violence against Wives," in Finkelhor et al., *The Dark Side of Families*, pp. 72-78.
22. Richard J. Gelles, "Violence in the Family. A Review of Research in the Seventies," *Journal of Marriage and the Family* 42 No. 4 (November 1980), 873-885.
23. Jacqueline Fawcett, "The 'What' of Theory Development," in *Theory Development: What, Why, How?* (New York: National League for Nursing, 1978), p. 25.

24. R. Emerson Dobash and Russell P. Dobash, "Social Science and Social Action," *Journal of Family Issues* 2 (December 1981): 439-63.

25. Jo Ann Ashley, "Foundations for Scholarship: Historical Research in Nursing," *Advances in Nursing Science* 1, (October 1978): 25-36.

26. Sherry L. Shamansky and Cherie L. Clausen, "Levels of Prevention: Examination of the Concept," *Nursing Outlook* 28 (February 1980): 104.

27. Ibid., p 106.

28. Ibid.

29. Ibid.

30. Ibid.

31. Ibid.

Theories of Violence

Jacquelyn Campbell

Joanne Dewey

as a young girl i played
with my cousins
in sun lit country fields
amazons in the jungles
fearless women
brave and strong
no harm could ever come to us
in these journeys that we made
through forests fields and over mountains
across the horizon as far as we could see
sometimes we were birds
flying floating gliding free as the wind
until
we came upon a country grave yard
a picture on a grave stone
stared out from the lonely plot

oh the solemn eyes
of the dark haired spirit staring
i remembered a story
that the news papers carried
of a young girls body
found by hunters in a stream
joanne dewey murdered
raped is what they said
etched beneath the picture
in the cold marble stone
here lies joanne dewey
born 1937 died 1953
and we as young girls ran
ran for our lives
birds with broken wings
freedom left behind

Susan Venters

Reprinted from *Every Twelve Seconds*, compiled by Susan Venters (Hillsboro, Oregon: Shelter, 1981) by permission of the author.

Violence in the family cannot be fully understood without analysis of the broader picture of violence in general. Suzanne Steinmetz and Murray Straus attest that "any social pattern as widespread and enduring as violence must have fundamental and enduring causes."[1] The purpose of this chapter is to provide a holistic background of the major theoretical frameworks found in the current literature and used to explain violence in our society. Concept analysis, historical background, and a summary of the perspectives on violence from biology, psychology, sociology, and anthropology will be presented as a basis for nursing conceptualization of violence as a health problem.

One way to estimate the magnitude of the health concern that violence represents is to examine homicide statistics. In the United States homicide is the eleventh leading cause of death, the second highest cause of mortality in adolescents (age fifteen to twenty-four), and the number one reason for the death of young black men and women (age fifteen to thirty-four).[2] If nursing identifies prevention of health problems as a major area of concern, an examination of causes of violence is mandated. In order to approach the research literature on the causes of violence, an examination of the concepts involved is necessary.

CONCEPT ANALYSIS

Peggy L. Chinn and Maeona K. Jacobs emphasize the importance of concept analysis as "the beginning examination of phenomena important to the area of inquiry."[3] That is to say, what seem to be relatively simple ideas, used frequently in common language, need to be carefully scrutinized as the basis for further study. When one examines the violence literature, one is struck by the disagreement among authors about definitions of even the most frequently used terms and more importantly, the values and connotations attached to them. Is aggression bad or good? Can violence be useful in achieving moral human aspirations or is it always negative? An abbreviated concept analysis will be presented of those two most important ideas in understanding this field—aggression and violence.

Aggression

Aggression is defined in *Webster's Third New International Dictionary* as "an offensive action or procedure." The root is Latin from the word *aggressus* which means attack.[4] From these beginnings there is a wide variety of definitions used in the literature and in common usage. The viewpoint that aggression is an instinct or drive common to all human beings softens the negative connotations of the definition. Psychoanalytic perspectives allow for healthy expressions of aggression as drives for accomplishment and mastery. Modern Western culture has traditionally conceived of aggression as a healthy attribute, at least for men. The synonyms listed for the adjective form, aggressive, reflect two very different perspectives. There is on the one hand: hostile, belligerent, assailant, pugnacious, vicious, contentious, then the second group: self-assertive, forceful, bold, enterprising, energetic, zealous. The disparate definitions reflect the ambivalence about aggression in American society.

The majority of scientists studying aggression today conceptualize the behavior as less innate. A representative definition of this school of thought is K. E. Moyer's description of aggression as "overt behavior involving intent to inflict noxious stimulation or to behave destructively toward another organism."[5] These scholars include psychological injury as one of the possible results of aggression. Nursing is also beginning to address aggression in the work attempting to distinguish assertiveness from aggression. Sonja J. Herman's book, *Becoming Assertive: A Guide for Nurses*, describes aggression as getting what is wanted at the expense of others. Aggressive behavior is seen as dominating, depreciating, humiliating, and embarrassing to others while "assertion is the direct, honest, and appropriate expression of one's thoughts, feelings, opinions and beliefs ... and without infringing on the rights of others."[6] This kind of distinction seems useful and will be accepted as a basic premise of this book. Aggression will therefore be seen as destructive in intent either physically or psychologically and as infringing on the rights of others.

Violence

Aggression can be seen on a continuum with violence at the extreme end, encompassing destructive results as well as aggressive intent. Webster defines violence as the "exertion of any physical force so as to injure or abuse."[7] The word originates from the Latin *violare*, to violate, rape, injure. Consistent with the official definition and its Latin root, common associations with violence are much more negative. Sandra Haber and Bernard Seidenberg conducted a small survey in which they found the following associations included in a list elicited by the word violence: "murder, crime, gangs, men, torture, hate, uneducated, unsocialized, disgusting animals."[8] Yet we still find that much violence is socially tolerated; for instance, police violence, war, self-defense, and in some cases, riots. As Haber and Seidenberg point out, whether violence is deemed appropriate depends on the agent, the circumstances, the status of the victim, and the degree of harm inflicted. Some authors have even insisted that violence is necessary as a reflection of conflicting groups and interests in any society. Yet there are cultures that are totally nonviolent and wherein violence in any form is absolutely disallowed.[9]

American culture officially condemns violence, but it is covertly sanctioned in many ways. Violent characters are glorified on television and in books; we threaten to hurt and kill each other in jest as a constant part of common language. Marvin Wolfgang states, "When war is glorified in a nation's history and included as part of the child's educational materials, a moral judgement about the legitimacy of violence is firmly made."[10] American society is not sure if hitting a child is legitimate punishment or a form of violence. The ambivalence that we as a society have about our attitudes and values toward violence are undoubtedly reflected in our high rate of violent crime and in our problems with violence in the family.

HISTORICAL BACKGROUND

Anthropologists are uncertain as to the prevalence of violence in early civilizations. Some scholars have used the historical record to argue in favor of the inevitability of violence. For instance, Lawrence Kolb observes that "at best, only ten generations in the era of recorded history have avoided war."[11] Derek Freeman argues that peoples of peace are relatively rare in the ethnographic record and says they were usually backward and submissive to a powerful and overtly aggressive neighbor.[12] In refutation, Bronislaw Malinowski shows that wars cannot be traced back to the earliest beginnings of human culture, only to the start of written history.[13] Stanislau Andreski adds that only a small percentage of the population took part in the early wars and that people have to be indoctrinated for war.[14] As for the contention that peaceful peoples were always in the minority, we can turn to evidence that the preponderance of the peoples living in the "cradle of civilization" (Asia Minor) from approximately 9000 to 5000 B.C. were hunter-gatherers and apparently lived in a predominantly peaceful manner. For the 800 years so far explored in the excavations of the Catal Hüyük neolithic peoples, "among the many hundreds of skeletons unearthed, not a single one has been found that showed signs of violent death." Far from being backward, this culture was one of the most advanced of its time.[15]

It has often been noted that the United States has a long history of violence used as a means to achieve socially acceptable ends. The favorite period of many Americans is the era of the "old West" which is characterized as violent as much as anything else. In a survey for the National Commission on Violence, Louis Harris found that 51 percent of Americans agreed or strongly agreed with the statement: "Justice may have been a little rough and ready in the old West, but things worked better than they do today with all the legal red tape."[16] Americans also tend to romanticize our early wars and to admire the violent heroes of the past. Some scholars have correlated our fascination with the violent past with the fact that there are only four countries that have a higher homicide rate (per 100,000 population) than the United States.[17] American rates have been traditionally high in comparison to other developed nations.

Thus, historical examination of violence shows a predilection for violence amongst human beings from at least very early in civilization, but a propensity that is by no means equally distributed among cultures nor among all periods of time. Historical background gives an overview to the problem of violence, but does not illuminate causation.

THEORETICAL FRAMEWORKS EXPLAINING VIOLENCE

The theoretical frameworks that attempt to illuminate the causative factors of violence can be divided in a variety of ways. The broad categories chosen to organize this material for this text are biological, psychological, sociological, and anthropological. This review of theoretical frameworks cannot be considered exhaustive, but will indicate the problems with determining causality of problems of violence and point out some of the inconsistencies, gaps, and difficulties in the traditional theoretical field. It will also serve to underpin the theoretical information concerned with specific aspects of violence in the family.

THE BIOLOGICAL PERSPECTIVE

The biological theories of violence can be explored in two main sections: instinctivist and neurophysiological. The two frameworks, although derived from at least two very different disciplines, hold in common the idea that violence is biologically determined and both draw heavily from studies of animals (ethology).

Instinctivist

Konrad Lorenz's theory on aggression is the best known in the field. He sees aggression as a fighting instinct which is common to men and animals and serves important species preservation functions by favoring genes for strength and preventing too much population density.[18] Robert Ardrey, who also sees aggression as innate and within species, uses observations of animals to postulate that dominance and subordination are inevitable, and aggression and competition insure the genetic transmission of useful traits. He believes that humans and animals are fundamentally motivated by aggression and the acquisition and defense of territory.[19]

Much time and space has been used to refute the simplistic theories of Ardrey and Lorenz from all perspectives. Suffice it to say here that they have been criticized severely for poor scholarship, for anthropomorphizing, for equating hunting with aggression, for ignoring evidence of cultures where violence is unknown, for failing to recognize that the fighting of animals of the same species (highly ritualized, defensive, stereotyped, and seldom fatal) cannot be compared to the cruel, destructive, and attacking violence of humans, and for disregarding the evidence that the early hunting and gathering populations were predominantly peaceful.[20] It has also been found that in nonhuman primates, male aggression, territoriality, and dominance battles are a minute fraction of the total interactions, and the group cohesively strives to keep these disruptive incidents to a minimum.[21] Craig Wallace points out that there are many animals who are almost entirely passive and yet are thriving as species.[22] Aggression leading to violence has been shown by more recent anthropologists to be maladaptive in early human civilizations and thereby hardly genetically favored.[23]

Neurophysiological

In contrast to the instinctivist theories, the neurophysiological branch is characterized by controlled laboratory research and generally by a recognition that many factors, both environmental and physical, contribute to violence. Neurophysiologists also draw extensively from studies of animals, but these have been conducted in the laboratory, mainly because of the ethical considerations involved in research with human subjects, not because they fail to grasp the problems in generalizing findings to human beings. Neurologists also point out that the neuroanatomically specific pathways in the human brain involved in the integration of aggressive behavior do not differ substantially in "distribution and general topography" from those of experimental animals.[24] This perspective is important in addressing violence from a holistic viewpoint because it explains the physical basis of the aggression and violent behavior that is seen. The literature in this area is frequently technical in nature and relies a great deal on graphs, charts, and schematic drawings of the brain. The reader may want to refer to anatomy and physiology texts for a more detailed clarification of neurophysiology.

One of the most comprehensive overviews of the subject is provided by K. E. Moyer in his book *The Psychobiology of Aggression*. Moyer maintains that aggression is "determined by an interwoven complex of internal, external and experiential factors" which are constantly interacting.[25] Aggression equates with hostility for most of the neurophysiologists like Moyer and includes violence, as opposed to achievement or assertiveness. Moyer and other brain researchers are in general agreement that:

> impulses generated in the sensory systems, the cerebral cortex and still undetermined neural structures may activate triggering mechanisms that in turn excite visceral and semantic systems whose activities in concert provide physiologic expression of aggressive behavior.[26]

Moyer is careful to point out that the sensorimotor feedback is also important because changes in the stimulus will cut off aggressive behavior. This shows that aggression is "stimulus bound" in contrast to the conceptualization of the instinctivists who see it as spontaneous.[27]

Studies of animals seem to indicate that there are several different neural systems for different kinds of aggression. In laboratory studies with animals, seven different kinds of aggression (predatory, competitive, defensive, irritative, territorial, maternal-protective, and sex-related) have been elicited by electrical stimulation in different neuroanatomical places.[28] Electrical stimulation of parts of the limbic system in humans has also produced evidence of different, although somewhat overlapping, neurological representations in the brain for different kinds of hostility.[29] Generalizing from these studies, brain researchers have concluded that many different neuroanatomical centers exist for specific types of human aggression also.[30]

Theories of Violence

However, as neurologist Luigi Valzelli cautions, "electrical stimulation of the brain produces no strange or distorted behavior but acts only as a trigger or modulator of cerebral functions by influencing the processing of sensory inputs and the release of previously acquired behavior patterns."[31]

Appropriate stimulus (that is, pain, danger) when perceived, activates the sensory system involved and alerts the animal (or person), leading to a generalized state of arousal which includes increased sensitivity of the sensory systems (greater responsiveness to the environment) and increased muscle tone. When one of the specific neural systems is active, all neural activity in one area is facilitated. Such substances as amphetamines enhance the activity in the area, but do not by themselves initiate activity in the aggressive systems. If any of the systems for aggression is active, the organism is more likely to respond aggressively to appropriate stimulus.[32]

Studies in animals indicate that there are both facilitory and inhibitory neural mechanisms for all different kinds of aggression. Both surgical interruption of the neural systems for aggression and electrical stimulation of inhibitory systems in humans have decreased the tendencies toward hostility resulting in neurologists making the same conclusions about our species. The activation of one system may involve the inhibition of another, as in animals where stimulation of the escape system inhibits aggression. Other neural systems (that is, higher brain centers in humans) are constantly interacting with the aggressive system, and the "ultimate behavior is a function of those interactions" not under control of the limbic system alone.[33]

Hormonal Influences

Blood chemistry is also responsible for both inhibiting and facilitating the aggressive neural systems. Again, in animals at least, levels of certain endocrines (that is, norepinephrine, acetylcholine, dopamine and serotonin) seem to affect selectively different kinds of aggression. Murray Goldstein has concluded that the "specific neural systems in the central nervous system that synthesize, store and release these agents are differentially engaged" for different kinds of aggression.[34] The action of these agents may explain the relationship of stress to aggression since both norepinephrine and acetylcholine have been identified as part of the stress reaction.[35] Deprivation states (that is, food and sleep deprivation and morphine withdrawal in addicted rats) have been associated with increased aggression and also cause a stress reaction. Although there has been no experimental verification as yet, Moyer also hypothesizes:

> It may well be that frustration induced irritability results from the sensitization of irritable aggressive systems in the brain by the particular hormone balance that characterizes the stress system.[36]

Other hormones affect both the facilitating and inhibitory mechanisms. It has been shown that testosterone sensitizes the brain system involved with inter-male aggression in animals so that it is more easily activated by adequate stimuli. However, the evidence supporting the facilitating effects of testosterone on humans is scarce and mixed. Human castration has decreased the problematic behavior of sexually deviant men, but has neither inhibited the aggression of severely violent prisoners nor helped their resocialization.[37] A plasma testosterone suppressing agent (Medroxyprogesterone Acetate) was administered to a small group of intractably violent prisoners with mixed results.[38] In another study, twenty-three girls who were accidentally androgenized postnatally, showed no difference in aggressive behavior from normal females although an increase in "tomboyishness" was noted.[39]

Testosterone levels are equal in preadolescent girls and boys, but boys are still more aggressive.[40] The relationship between high violent crime rates and adolescent boys has often been noted even though the testosterone levels have started to fall during the period of highest violence (age eighteen to twenty-five).[41] The correlations between testosterone levels, hostility, aggression, and dominance found in young men and in criminal populations, as well as the high serum testosterone levels found in especially aggressive hockey players have led some researchers to postulate that although gonadal hormones do not regulate aggressive behavior, they may play a role in sustaining these actions.[42]

Progesterone, as an androgen inhibitor, and estrogen have also been studied in relation to aggression. Feelings of irritability and hostility and reports of increased violence in women have been linked to the fall of progesterone premenstrually in women.[43] However, Rudolf H. Moos and his associates found that premenstrual symptoms are not the same across all women, that the mood changes were consistent with the general personality. Only generally more aggressive or irritable women showed consistent increases in these affective states premenstrually.[44]

Because of the contradictory evidence, most neurophysiologists and ethologists are cautious about their conclusions regarding hormonal influences on aggression. David A. Hamburg concludes that androgens may predispose an individual to the development of aggressive behavior later, but that hormonal effects interact with the conditions of social environment.[45] Arnold Klopper states that "previous conditioning determines behavioral responses to testosterone and estrogen".[46]

The Role of Alcohol

Other substances in the blood can affect the inhibitory or facilitating neural mechanisms for aggression. The role of alcohol in this regard is not completely clear. Approximately one-half the victims and perpetrators in studies of homicide are found to have been drinking, but murderers are seldom diagnosed as alcoholics.[47] However, A. R. Nicol et al. found persistent criminal behavior associated with alcoholism (as well as unemployment, marital failure, and psychiatric abnormalities) in prison inmates.[48] Lowell Gerson and Donald A. Preston analyzed the correlations between violent crime, age, sex, income, population density, and sales of alcohol in urban areas. The alcohol sales accounted for only 16 percent of the rate variations in violent crime.[49] Laboratory experiments have shown increased aggression with alcohol ingestion, but there is variability in the studies and not all subjects react the same. Kathryn Graham, in her careful review of the literature, has concluded that research has not substantiated a "direct cause paradigm," the theory that alcohol directly causes aggression by disinhibition.[50] However, alcohol does produce psychological and physiological changes that seem to increase the probability of aggression under certain conditions. Because al-

Theories of Violence

cohol is frequently implicated in family violence, some examination of these changes is warranted.

The cognitive effects of alcohol ingestion have been examined in several studies. Not all research shows intoxication resulting in decreased intellectual functioning, but a decrease in verbal fluency is well established, an increase in expectation of attack from others has been noted in several studies, and higher doses of the substance do result in a variety of impairments.[51] Increased risk taking, time distortions, and a decreased awareness of the drinker's own actions and environment have also been documented.[52] It is more difficult to establish a direct relationship between those changes and aggressive behavior.

Physiological results of long-term ingestion such as brain damage, disruption of rapid eye movement or REM sleep, and poor nutrition leading to hypoglycemia have all been related to aggression in themselves, but not directly in relation to alcohol ingestion.[53] The immediate effects of alcohol are both sedative and arousing, depending on both internal and external circumstances. It has been hypothesized that increased testosterone levels interact with alcohol to produce increased facilitation of aggression, but this has not been corroborated in research.[54] Alcohol has been shown to cause temporal lobe dysrhythmia, which has been associated with aggressivity under laboratory conditions, but the subjects had all committed acts of violence previously.[55] The substance has also produced abnormal electroencephalograms (EEGs) in some men with ordinarily negative readings.[56] George Bach-Y-Rita et al. found twenty-five of thirty violent criminals hospitalized for psychiatric illness to have problems with "pathological intoxication" which he characterizes as loss of control early in the course of intoxication and leading to an outburst of explosive violence for which the man was amnesic afterwards, suggesting neurologic predisposition.[57] From these findings, it has been hypothesized that the aggression apparently stemming from physiological causes is related to a prior susceptibility to alcohol's effects or an already neurologically or environmentally established tendency to aggression.[58] Such pathological intoxication seems very rare and stressful environmental conditions appear necessary for such states to result in violence.[59]

The emotional lability sometimes cited as stemming from alcohol consumption and facilitating aggression is not well documented in research. People seem to drink for a variety of reasons, including a desire to reduce anxiety and tension which does not fit with an aggressive behavior model. However, some men have been documented to drink in order to feel stronger or increase their sense of personal power which may be then expressed in sexual and aggressive conquests. A subset of the population may be predisposed to aggression and use drinking occasions as an acceptable time to express this behavior. Again, there is ambivalence in our culture about whether people are less guilty for violent acts when drunk.[60] Richard Gelles has observed that there are other cultures where drunkenness is not followed by so-called disinhibited behavior, concluding that "drunken deportment is situationally variable and essentially a learned affair."[61]

Although alcohol ingestion and aggression and violence are linked in our society, cause and effect are not directly established. Such factors as preexisting physical and personality factors, dosage, expectations, settings, and other circumstances surrounding the drinking are as important as the neurophysiological effects of the substance.

Effects of Heredity

The effects of heredity on the neural bases of aggression are in an equally debatable state. Animal breeding for aggression has been done successfully in bulls and fighting cocks in natural settings and in mice in the laboratory.[62] Valzelli uses these findings plus his research on brain levels of serotonin, which is a genetically determined characteristic related to emotional stability, to conclude that there are multiple genetic determinants to aggression.[63] There may be genetic variability in the sensitivity of specific neural systems and in the determination of hormonal levels in humans, but research has not definitely established the connections.[64] In the 1960s there was great excitement when the XYY and XXY karotypes were discovered to be prevalent in imprisoned men.[65] However, more recent research has found (1) a great deal of selection bias in the earlier studies, (2) studies of prevalence in normal populations varied widely, (3) lab procedures for testing also varied, (4) the XXYs and XYYs could not be identified on the basis of violent crimes, and (6) the differences could probably be better explained by lower intelligence levels in these men resulting in lower socioeconomic class, thereby increasing probability of incarceration.[66]

Brain Disorders

The interaction between epilepsy and aggression has been carefully studied. Usually aggressive acts are *not* part of temporal lobe seizures. When they do occur, they are described as "bad moods" rather than destructive or assaultive behavior (occurring in only about 5 percent of epileptics) which, when it does occur, is frightening to the family, but rarely results in criminal acts and does not occur without provocation.[67]

The periodic or episodic dyscontrol syndrome has been associated with violence. Russell R. Monroe defines the disorder as

> precipitously appearing maladaptive behavior that interrupts the life style and life flow of the individual; the behavior is out of character for the individual and out of context for the situation.[68]

This behavior is contrasted with psychopathic behavior which is a way of life for an individual. Monroe characterized the syndrome as the result of both "faulty learning and faulty equipment." The neurological basis is theorized to be excessive neuronal discharges in the limbic system which often do not appear on routine (scalp) EEGs, but may be manifested using deeply implanted electrodes.[69]

"Soft" neurological signs such as impaired psychomotor and perceptual ability, history of altered status of consciousness, history of febrile convulsions, and headaches have been associated with episodic dyscontrol.[70] In addition, hyperactivity has been associated with aggressiveness in children. Violent male criminals frequently describe a history of this indication of minimal brain damage.[71] Richard Allen, Daniel Safer, and Lino Covi, however, point out that aggressiveness may be only secondary to the effects of overactivity and may only reflect the way these boys have been dealt with and/or their need for constant stimulation and ways to expend their energy.[72] The favorable response of some patients to anticonvulsant medications has been used as evidence for the neurological epileptic-like basis for the episodic dyscontrol syndrome.[73] However, most of the studies were not blind, and in one study that was, there were few dramatic changes with anticonvulsant medication and the most therapeutic response was from the placebos.[74]

It has been definitely established that some serious brain damage may cause otherwise unexplainable violent and aggressive behavior (that is, brain tumors in the limbic system and temporal lobes, brain trauma, and encephalitis) showing that human beings' "neural systems for aggression can be activated by internal physiologic processes."[75] It is therefore theorized that minimal brain damage can do the same, but the exact neural mechanisms have been variously explained as lack of integration of the nervous system, extra activity in the neural cells responsible for aggression, increased sensitivity to aggressive cues because of general arousal, destruction of inhibitory systems, or destruction of learning systems.[76] The results could also be explained by a combination of two or more of the above. Moyer describes four variables which may interact in some not yet completely understood manner to explain chronic behavioral tendencies toward aggression: (1) a lowered threshold for activation of the neural systems of aggression (caused by heredity); (2) normal threshold, but increased sensitization of neurons (by hormones, activation from other systems, blood chemistry changes from stress and frustration, structural damage) facilitating their activation; (3) normal aggression system activation with decreased inhibition system activation (from decrease in some hormones and other blood substrates and alcohol); and (4) learning.[77] Most of the researchers on episodic dyscontrol have noted other psychological and sociological correlates with the syndrome.[78] Researchers in aggressive neurophysiology usually stress the importance of the interaction of social, environmental, and hereditary influences.[79] They are all convinced of the aggressive potential in all human brains, but as Moyer states:

> Man, of course, learns better and faster than any other animal. It is therefore reasonable to expect that the internal impulses to aggressive behavior would be more subject to modification by experience in man than in any other animal. In addition, because of man's additional ability to manipulate symbols and to substitute one symbol for another, one would expect to find a considerable diversity in the stimuli that elicit or inhibit activity in the aggression system. One would expect that the modes of expression would be more varied, diverse and less stereotyped in man than in other animals.[80]

Only a few of the brain researchers imply that most violence could be stopped by surgery, pharmacological agents, or electrical pacemakers, or that violence is completely determined by biological mechanism. The few that do, for instance Vernon H. Mark and Frank R. Ervin, are severely criticized by the rest, as well as by social scientists.[81] It must be kept in mind that the biological mechanisms detailed underlie aggression, not necessarily violence. When applied to violence, these mechanisms may only explain potential for problems, not the violent behavior itself.[82] Aggressive people are rarely always aggressive and their hostile behavior may or may not be superimposed on a background of hostility.[83] There are also no automatically elicited behavior patterns of aggression from environmental or electrical stimulus for humans as there are for animals.[84] Lawrence Kolb points out that the neocortex in humans has "both a facilitory and inhibitory influence on aggressive behaviors characterized by rage" and that it also influences the direction and timing.[85]

Limitations of the Neurophysiological Approach

It should be pointed out that most of the brain research has been conducted with men, that men are inexplicably more likely to display episodic dyscontrol, and that the researchers use "man" in all of their descriptions of human beings. It is difficult to tell if they are referring only to the male sex in describing conclusions. Except for the evidence on the influence of hormones which we have seen is fragmentary and not totally conclusive, the neurophysiologists have not adequately explained the differences between male and female behavior. Females of all species are generally more difficult to stimulate to aggression and once stimulated, express hostility somewhat differently.[86] It has been found that previous social experience and acquired learning of hierarchical rules are more important than sexual hormones in aggressiveness and dominance pattern formation in monkeys.[87] The single largest determining factor in aggressive behavior in humans is gender and although gender is obviously a physical factor, the explanation of that difference is mainly found in the fields of sociology and psychology.

Sociologists and psychologists generally acknowledge the neuronal and blood chemistry basis for aggression, but differ in their perspectives on the major determinants of violence. Sociologists point to the peaceful cultures that exist, and wonder why persons with minimal brain damage in those societies do not behave aggressively if socialization is not more important than brain disorders. Josi M. R. Delgado asserts that patients with implanted electrodes display hostility when stimulated, "but it is always expressed according to the subject's previous experience and evaluation of his present environment."[88] Brain researchers have also been criticized for diverting attention from our social dilemmas which "contributes to unwillingness to undertake the political solutions to violence which promise to achieve much more."[89] However, neurophysiological bases for aggression are important for holistic understanding and can be viewed as background for psychological, sociological, and cultural influences which may lead to violent expression of the aggression.

PSYCHOLOGICAL THEORIES OF VIOLENCE

Psychological explanations of violence vary a great deal. Many psychologists echo Sigmund Freud's theories that aggression is a basic instinct or drive.[90] Others deemphasize or refute that view and identify other psychological traits that characterize the violent person. The basic premise of most psychoanalytic frameworks is that in the violent individual, some basic need or needs have been thwarted, usually by some form of faulty childraising.[91] The other major branch of psychological theories is derived from behavioral psychology. This includes Albert Bandura's social learning theory and Hans Eysenck's biologically rooted conditioning framework.

Theories of Violence

Psychoanalytic Viewpoints

The psychoanalytic instinctivists derive their theories from basic Freudian concepts. Freud, of course, is not a modern theorist and his views have been analyzed extensively elsewhere.[92] Suffice it to say that by the end of his career he had reluctantly concluded that aggression was a basic instinct, as part of the death instinct and as opposed to eros.[93] His influence in this regard has pervaded psychoanalytic thought.

John M. MacDonald, a relatively modern psychoanalyst, also writes from the same perspective of an "internal need to discharge hostility." He theorizes that murderers are likely to have ego weaknesses resulting in erratic control over aggressive impulses.[94] David Abrahamsen postulates that human behavior has four roots: (1) society at large, (2) community and its subcultures, (3) family, and (4) individual (psychological and physical). Thus, he acknowledges the multiplicity of causative factors for criminal behavior, but still insists that all people have "criminal tendencies," "murderous impulses," and "hidden violence," which are activated when acted upon by internal and external events.[95]

A corollary of the psychological instinctivists is that frustration is the instigation or stimulus which leads to the expression of aggression. This part of the theory was first advanced in 1939 and was linked to early behavioral psychology language. It was hypothesized by John Dollard and his associates that the occurrence of aggression always presupposes frustration.[96] Since then it has been determined in research that frustration does not always lead to aggression and that aggression does not always stem from frustration, nor is it the most potent instigator.[97] There is also ambiguity about the meaning of Dollard's terms. However, this concept has been adopted widely because of its simplicity, and there are references to it in sociological literature.

One of the basic premises of the drive theory is that since aggression is a basic instinct, its appearance in behavior will reduce accumulated hostility and decrease the amount of aggression shown in response to further frustration.[98] This is the catharsis premise first formulated by Freud and conceptualized by Jack E. Hokanson as "the idea that the expression of aggression reduces the aggressor's internal state of anger and his general level of physiological tension."[99] The catharsis theory is one aspect of psychoanalytic theory which lends itself to empirical testing, and the literature abounds with such research. Discriminatory studies have shown "clearly that overt aggression does not inevitably lead to either physiological tension reduction or a reduction in subsequent aggression."[100] Evidence against the catharsis hypothesis comes from other perspectives. The neurophysiologists are represented by Moyer who states that "a continuing accumulation of aggressive energy relievable only by the expression of aggression is not in keeping with the physiological evidence."[101] In both experimental and natural settings, verbal aggression has not been shown to decrease subsequent physical attack; in fact, the opposite tends to occur.[102] The watching of violent films, seen by catharsis proponents as a substitution for aggressive behavior, has been shown to increase rather than decrease later aggression.[103] It has also been observed that watching violent sports tends to instigate aggression rather than lessen it.[104] One of the weakest points of the psychoanalytic view of aggression as a drive which must be expressed is therefore the catharsis assumption.

One of the outgrowths of the catharsis concept is Edwin I. Megargee's concept of "over-controlled personality types" who display extreme violence. Megargee theorizes that these persons are instilled with such excessive inhibitions against aggression in childhood that their hostile impulses build up. Although the instigation for aggression must be much stronger finally to elicit aggressive behavior, when it does appear it is likely to be excessively violent.[105] Much work has been done to identify these overcontrolled personalities. Behavioral and psychological tests in prison populations of murderers and violent criminals have been developed, and a subscale of the Minnesota Multiphasic Personality Inventory (MMPI) was developed (OH—"overcontrolled hostility"—scale) for identification.[106] The OH scale has not proved to be valid and the whole catharsis concept is controversial, so this explanation of violence must be highly questioned.[107]

Limitations of the Psychoanalytic Perspective

It is difficult not to be alienated by the blaming of mothers for violent sons rampant in psychoanalytic literature. Whether it is because of a "loveless" home, "emotional deprivation," "maternal symbiosis," "mother domination," "maternal deprivation," or "parental neglect," the implication is that the mother has the primary responsibility for childrearing and she has failed in her task.[108] These theorists also note that the violent men have also frequently been exposed to abusive and alcoholic fathers.[109]

The mechanisms the psychoanalysts believe to be operating here vary. The general theme is that the violent individual is acting out some form of emotional problems. Terms such as "psychotic," "neurotic," "psychopathic," "personality disorder," "passive aggressive," "self-destructive," "paranoid," and so forth, are used to describe almost every violent individual evaluated in psychoanalytic literature.[110] The triad of youthful enuresis, fire setting, and cruelty to animals has been identified as common in the childhood of habitually violent men.[111] The "individual psychology of the murderer" or violent person is considered the most important factor, and as Abrahamsen states, "emotional disturbances are always at the root of antisocial or criminal behavior."[112]

There are problems with this conceptualization. The theories are usually derived from small case studies of violent men (rarely any women), and research involving larger groups often uses psychiatric hospital patients as controls (if there are any controls at all) when identifying psychological traits "causing" violence.[113] The prisoners given psychiatric diagnoses by psychoanalysts have seldom been identified as mentally ill by the courts or other psychiatrists; the literature often indicates attempts to make the men "fit" into categories even when symptoms and testing show minimal aberrations.[114] It has been found that the rates of violence for those patients labeled criminally insane (by the courts) are "not remarkably different" from the normal population, and the actual psychiatric pathology in criminal populations is estimated at only 18 percent.[115] If vio-

Theories of Violence

lence and psychiatric illness are so interwoven, it is difficult to explain why former mental patients commit fewer crimes, including violent crimes, than the normal population.[116] Psychiatrists and psychologists have not been able consistently and accurately to predict dangerousness or violence using psychological tests, psychiatric examination, or identification of the childhood "triad."[117] The theories do not account for the preponderance of males committing violent offenses, and they share the assumption of the instinctivists (although not as forcefully) that aggression is an innate drive.

Derivations of Psychoanalytic Theory

A derivative branch of psychoanalytic theory is represented mainly by Erich Fromm, Rollo May, and Howard B. Kaplan. They each conceptualize aggression as a result of the thwarting of some basic human need, differing somewhat in the need identified. These three theorists have moved away from the instinctivist position.

Erich Fromm considered benign forms of aggression which are biologically adaptive and life serving (that is, self-assertive aggression, defensive aggression), to be innate while malignant aggression (sadism and necrophilia) is not. The basic need which Fromm considers as thwarted when malignant aggression appears is the need "to transcend the triviality of life" to find greater meaning. He feels that although pathological childrearing and genetics can play a part, the main determinant of malignant aggression is the "dry, banal, pedantic, dishonest, unalive atmosphere" characterizing many families and social situations.[118] Fromm's analysis is more philosophical in nature than research oriented. The ideas are interesting and useful for approaching the meaning of violence, but difficult to apply to specific situations.

Rollo May also talks about the basic need for a sense of significance, but in terms of self-affirmation and self-assertion. His theory can be summed up in the following quote:

> Deeds of violence in our society are performed by those trying to establish their self-esteem, to defend their self-image and to demonstrate that they, too, are significant.

May characterizes aggression as "moving into position of power or prestige" and feels that violence is the expression of powerlessness. He sees power on a continuum from energy to force to violence depending on the amount of blockage the person encounters.[119]

Howard Kaplan's theory is very close to May's in that he ascribes a basic need for self-esteem to human beings and feels that when a person has a history of low self-esteem and self-devaluing experiences, he is more likely to develop hostile and retreating defenses.[120] People with "negative stable self-attitudes" are "predisposed or motivated to seek out and adopt deviant patterns." The deviant patterns alleviate the subjective distress associated with what the person sees as the critical attitude associated with the normative environment. They also satisfy the need for self-esteem by the "avoidance of, attacks upon or substitution for the normative environment." The person reacting to a history of self-devaluing experiences with hostile defenses is suspicious of and lacks identification with others and is thereby more likely to use violence.

Kaplan cites Hans Toch's study of sixty-nine male inmates and parolees as support for his theory. Toch found that almost one-half of the offenders had used violence to buttress feelings of inadequacy in one way or another. Even though their self-esteem was considered normal, another large group showed evidence of dehumanizing their victims which is associated with Kaplan's hostile defenses.[121] Kaplan maintains that many criminals will not show low self-esteem, because their deviant behavior has resulted in a reduction of negative self-feelings.[122] Thus, it is difficult to prove or disprove his theory by looking at criminal populations. Paul Yelsma and Julie Yelsma gave the Coopersmith self-esteem inventory to sixty-two inmates (sixty male, two female) of a county jail and a forensic center. They found that those who were destructive only to themselves (convicted of alcohol-related charges) had the lowest scores; those directly violent to others (murder, rape, or robbery) also had lower than normal scores, while those who were only indirectly destructive (forgery, drug sales) had higher than normal scores.[123] From this evidence it can be postulated that there is some support for Kaplan's association of deviance and retreating defenses with low self-esteem, but the reason that the behavior had resulted in more positive self-concept for some and not for others is unclear. A small study of ten homicidal adolescents (nine male, one female) found "vacillations" in self-esteem and a "lack of cohesion of self."[124] Other psychologists postulate that negative self-concept accounts for violence in some violent individuals but not in others, or that threatened self-esteem always results in aggression, but the aggression is not necessarily destructive.[125]

Other psychoanalytic formulations about aggression need to be mentioned briefly. Alfred Adler saw the drive for power as a source of aggression, postulating that those who needed to attack in order to get power usually were acting out of inadequacy. Carl Jung saw violence as the "unleashing of primordial archetypical behavior inherent in the collective unconscious." Karen Horney conceptualized destructive aggression as part of the behavior of those who "move against" rather than those who "move toward" or "move away." Harry Stack Sullivan was more apt to see violence and aggression arising from disturbances in interpersonal relationships.[126]

Many ego psychologists do not conceptualize aggression as an independent drive and clearly differentiate benign aggression, a trait similar to what has been defined here as assertion, from malignant aggression or violence. They maintain that the healthy individual has strong ego boundaries which allow for the use of "reality testing, accurate appraisal of threat, learning, conflict resolution and the use of defense mechanisms" by the ego to make sure that aggression is dealt with without harming others.[127] These conceptualizations are all useful in understanding the emotional context of violent behavior but have generally not been operationalized for empirical testing.

As has been seen, the psychoanalytic theories and those derived from this framework are characterized by less support from empirical research than those of the biologists and a general reliance on some of the highly disputed assumptions of Sigmund Freud. They generally fail to account for the preponderance of males committing violence, suffer from a primarily male orientation, and do not explain predominantly peaceful cultures.

Theories of Violence

The emotional conditions supporting violence are important in a holistic framework, but the psychoanalytic viewpoint has failed to prove that psychological mechanisms are mainly responsible for causing violence. However, there are violent individuals who must be considered mentally ill. Although "the incidence of psychosis among murderers is no greater than the incidence of psychosis in the total population," occasionally psychotic individuals, especially paranoid schizophrenics, are directed by auditory hallucinations or other delusionary systems to act violently. Even in these cases, psychological and sociological mechanisms affecting the "normal" murderer also influence the one who is labeled insane.[128]

Social Learning Theory

Albert Bandura is the originator and best known proponent of social learning theory as an explanation for aggression. He himself calls the theory psychological because it grows out of the school of behavioral psychology, yet it obviously also combines aspects of sociological frameworks.[129] In a review of the literature by Alan Newcombe in 1978 it was found that the "majority of social scientists" agreed that aggression and violence are learned rather than instinctive.[130] It is also not uncommon to find theorists combining aspects of the social learning theory with neurophysiological research.[131]

Bandura defines aggression as "behavior that results in personal injury and in destruction of property," including that the injury "may be psychological." He also notes that the behavior must be labeled as aggressive by society, this labeling determined by the action's intensity, the intentions attributed to the performer by others, and the characteristics of the labelers.[132] Bandura feels that aggressive behavior may be considered adaptive or destructive depending on the situation in which it is employed. He acknowledges the role of biological subcortical structures in producing destructive behavior, but believes that the social situation is most important in determining the frequency, form, circumstances, and target of the action.[133] Bandura states:

> In the social learning view, people are endowed with neurophysiological mechanisms that enable them to behave aggressively, but the activation of these mechanisms depends on appropriate stimulation and is subject to cognitive control.[134]

Bandura postulates that rather than arising from instinct or frustration, aversive experiences result in emotional arousal, which is perceived in the individual as fear, anger, sorrow, or even euphoria depending on their prior learning, cognitive interpretation, and other people's reaction to the same experience. Moreover, "frustration or anger arousal is a facilitative but not a necessary condition for aggression."[135] Bandura has concluded that the majority of events that stimulate aggression (that is, insults, status threats, unjust treatment) "gain activating capacity through learning experiences." To illustrate this, Bandura points to the many people who have experienced broken homes, parental rejection, poverty, mental illness, brain damage, and so forth, who have never become violent. He sees motivation for aggression as reinforcement based, not biologically determined.

> The social learning theory of aggression distinguishes between acquisition of behaviors

that have destructive and injurious potential and factors that determine whether a person will perform what he has learned ... because not all that people learn is exhibited in their actions.[136]

The acquisition of aggressive behavior can be learned through modeling or observational learning or by direct experience or practice.[137] Performance is determined by both internal (biological and cognitive) and external instigators.[138] This has been confirmed in laboratory experiences with children.[139]

Models for aggressive behavior are to be found in the family, the subculture, and the media. Using analysis of a nationwide self-report sample of violent behavior and attitudes toward violence, Straus and Owens concluded that the more a child sees or is the victim of violence in his or her home or social structure, the more violence the child will perform as an adult, since he or she has seen the behavior modeled.[140] Observation of others' behavior also gives clues as to whether the action will be rewarded or punished when it occurs. If a child sees a parent or peer gain status, dominance, resources, or power by using violence, he or she will be more likely to use it.[141] It has often been noticed that violent men are more likely to have been abused as children, and these ideas also help to explain why some peer groups (that is, gangs) and subcultures are known for violence.[142] Bandura found that parents of aggressive boys from middle-class homes, although they neither abused their children or displayed antisocial violence, "repeatedly modeled and reinforced combative attitudes and behavior."[143] The long-term effects of modeling were shown in an experiment where nursery school boys could imitate aggressive behavior shown six months previously. The girls, however, showed much less imitative behavior in this study.[144] Parents' use of physical punishment is also considered a strong model for the use of force in other contexts. A recent study done by Jerry Neopolitan suggests that the more juvenile males identify with their fathers, the greater the correlation between aggressive behavior and frequent use of physical punishment by male parents.[145]

The part that the media and especially television plays in modeling aggressive behavior has often been noted in theories of violence. Empirical evidence is beginning to show considerable substantiation. Elizabeth D. McCarthy and her associates did a five-year follow-up on a random sample cross section of 732 children in Manhattan and Houston. She found that heavy viewing of violent programs was associated with two (of three) measures of aggression, fighting, and delinquency, as well as with regressive anxiety, mentation problems, and depression.[146] However, Stanley Milgram and R. Lance Shotland found no more imitative results from a television program showing a man stealing watched by male adult subjects who were then given an easy opportunity to do the same, in comparison to a matched control group who watched a neutral film. Several other studies have shown no effects or unreliable effects of television on violence or aggression.[147] The effects of violent television viewing seem to be more apparent in children suggesting that there is a critical period when aggressive patterns are being learned and when television has the most impact. Jerome Singer and Dorothy Singer found impressive correlations between extensive violent television watching and aggressive behavior in preschoolers.[148] Leonard Eron's longitudinal study of more than 400 children showed that the single best predictor of the boys' aggressive behavior at age nineteen was how much violent television they were watching at eight years old.[149] In an extensive review of literature (1956–76) of 153 studies, F. Scott Andison found a weak positive overall correlation between viewing violence and subsequent aggressive behavior and noted that the more recent studies are showing increasingly positive results.[150] This may be due to a cumulative effect of increasingly violent television watching, more emphasis on the effects on children, and/or better methods used in the later studies.

There is no doubt that a great deal of television programming, especially children's programs, depicts violence, and shows violent males as heroes who gain power by its use.[151] Researchers postulate that in addition to the modeling effect, heavy violence viewing disinhibits aggressive behavior by showing good triumphing over evil with the use of violence, and by desensitizing and habituating people to violence.[152] Jeffrey Goldstein's study of people exposed to more violence in real life showed that they also were more likely to prefer violent portrayals in media.[153] A study by Allen Fenigstein suggested that previous aggressive thoughts and actions increase preferences for viewing violence which in turn further increases aggressive behavior.[154] Jacque-Phillipe Leyens and his associates found that only previously aggressive boys in their study were increasingly aggressive after watching filmed violence; the less aggressive boys were not. However, the more violent boys showed a modeling effect, because their physical aggression closely paralleled the types shown in the movies.[155]

The other postulated effect of televised violence is the production of a concept of the world as a dangerous place. Viewers who watch television heavily have shown to have more feelings of mistrust and suspicion which may increase their tendencies to use violence in marginally appropriate situations.[156] George Gerbner, who has done extensive research on the results of television watching, concludes that only 1 to 2 per 1,000 heavy watchers will actually imitate the violence on television and threaten society, but that the large majority become more fearful, insecure, and dependent on authority.[157]

Bandura explains that behavior learned from models is reinforced if the imitative actions are seen to be useful to the person.[158] Twenty-four male subjects were more aggressive toward experimental victims when they were verbally reinforced for doing so.[159] Henri Laborit explains that if aggression is successful and dominance achieved by it, "then the aggression will in itself constitute reinforced behavior because of the gratification that followed."[160] This mechanism was illustrated in a study showing that fifth grade boys who were measured as aggressive were more likely to reward themselves with tokens for aggressive behavior even when the victim expressed pain, than those who showed low aggression on the inventory.[161] Laborit also notes that "society's rewards tend to go to the least compassionate members" which is a strong reinforcement for aggression."[162] There are problems with extending this model to women; however, the social learning theorists postulate that aggressive behavior is a product of the cognitive structure which either inhibits or disinhibits the performance of the activity.[163] They feel that the socially learned inhibitors to aggression are much stronger for women and that violence is less useful to women.[164]

Empirical Verification

Much laboratory research has been done to identify and determine the relative strength of the inhibitors, disinhibitors, and facilitators of learned aggressive behavior. Most of the studies involve subjects being given the opportunity to aggress by using shock machines. The intensity, duration, and number of shocks given is measured to determine the amount of aggression shown. There is much controversy among the researchers as to what conditions are the most powerful in affecting aggression. Most of the studies use male college students, and it is questionable whether these laboratory results can be generalized to the rest of the population.[165] For the purposes of this review we will summarize these studies by saying that the effects of: (1) generally arousing films (not necessarily violent), (2) the presence or firing of guns, (3) violence depicted as justified, (4) lowered responsibility for actions, (5) dehumanization of victims, (6) continued aggressive action as self-reinforcement, (7) competition, (8) sexual arousal especially when subjects are angered, (9) pain cues given by the victim, (10) anticipated punishment, (11) empathy, and (12) prior social contact with the victim have all been studied.[166] The relative strengths of these factors are controversial, but the evidence suggests that the first eight may facilitate or disinhibit aggression and the last three have at least some inhibiting effect. Pain cues or other signs of victim suffering seem to increase aggression when the subject is angered or reinforced for such behavior.[167]

The social learning theory does incorporate biological, psychological, and sociological factors of causation of violence. Other theorists have modified and/or amplified Bandura's basic propositions, but the thrust of the arguments remains the same.[168] These authors feel that aggressive behavior, the instigations for hostile activity, the factors that facilitate or inhibit its expression, the appropriate targets, and the mechanism used to display aggression are all learned although somewhat influenced by neurophysiological and psychological mechanisms. As we have seen, there is much empirical evidence to support these conclusions, although the details have not yet been conclusively established. These theories account for the effects of different sociological factors in terms of learning.

SOCIOLOGICAL FORCES AFFECTING VIOLENCE

The sociological theories of violence generally take into account some of the biological and psychological aspects of causation, but their basic proposition is that social structure and conditions are more important.[169] They vehemently reject the idea that aggression is an instinct or drive, and postulate that most violent offenders are basically normal and generally do not act destructively.[170] Other than in these areas of agreement, the sociologists vary widely in their approach. There are theorists who emphasize any one of the following aspects: cultural attitudes fostering violence, the structural violence inherent in our society, social frustration, social disorganization, population density, the influence of poverty, a subculture of violence, machismo, and roles.

Cultural Attitudes Fostering Violence

The United States has a long history of violence being used as a means to achieve socially approved ends. American culture reflects at least a covert acceptance of violence in the media, in attitudinal surveys, and in our choice of heroes. Monica Blumenthal and her associates interviewed 1,374 American men with a variety of socioeconomic characteristics and found that one-half to two-thirds of them could justify the police shooting in situations *not* involving self-defense or protection of innocent people from bodily harm, situations only requiring social control (conditions like campus protests or riots or gangs inflicting property damage). Twenty to thirty percent would advise the police to shoot to kill in these instances. These researchers feel such attitudes are a "covert message that it is socially acceptable to use violence for instrumental reasons."[171] A variation on this theme in different terminology is Henry P. Lundsgaarde's view of homicide as reflecting the sanctions in a culture. "A sanction is a reaction on the part of a society or a considerable number of its members to a mode of behavior which is thereby approved (positive sanctions) or disapproved (negative sanctions)." Lundsgaarde used an analysis of homicide in Houston, Texas, in 1969 to show that official negative sanctions (the police, courts, and laws) against killing can be overcome by covert positive sanctions defining homicide as more permissible in such cases as husband-wife killings or homicides among friends and associates or those among the poor and black.[172]

Structural Violence of Society

A closely related theme to the one above is the idea that violence in America reflects the violence inherent in our way of life. David G. Gil points out that the structure of our society results in "acts and conditions which obstruct the spontaneous unfolding of innate human potential, the inherent drive toward development and self-actualization."[173] He feels that capitalism fosters an "all pervasive, exploitative attitude" which is necessary to get ahead in the system, and that families act as agents of the structure in their stress on hierarchical patterns and arbitrary authority, which transmits those violent attitudes to each succeeding generation.[174] Bernard Bergen and Stanley Rosenberg echo these sentiments when they talk about our culture as "brutalizing" and our society represented by "competitive striving and lust for power and control over one's fellows, and mutual exploitation."[175] Marvin Wolfgang also speaks of the society legitimizing violence by "the labels of virtue" it attaches to methods of social control and the use of military force.[176]

Social Frustration or Strain Theories

The sociological theories grouped together under the label of strain theory generally postulate that crime and delinquency results when "socially approved ends (e.g., material possessions) cannot be achieved through conventional channels and illegal activities are chosen as alternative means of obtaining desired ends."[177] These theories are some of the oldest in sociology and were first expressed by Robert K. Merton in 1938.[178] He used the theory to explain the association between poverty and crime and first used the word "anomie" to describe the discrepancies between aspirations and opportunities.[179] Richard A. Cloward and Lloyd E. Ohlin studied male delinquent gangs in the 1950s and found that gang members anticipated that legitimate channels to goals would be limited or closed to them. The boys' sense of injustice led them to attribute legitimacy to delinquent acts.[180]

Social Disorganization

J. P. Scott theorizes that agnostic behavior (which may or may not lead to violence) is adaptive behavior for conflict situations. He feels that violence developing from agnostic behavior increases as social systems become disorganized on any level.[181] For example, Scott feels that although violence may be used to establish dominance-subordination relationships, it decreases once they are established and will only increase if threatened. The term "anomie" is also used in the social disorganization context. In this case it is used to describe normlessness or confusion of values which can also occur at any level of society, including the family.[182] "Anomie" rarely appears in recent literature or research, but the concept of social disintegration is woven into other sociological perspectives.

Population Density

The idea of population density leading to violence was derived from animal studies of crowded behavior and the observation that homicide (and other violent crimes) are much more likely to occur in the nation's larger cities.[183] No significant association has been found in studies measuring population density (population per square mile) and crime when socioeconomic status and ethnic background are controlled.[184] However, one study did find such a relationship with juvenile delinquency when people per room of housing was used as the measure of crowding.[185] Another study failed to find a relationship using the same measure of density with the incidence of violent crime.[186] A longitudinal study of Buffalo and Boston showed murder decreasing as city size increased and failed to find any general relationship between city growth and homicide rates.[187]

Poverty

In an effort to further explain the greater amounts of urban violence, especially among poor young black men, sociologists have theorized extensively.[188] Lynn A. Curtis in a study of the seventeen largest U.S. cities found that reported urban criminal homicide and aggravated assault is most frequently committed by black males in their teens and twenties who are victimizing other black male friends, acquaintances, or strangers, the same age or older, living in close proximity, in the course of relatively trivial altercations.[189] Rather than postulating that any one factor causes this violence, the social scientists tended to criminal homicide in Philadelphia were used to substantiate the subculture of violence thesis, but these were only descriptive in nature and the subculture of violence theory has been criticized for its lack of explanatory power.[206] The problem with blaming the culture of a race or class for violence without identifying the antecedents of that culture is that it becomes a way of subtly blaming the victims (and perpetrators) for creating the culture.[207] It can be argued that any subculture of violence in the lower class and/or black culture is due to the systematic denial of opportunity by the majority of society.

Richard Moran synthesized the subculture hypothesis with the idea that "the more fully low status groups or individuals seek to occupy or maintain status positions based on achievement, the more likely they are to commit criminal homicide." Using homicide data from Boston (1962–66), Moran found that age had a stronger relationship to homicide than sex or race, suggesting that in low-status populations the age group twenty to twenty-nine, which commits the largest proportion of homicides, does so because this is the age group which has the most emphasis on achievement. When he looked at homicide rates among ethnic groups, he found that the association between gender and homicide was stronger than that between race and homicide and felt that this "suggests the presence of a subculture of violence among males." Moran's conclusion was that "a subcultural normative system sanctioning the use of violence during social interaction exists mainly among low status groups of individuals experiencing subjective external restraint."

Moran accounts for gender differences in homicide in terms of males being more frustrated by occupational status blocking than females. He feels that black women are more achievement oriented than other ethnic groups which is why, according to Moran, those women commit more homicides than white, Italian, Puerto Rican, or Irish females.[208] In the face of evidence that black women are the lowest paid group in the United States, and considering their supposed achievement orientation, it is difficult to understand why their homicide rate is only one-fourth that of black men.[209] Moran also fails to account for a reason why the majority of low-status males do not act out the subculture of violence.

An interesting corollary to the subculture of violence theory is the controversy about the existence of a southern version of these values which has diffused into the urban centers by way of migration patterns. Raymond Gastil first advanced this idea by noting the high statistical rates of homicide in the South and by linking this with the southern values of exaggerated sense of honor and a historical predilection for violence, which is usually only lightly punished.[210] Much controversy was raised about whether southerners actually were more likely to own guns (versus handguns), whether less available and lower-quality medical care in the South accounts for the higher homicide rates, and whether it was southerners who had migrated who were committing northern urban violence.[211] The conclusions reached varied widely according to the measures used to indicate southernness and violence approval, the statistical methods employed, and the populations studied, making meaningful comparisons difficult.

Lynn Curtis uses the subculture of violence concept as a base and goes on to develop a theory which perhaps best explains sociologically the preponderance of poor black urban males committing homicides.[212] Curtis joins the other subcultural theorists in noting the strong influence of violence as a characteristic of the masculine ethic.[213] (See Chapter 4 for further explanations of the role of machismo in wife-beating.)

Role Theory

Stuart Palmer explains violence in terms of roles. His theory has elements of all of the sociological viewpoints expressed thus far, somewhat rearranged and with different terminology. Roles for Palmer are behaviors that accompany a person's status. His term "reciprocity" is used to describe "social interactions as a constant process of giving and receiving." Reciprocity is denied lower classes by the upper classes and is decreased when there is social disintegration or a lack of agreement about "basic life values." Reciprocity is increased when there is mutual facilitation of role performances and thereby tension in the social situation decreases. Tension increases and causes a greater likelihood of homicide when each person thinks that the other is blocking his or her role performance. Therefore, reciprocity and homicide would be inversely related.[214]

There are other sociological frameworks which look at violence in terms of large groups, organizations, and societal conflict. These postulations are beyond the scope of this book, since the main interest is in how social forces affect individuals within a small group, the family. Most of the theorists in the field of family violence are sociologists, and the application of sociological formulations on violence in the family will be addressed in subsequent chapters. This review has laid a theoretical background explaining the social systems and structures that this field of study sees as important regarding their effects on violent behavior.

INSIGHTS FROM ANTHROPOLOGY

The studies of anthropologists have rarely been directly focused on the problem of violence cross-culturally. Rather, an anthropologist is likely to observe and record all the characteristics of one culture. However, the study of peaceful societies offers some tantalizing clues as to what factors of socialization tend to promote or discourage violence. The fact that there are such cultures is powerful evidence that cultural forces and learning are more important than biology in explaining the occurrence of violence.[215] A limited selection of anthropological works regarding these peaceful cultures will be examined, noting consistent themes.

Cultures Without Violence

Erich Fromm has devised a classification system that will be used in looking at the cultures.[216] He divides cultures on a continuum wherein System A stands for "life-affirming societies" which are characterized by "a minimum of hostility, violence or cruelty among people, no harsh punishment, hardly any crime and the institution of war is absent or plays an exceedingly small role." System B includes societies which are not basically destructive, but "aggressiveness and war, although not central are normal occurrences and competition, hierarchy and individualism are present." The cultures of System C demonstrate "much interpersonal violence, destructiveness, aggression and cruelty, both within the tribe and against others, a pleasure in war, maliciousness and treachery." Fromm analyzed thirty nonindustrial cultures in this conceptualization and noted that in System A, "women are in general considered equal to men, or at least not exploited or humiliated," while System B is more "imbued with a spirit of male aggressiveness and individualism," and System C is characterized by extreme competition and "strict hierarchies," especially of men over women. He also noted that in System A, societies treat children with kindness and an absence of corporal punishment, sex is treated permissively and affirmatively, and more cooperation between the sexes and among men is fostered in comparison to B and C. Fromm also found that System A groups had a variety of economic circumstances, that some lived in areas of scarcity and hardship, and they represented gathering, agricultural, and hunting means of food acquisition.

Original anthropological writings on fifteen basically peaceful peoples were reviewed for this text. There was evidence in each of the societies that at least direct expressions of violence against women (such as rape, wife abuse, female genital mutilation) were virtually absent although the status of women varied from female superiority in some aspects of societal structure (that is, Mbuti) to virtual equality (that is, Zuni Indians) to relative submission (Utku Eskimos).[217] Even in those cultures where the female is under male control in one respect or another, there is evidence that women have an important and highly respected role in that society. For instance, the wife in the Utku Eskimo society obeys her husband's wishes, but participates almost equally in physical labor and is recognized as being equally important for economic survival.[218] In all these groups where such information was noted, there is also a consistent theme of the father being close to as involved in childrearing as the mother.[219]

The most striking feature of all the peaceful cultures is the way children are raised. Physical punishment is almost never used, and children are treated with affection. Both girls and boys are taught that force is abhorrent; jealousy is unacceptable; and competition frowned upon; while cooperation is regarded as a prime virtue; gentleness is emphasized; nature is glorified; and caution, fear, and timidity are either encouraged or considered healthy.[220]

An example of Fromm's System B, which can be used for comparison to the peaceful societies, is that of the Australian Aborigines. They are characterized as relatively unaggressive but not totally, because small-scale warfare between males does exist.[221] In this culture marriages are arranged, often in infancy and usually without regard for the women's wishes. Authority is vested in male elders. However, women play a significant part in all important sacred rituals, the predominant spiritual focus is female deities, and although children belong to the father's religious group and tribe, they belong to the mother's social group.[222] In aboriginal society both fathers and mothers have an important role in parenting, but the mother is most central the first three or four years.[223] There is religiously oriented competition although the main stress is on economic cooperation.[224] Thus, we have a society in which aggressiveness is played down, but has not been eliminated.

John Paddock examined two small towns in Mexico in the early 1970s with the same ethnic composition and located only ten miles apart.[225] They represent very different points on the continuum of violence versus nonviolence. Both communities were characterized by low educational levels, low population density, low social disorganization, poverty, and high consumption of alcohol. Yet one town was free of homicide (Town A), while the other had very high rates (Town B). Four differentiating characteristics were noted:

1. Childrearing was nonviolent in Town A (although discipline was firm and consistent) while in Town B there was "greater belief in the efficacy of striking a child."[226]

2. Local custom did not allow women to vote in either community, but in Town A fourteen-year-old girls were found to be "psychically and socially stronger" than in Town B.

3. "Machismo was all but absent" in Town A and children were taught to leave or avoid fights, while Town B emphasized traditional masculine behavior and such signs of machismo as cockfights were prevalent.[227]

4. Town A had less marital conflict.[228] (Paddock does not mention wife abuse specifically.)

Evidence for the idea that violence can be linked with strong machismo attitudes, forceful domination of women, and the use of physical punishment with children can be found in other anthropological studies. Leopold Bellak and Maxine Antell observed interactions between adults and children and between children on playgrounds in Frankfurt, Florence, and Copenhagen.[229] They found that both verbal and physical aggression was by far the highest by adults toward children in Frankfurt, as was violence between children. The rate of homicide is also much higher in Frankfurt than in Copenhagen, and a survey revealed that 60 percent of German parents believe in beating, "not slapping or spanking, but beating their children." The status of women is also much higher in Denmark.

Shirley A. McConahay and John B. McConahay used a random sample of seventeen nonindustrial cultures and found a significant correlation between sex role rigidity and violence, measured by punishment in childrearing, the prevalence of rape and murder, and the extent of war.[230] William Tulio Divale and Marvin Harris found that "frequent warfare is significantly correlated with patrilocal residence, patrilineal inheritance, polygyny, marriage by capture, brideprice, post-marital sexual restrictions on women and male secret societies." These authors conclude that "hostility between males is an integral part of the male supremacist complex."[231] James W. Prescott in a cross-cultural review found violence significantly associated with slavery, polygyny, inferior status of women, low levels of physical affection shown to infants, rigid values of monogamy, chastity and virginity, low overall infant indulgence, low invidious display of wealth and low religious activity.[232] In a study of fifty-seven cultures, Martin G. Allen found high crime rates in communities where there were also high levels of social and class stratification.[233] Beatrice B. Whiting studied six modern cultures ranging from nonindustrialized to highly industrialized. The two with the highest incidence of homicide and assault (Khalaphur,

Theories of Violence

India, and Nyarsongo, Kenya) both have a warrior and cattle thieving tradition in men; have little participation of fathers in childcare; and have customs separating men and women for sleeping, eating, working and playing.[234] Both cultures also practice violence against women: rape and genital mutilation are prevalent in Kenya and the women in this Indian region are kept in purdah (strict isolation and veiling in public) and are forced to "get down on the floor and cover their heads every time a man enters the courtyard."[235]

There are other anthropological views regarding the cultural origins of violence. Melvin Ember also found a significant relationship between polygyny and warfare, but postulates that polygyny is a result of the high male mortality rate in war.[236] Allen G. Pastron theorized that the violence that occurred regularly and frequently in an Indian culture in Mexico was because of the sanctions against verbal outlets for aggression since nonviolence is idealized. However, he also noted "minimal" involvement with machismo, frequent wife-beating, and violence based on jealousy. Pastron also found that children were "rarely hit," but this method of discipline was used occasionally.[237] Rather than classifying this culture as nonviolent as Pastron does, it seems reasonable to put it further along the continuum toward the violent end.

There was one anthropological study that found no association between the status of women and militarism.[238] However, it can be argued that the status of women cannot be measured simply. Martin King Whyte identified sixty-one measures of female position in a culture and found only weak correlations among them when applied to ninety-three randomly selected past and present cultures.[239] David Lester correlated rates of wifebeating in seventy-one nonliterate primitive societies and found it significantly related to inferior status of women, torturing enemies, aggressiveness with drinking, and "other indices of aggression in the society." It was less common where love-oriented techniques of disciplining children were more frequently used.[240]

These insights from the field of anthropology on the roots of violence in our society are useful for theoretical formulations but do not hold explanatory power in themselves. There is need to try and synthesize perspectives as a background for holistic nursing care.

Summary

Causative factors identified by various disciplines for violence have been seen to be complex, multifaceted, and not thoroughly substantiated by empirical research. It is evident that the problem of violence is deeply rooted historically, not easily delineated, nor casually approached. The corollary to such an observation is that if the answers were easy, we would have made more progress toward eliminating violence from our society! Various branches of scholarly endeavor have approached the problem and give important information from which to derive both societal and nursing approaches to solutions directed at prevention. The neurophysiologists have accumulated persuasive evidence about the neurological mechanisms with which human beings are born that make violence possible. They have pointed out that such factors as alcohol, stress, male hormones, and certain neurological defects can either enhance activity in the centers for aggressive behavior in the brain or partially counteract the normal physiologic inhibition processes for aggressive behavior. However, they are generally careful to point out that the neurological basis explains aggression mechanisms, not violent behavior, and that other factors are stronger in governing the incidence of that behavior.

Emotional states are one such factor and psychologists have postulated some of the affective conditions under which violence is more likely to occur. Low self-esteem, emotional deprivation, problems in interpersonal relationships, poorly developed ego functions, and frustrated goals can all be seen as psychological predispositions to violent behavior. Yet intrapsychic factors have not been shown to be the whole answer to who commits violent acts nor why they are committed. Another determinant of violence is undoubtedly learning, examined in detail by the social learning theorists. There is impressive evidence that aggression can be learned, but the exact behavioral response to that learning cannot be predicted in individuals. The sociologists have identified social factors that tend to accompany violence, yet these circumstances do not lead to violence in most people who experience them. Both sociological and anthropological studies have shown the importance of cultural sanctions for violence. The overview of comparatively violent and nonviolent cultures has afforded some clues to societal practices which are related to aggressive behavior. None of the disciplines claims to have discovered all the answers, and there needs to be an awareness of all the approaches to derive a meaningful synthesis.

Synthesis of theories is necessary for nursing as a background for understanding and approaching violence in the family. All the factors which influence violence in general can be brought to bear on the problems of child abuse, wife abuse, and abuse of other family members. With this kind of holistic theoretical representation, we can move forward to examine the issues which affect families in general and the specific causes of violence in the family as the basis for nursing practice.

Chapter 2

1. Murray Straus, "Violence Research, Violence Control, and the Good Society", in *Violence in the Family*, ed. Suzanne K. Steinmetz and Murray Straus (New York: Harper & Row. 1974), p. 321.

2. Juanita Kreps, *Social Indicators*, 1976 (Washington, D.C.: U. S. Department of Commerce, 1977), p. 195.

3. Peggy L. Chinn and Maeona K. Jacobs, "A Model for Theory Development in Nursing," *Advances in Nursing Science* 1, no. 1 (October 1961): 41.

4. *Webster's Third New International Dictionary*, s.v. "aggression."

5. Kenneth E. Moyer, The Psychobiology of Aggression (New York: Harper and Row, 1976) pp. 2, 3.

6. Sonja J. Herman, *Becoming Assertive: A Guide for Nurses* (New York: Van Nostrand Co., 1978), pp. 19, 17-18.

7. *Webster's Third New International Dictionary*, s.v. "violence."

8. Sandra Haber and Bernard Seidenberg, "Society's Recognition and Control of Violence," in *Violence: Perspectives on Murder and Aggression*, ed. Irwin L. Kutash et al. (San Francisco: Jossey-Bass Publishers, 1978), pp. 462, 463-465.

Theories of Violence

9. Bronislaw Malinowski, "An Anthropological Analysis of War," in *Aggression, Hostility and Violence*, eds. Terry Maple and Douglas R. Matheson (New York: Holt, Rinehart and Winston, 1973), 76–100. p. 86.
10. Marvin Wolfgang, "Violence in the Family," in Kutash et al. eds. *Violence: Perspectives on Murder and Aggression*, p. 469.
11. Lawrence Kolb, "Violence and Aggression: An Overview," in *Dynamics of Violence*, ed. Jan Fawcett (Chicago: American Medical Association, 1971), p. 7.
12. Derek Freeman, "Human Aggression in Anthropological Perspective," in *The Natural History of Aggression*, eds. J. D. Carthy and F. J. Ebling (London: Academic Press, 1964), 109–116, p. 112.
13. Malinowski, "An Anthropological Analysis of War," p. 23.
14. Stanislau Andreski, "Origins of War," in *The Natural History of Aggression*, ed. J. D. Carthy and F. J. Ebling (London: Academic Press, 1964), p. 130.
15. Erich Fromm, *The Anatomy of Human Destructiveness* (New York: Fawcett, 1973), pp. 169–86; Ruby Leavitt, *Peaceable Primates and Gentle People: Anthropological Approaches to Women's Studies* (New York: Harper & Row. 1975), pp. 17–20, 179–80.
16. Donald J. Mulvehill and Melvin M. Tumin, *Crimes of Violence*, vol. 12. A Staff Report Submitted to the National Commission on the Causes and Prevention of Violence (Washington, D. C.: U.S. Government Printing Office, 1969), p. 481.
17. Henry P. Lundsgaarde, *Murder in Space City* (New York: Oxford Press, 1977). p. 11.
18. Konrad Lorenz, *On Aggression* (New York: Bantam Books, 1966), p. ix.
19. Robert Ardrey, *The Territorial Imperative* (New York: Antheneum. 1966), pp. 252–75.
20. Ashley Montagu, *The Nature of Human Aggression* (New York: Oxford University Press, 1976); Fromm, *Anatomy of Human Destructiveness*, pp. 22–54; Alexander Alland, *The Human Imperative* (New York: Columbia University Press, 1972), pp. 25–99.
21. Leavitt, *Peaceable Primates*, p. 3; Montagu, p. 87.
22. Craig Wallace, "Why Do Animals Fight?", in *Aggression, Hostility and Violence*, ed. Terry Maple and Douglas R. Matheson (New York: Holt, Rinehart and Winston, 1973), pp. 65–76.
23. Leavitt, *Peaceable Primates*, p. 36.
24. Luigi Valzelli, *Psychobiology of Aggression and Violence* (New York: Raven Press, 1981), p. 44.
25. Moyer, *The Psychobiology of Aggression*, p. XIII.
26. Murray Goldstein, "Brain Research and Violent Behavior," *Archives of Neurology* 30 (January 1974): 2.
27. Moyer, *Psychobiology of Aggression*, p. 6.
28. Valzelli, *Psychobiology of Aggression and Violence*, p. 75.
29. Goldstein, "Brain Research" p. 8; Kenneth E. Moyer, "The Physiology of Aggression and the Implications for Aggression Control," in *The Control of Aggression and Violence* ed. Jerome Singer (New York: Academic Press, 1971), p. 62.
30. Moyer, *Psychobiology of Aggression*, p. 8.
31. Valzelli, *Psychobiology of Aggression and Violence*, p. 54.
32. Moyer, *Psychobiology of Aggression*, pp. 6–7.
33. Ibid., pp. 8, 10, 57.
34. Goldstein, "Brain Research," p. 13.
35. Hans Seyle, *The Stress of Life* (New York: McGraw-Hill, 1956), pp. 118, 119.
36. Moyer, *Psychobiology of Aggression*, pp. 8, 11.
37. Goldstein, "Brain Research," p. 16.

38. Dietrich Blumer and Claude Migeon, "Hormones and Hormonal Agents in the Treatment of Aggression," *Journal of Nervous and Mental Diseases* 160 (January 1975): 128.

39. John Paul Scott, *Aggression* (Chicago: University of Chicago Press, 1958 and 1975), p. 144.

40. Steven Goldberg, *The Inevitability of Patriarchy* (New York: William Morrow & Co., 1973), p. 108.

41. H. Persky, K. D. Smith, and G. K. Basu. "Relationship of Psychologic Measures of Aggression and Hostility to Testosterone Production in Men," *Psychosomatic Medicine* 33 (1971): 265.

42. Valzelli, *Psychobiology of Aggression and Violence*, p. 119.

43. Moyer, *Psychobiology of Aggression*, pp. 67, 69.

44. Rudolf H. Moos et al., "Fluctuations in Symptoms and Moods During the Menstrual Cycle," *Journal of Psychosomatic Research* 13 (March 1969): 43.

45. David A. Hamburg, "Recent Research on Hormonal Factors Relevant to Human Aggressiveness," *International Social Science Journal* 23 (1971): 41.

46. Arnold Klopper, "Physiological Background to Aggression," in *The Natural History of Aggression*, ed. J. D. Carthy and F. J. Ebling (London: Academic Press, 1964), p. 70.

47. Donald Goodwin, "Alcohol in Suicide and Homicide," *Quarterly Journal of Studies on Alcohol* 34 (March 1973): 153.

48. A. R. Nicol, "The Relationship of Alcoholism to Violent Behavior Resulting in Long-Term Imprisonment," *British Journal of Psychiatry* 123 (1973): 47–51.

49. Lowell Gerson and Donald A. Preston, "Alcohol Consumption and the Incidence of Violent Crime," *Journal of Studies on Alcohol* 40 (March 1979): p. 311.

50. Kathryn Graham, "Theories of Intoxicated Aggression," *Canadian Journal of Behavioral Science* 12, no. 2 (April 1980): 143.

51. Ibid, p. 144; Gregory Schmutte, Kenneth Leonard, and Stuart Taylor, "Alcohol and Expectations of Attack," *Psychological Reports* 45 no. 1 (August 1979): 164.

52. Graham, "Theories of Intoxicated Aggression," p. 145; Robert J. Powers and Irwin L. Kutash, "Substance Induced Aggression," in Kutash et al., *Violence: Perspectives on Murder and Aggression*, p. 322.

53. Graham, "Theories of Intoxicated Aggression," p. 147.

54. Graham, "Theories of Intoxicated Aggression," p. 147; Jack M. Mendelson and Nancy K. Mello, "Alcohol, Aggression, and Androgens," in *Aggression*, ed. Shevert H. Frazier (Baltimore: Williams & Wilkins Press, 1974), pp. 226, 237, 244.

55. Ernest L. Abel, "The Relationship between Cannabis and Violence: A Review." *Psychological Bulletin* 84 (March 1977): 204.

56. Mortimer A. Gross, "Violence Associated with Organic Brain Disease," in *Dynamics of Violence*, ed. Jan Fawcett (Chicago: AMA, 1971), p. 87.

57. George Bach-Y-Rita et al., "Episodic Dyscontrol: A Study of 130 Violent Patients," *American Journal of Psychiatry* 127 (May 1971): 1475.

58. Abel, "Relationship between Cannabis and Violence"; p. 207. Gross, "Violence Associated with Organic Brain Disease," p. 81.

59. Powers and Kutash, "Substance Induced Aggression," p. 323.

60. Graham, "Theories of Intoxicated Aggression," pp. 148, 151, 152, 153.

61. Richard Gelles, *The Violent Home* (Beverly Hills: Sage Publications, 1972), p. 114.

62. Moyer, *Psychobiology of Aggression*, p. 12.

63. Valzelli, *Psychobiology of Aggression and Violence*, pp. 99, 112.

64. Ibid., p. 13.

Theories of Violence

65. Goldstein, "Brain Research," p. 17.

66. Ibid., pp. 17, 18; David Owen, "The 47, XYY Male," *Psychological Bulletin* 78 (September 1972): 209–233, 210, 226; Herman A. Witkin et al., "Criminality in XYY and XXY Men," *Science* 193 (13 August 1976): 550, 551.

67. Dietrich Blumer, "Epilepsy and Violence," in *Rage, Assault, and Other Forms of Violence*, ed. Denis J. Madden and John R. Lion (New York: Spectrum Publications, 1976), p. 209.

68. Russell Monroe, *Brain Dysfunction in Aggressive Criminals*, (Lexington, Massachusetts: D.C. Heath and Company, 1976), p. 1.

69. Ibid., p. 6.

70. Ibid, p. 88. Barry M. Maletzky, "Episodic Dyscontrol Syndrome," *Diseases of the Nervous System* 34, (March 1973), pp. 178–185, p. 179; Frank Spellacy, "Neuropsychological Difference between Violent and Nonviolent Adolescents," *Journal of Clinical Psychology* 33 (October 1977): p. 168; Frank Elliott, "The Neurology of Explosive Rage," *Practitioner* 217 (July 1976): pp. 51–59, p. 54. James R. Morrison and Kenneth Minkoff, "Explosive Personality as a Sequel to the Hyperative-Child Syndrome," *Comprehensive Psychiatry* 16 (July/August 1975): p. 346.

71. Lion and Penna, p. 169; Bach-Y-Rita, "Episodic Dyscontrol," p. 1477; Elliott, p. 54; Morrison and Minkoff, "Explosive Personality," p. 346.

72. Richard Allen, Daniel Safer, and Lino Covi, "Effects of Psychostimulants on Aggression," *Journal of Nervous and Mental Diseases* 160 (February 1975): 138–145.

73. Bach-Y-Rita, "Episodic Dyscontrol," p. 1478; Russell R. Monroe, "Anticonvulsants in the Treatment of Aggression," *Journal of Nervous and Mental Diseases* 160 (January 1975): 125.

74. Maletzky, "Episodic Dyscontrol Syndrome," p. 183; Monroe et al., *Brain Dysfunction*, p. 164.

75. Moyer, *Psychobiology of Aggression*, pp. 38, 32.

76. Frank Spellacy, "Neuropsychological Discrimination between Violent and Nonviolent Men," *Journal of Clinical Psychology*, 34 (January 1978): 50; Gross,"Violence Associated with Organic Brain Disease," pp. 87, 90; Moyer, *Psychobiology of Aggression*, pp. 10, 28; Kolb, "Violence and Aggression," p. 10.

77. Moyer, *Psychobiology of Aggression*, pp. 18–20.

78. Maletzky, "Episodic Dyscontrol Syndrome," p. 179; Monroe et al., *Brain Dysfunction*, p. 82.

79. Goldstein, "Brain Research," p. 18; Gross, "Violence Associated with Organic Brain Disease," p. 85.

80. Moyer, *Psychobiology of Aggression*, p. 18.

81. Vernon H. Mark and Frank A. Ervin, *Violence and the Brain*, (New York: Harper and Row, 1970) pp 155–160.

82. Gross, "Violence Associated with Organic Brain Disease," p. 90.

83. Lion and Penna, P. 168.

84. Moyer, *Psychobiology of Aggression*, p. 23.

85. Kolb, "Violence and Aggression," p. 10.

86. Scott, *Aggression*, p. 131.

87. Henri Laborit, "The Biological and Sociological Mechanisms of Aggression," *International Social Science Journal* 30 (1978): 738.

88. Josi M. R. Delgado, "The Neurological Basis of Violence," *International Social Science Journal* 33 (1971): 33.

89. Lee S. Coleman, "Perspectives on the Medical Research of Violence," *American Journal of Orthopsychiatry* 44 (October 1974): 685.

90. Sigmund Freud to Albert Einstein, 1932, "Why War?" in Maple and Matheson, *Aggression, Hostility, and Violence*, p. 21.

91. Marguerite Q. Warren and Michael J. Hindelang, "Current Explanation of Offender Behaviory," in *Psychology of Crime and Criminal Justice*, ed. Hans Toch (New York, Holt, Rinehart, & Winston, 1979), p. 172.

92. Fromm, *Anatomy of Human Destructiveness*, pp. 486-528; Irwin Kutash, "Psychoanalytic Theories of Aggression," in *Violence: Perspectives on Murder and Aggression*, pp. 8-57.

93. Freud, "Why War?"

94. John M. MacDonald, *The Murderer and His Victim* (Springfield, Ill.: Charles C. Thomas, 1961), p. 110.

95. David Abrahamsen, *The Psychology of Crime* (New York: Columbia University Press, 1960), pp. 15, 23, 25, 30; David Abrahamsen, *Our Violent Society* (New York: Funk & Wagnalls, 1970), p. 60.

96. John Dollard et al., "Frustration and Aggression," in *The Dynamics of Aggression*, ed. Edwin I. Magargee and Jack E. Hokanson (New York: Harper & Row, 1970), p. 25; Neal E. Miller, "The Frustration-Aggression Hypothesis," in Maple, and Matheson, *Aggression, Hostility, and Violence*, p. 104.

97. Fromm, *Anatomy of Human Destructiveness*, p. 92; Arnold Buss, *The Psychology of Aggression* (New York: John Wiley & Sons, 1961), p. 27.

98. Dollard, "Frustration and Aggression," p. 31.

99. Jack E. Hokanson, "Psychophysiological Evaluation of the Catharsis Hypothesis," in *The Dynamics of Aggression*, Megorgee and Hokanson, p. 75.

100. Ibid., p. 85; Leonard Berkowitz, "Experimental Investigation of Hostility Catharsis," *Journal of Consulting and Clinical Psychology*, 35, (February 1970): p. 6.

101. Moyer, *Psychobiology of Aggression*, p. 276.

102. Shanbaz K. Mallick and Boyd R. McCandless, "A Study of Catharsis of Aggression," *Journal of Personality and Social Psychology* 4 (November 1966): 596; Murray Straus, "Leveling, Civility, and Violence in the Family," *Journal of Marriage and the Family* 36 (February 1974): 18, 25.

103. Berkowitz, "Experimental Investigation," p. 3; Dolf Zillman, "Excitation Transfer in Communication-Medicated Aggressive Behavior," *Journal of Experimental Social Psychology* 7 (May 1971): 430; Donald P. Hartman, "Influence of Symbolically Modeled Instrumental Aggression and Pain Cues on Aggressive Behavior," *Journal of Personality and Social Psychology* 11 (1969): 285.

104. Montagu, *Nature of Human Aggression*, p. 77; Fillman, "Excitation Transfer," p. 430.

105. Edwin I. Megargee, "Undercontrolled and Overcontrolled Personality Type in Extreme Antisocial Aggression," *Psychological Monographs* 80 (1966): 3-20.

106. Ibid, p. 7; Charles Hanley, "The Gauging of Delinquency Potential," in Toch, *Psychology of Crime and Criminal Justice*, p. 259; Gary Fisher, "Discriminating Violence Emanating from Over-Controlled Versus Under-Controlled Aggressivity," *British Journal of Social and Clinical Psychology* 9 (February 1970): 55.

107. Megargee, "Undercontrolled and Overcontrolled Personality Type," p. 17; Hokanson, "Psychophysiological Evaluation," p. 85; Fisher, "Discriminating Violence," p. 56.

108. Abrahamsen, *Our Violent Society*, pp. 21, 230; Seyle, *Stress of Life*, p. 68; Anthony Storr, *Human Destructiveness* (New York: Basic Books, 1972), p. 37; Ismail B. Sendi and Paul G. Blongren, "A Comparative Study of Predictive Criteria in the Predisposition of Homicidal Adolescents," *American Journal of Psychiatry* 132 (April 1975): 425, 426; Abrahamsen, *Psychology of Crime*, p. 68.

109. Sendi and Blongren, "Comparative Study of Predictive Criteria," p. 425; Joseph Satten et al., "Murder Without Apparent Motive: A Study in Personality Disorganization," *American Journal of Psychology* 117 (1960): 49; Maletzky, "Episodic Dyscontrol Syndrome," p 179.

110. Storr, *Human Destructiveness*, pp. 37, 86; Sendi and Blongren, "Comparative Study of Predictive Criteria," p. 424; George Bach-Y-Rita and Arther Veno, "Habitual Violence: A Profile of Sixty-Two Men," *American Journal of Psychiatry* 131 (September 1974): 1016,

111. Bach-Y-Rita and Veno, "Habitual Violence," p. 1016.

Theories of Violence

112. Donald T. Lunde, *Murder and Madness* (San Francisco: San Francisco Book Co., 1976), p. 83; Abrahamsen, *Psychology of Crime*, p. 56; Leon Saul, "A Psychoanalytic View of Hostility: Its Genesis, Treatment, and Implications," *Humanitas* 12 (May, 1976) 171-182, p. 172.

113. Sendi and Blongren, "Comparative Study of Predictive Criteria," p. 424; Satten, "Murder Without Apparent Motive," p. 48; Bach-Y-Rita and Veno, "Habitual Violence."

114. Henley, "Gauging of Delinquency Potential," p. 256; Barry J. McGurk, "Personality Types among 'Normal' Homicides," *British Journal of Criminology* 18 (April 1978): 158, 159.

115. Alvin M. Mesnikoff and Carl D. Lauterbach, "The Association of Violent Dangerous Behavior with Psychiatric Disorders: A Review of the Research Literature," *Journal of Psychiatry and the Law* 3 (Winter 1975): 440.

116. John J. Brennan, "Mentally Ill Aggressiveness—Popular Delusion or Reality," *American Journal of Psychiatry* 120 (June 1964): 1184; Kolb, "Violence and Aggression," p. 12.

117. Mesnikoff and Lauterbach, "Association of Violent Dangerous Behavior," p. 439; James M. Mullen et al., "Dangerous and the Mentally Ill Offender," *Hospitals and Community Psychiatry* 29 (July 1978): 425; Jeffrey A. Buck and John R. Graham, "The 4-3 MMP, Profile Type: A Failure to Replicate," *Journal of Consulting and Clinical Psychology* 46 (April 1978): 344; Joseph J. Cocozza and Henry Steadman, "Some Refinements in the Measurement of Prediction of Dangerous Behavior," *American Journal of Psychiatry* 131 (September 1974): 1014.

118. Fromm, *Anatomy of Human Destructiveness*, pp. 299, 361, 482.

119. Rollo May, *Power and Innocence* (New York: W. W. Norton, 1972), pp. 21, 23, 35, 39, 99.

120. Howard B. Kaplan, *Self-Attitudes of Deviant Behavior* (Pacific Palisades, Calif.: Goodyear Publishing Co., 1975), pp. 10, 21, 67, 130.

121. Hans Toch, *Violent Men* (Chicago: Aldine Publishing Co., 1969), pp. 137, 188.

122. Kaplan, *Self-Attitude of Deviant Behavior*, p. 91.

123. Paul Yelsma and Julie Yelsma, "Self-Esteem of Prisoners Committing Directly Versus Indirectly Destructive Crimes," *Perceptual and Motor Skills* 44 (April 1977): 375, 378.

124. James B. McCarthy, "Narcissism and the Self in Homicidal Adolescents," *American Journal of Psychoanalysis* 38 (Spring 1978): 25.

125. Gregory Rochlin, *Man's Aggression* (Boston: Gambit, 1973), p. 2; Donald Grant, "A Model of Violence," *Australian and New Zealand Journal of Psychiatry* 12 (June 1978): 123.

126. Kutash, "Psychoanalytic Theories of Aggression," pp. 12-17.

127. Ibid., pp. 21-25.

128. Lunde, *Murder and Madness*, pp. 93, 75.

129. Albert Bandura, *Aggression: A Social Learning Analysis* (Englewood Cliffs, N.J.: Prentice-Hall, 1973), p. viii.

130. Alan Newcombe, "Some Contributions of the Behavioral Sciences to the Study of Violence," *International Social Science Journal* 30 (1978): 750-768.

131. Laborit, "Biological and Sociological Mechanisms."

132. Ibid., pp. 5-7.

133. Albert Bandura, "The Social Learning Perspective," in Toch, *Psychology of Crime and Criminal Justice*, p. 200.

134. Ibid.

135. Bandura, *Aggression: A Social Learning Analysis*, pp. 55-57, 58.

136. Ibid., p. 58.

137. Mullen et al., "Dangerous and Mentally Ill Offender," pp. 203, 204.
138. Bandura, *Aggression: A Social Learning Analysis*, p. 115; Bandura, "Social Learning Perspectives."
139. Albert Bandura, "Influence of Models' Reinforcement Contingencies on the Acquisition of Initiative Responses," *Journal of Personality and Social Psychology* 1 (June 1965): 590.
140. David J. Owens and Murray A. Straus, "The Social Structure of Violence in Childhood and Approval of Violence as an Adult," *Aggressive Behavior* 1 (1975): 195, 196, 210.
141. Bandura, *Aggression: A Social Learning Analysis*, pp. 128, 3.
142. Ibid., p. 193; L. B. Silver, C. C. Dublin, and R. S. Lourie, "Does Violence Breed Violence? Contributions from a Study of the Child Abuse Syndrome," *American Journal of Psychology* 126 (1969): 407.
143. Bandura, *Aggression: A Social Learning Analysis*, p. 94.
144. David J. Hicks, "Imitation and Retention of Film-Medicated Aggressive Peer and Adult Models," *Journal of Personality and Social Psychology* 2 (1965): 100.
145. Jerry Neopolitan, "Parental Influence on Aggressive Behavior: A Social Learning Approach," *Adolescence* 16 (Winter 1981): 831–840.
146. Elizabeth D. McCarthy et al., "Violence and Behavior Disorders," *Journal of Communications* 25 (Autumn 1975): 72, 77.
147. Stanley Milgram and R. Lance Shotland, *Television and Antisocial Behavior: Field Experiments* (New York: Academic Press, 1973), p. 46; Robert M. Kaplan and Robert D. Singer, "Television Violence and Viewer Aggression: A Reexamination of the Evidence," *Journal of Social Issues* 32 (Fall 1976): 62.
148. Jerome Singer and Dorothy Singer, "Television Viewing, Family Style and Aggressive Behavior in Preschool Children," in *Violence and the Family*, ed. Maurice R. Green (Boulder: Westview Press, 1980), pp. 37–65.
149. Leonard Eron, "Prescription for Reduction of Aggression," *American Psychologist* 35 (March 1980): 244–252.
150. F. Scott Andison, "TV Violence and Viewer Aggression: A Cumulation of Study Results, 1956–1976" *Public Opinion Quarterly* 41 (Fall 1977): 318, 319.
151. George Gerbner et al., "TV Violence Profile No. 8: The Highlights," *Journal of Communications* 27 (Spring 1977): 178; George Gerbner et al., "The Demonstration of Power: Violence Profile No. 10," *Journal of Communications* 29 (Summer 1979): 180.
152. Bandura, "*Social Learning Perspective*," p. 204; McCarthy, "Violence and Behavior Disorders," p. 72.
153. Jeffrey Goldstein, *Aggression and Crimes of Violence* (New York: Oxford University Press, 1975), p. 39.
154. Allen Fenigstein, "Does Aggression Cause a Preference for Viewing Media Violence?" *Journal of Personality and Social Psychology* 37 (December 1979): 2307–2317.
155. Jacques-Phillipe Leyens et al., "Effects of Movie Violence on Aggression in a Field Setting as a Function of Group Dominance and Cohesion," *Journal of Personality and Social Psychology* 32 (August 1975): 353.
156. Gerbner et al., "Demonstration of Power," p. 171; Bandura, "Social Learning Perspective," p. 204.
157. Gerbner et al., "Demonstration of Power," p. 196.
158. Bandura, "Social Learning Perspective," p. 207.
159. Russell G. Geen and David Stonner, "Effects of Aggressiveness Habit Strength on Behavior in the Presence of Aggression-Related Stimuli," *Journal of Personality and Social Psychology* 17 (February 1971): 149.
160. Laborit, "Biological and Sociological Mechanisms," p. 740.
161. David G. Perry and Kay Bussey, "Self-Reinforcement in High- and Low-Aggressive Boys Following Acts of Aggression," *Child Development* 48 (June 1977): 653, 655.
162. Laborit, "Biological and Sociological Mechanisms," p. 746.

163. Edwin I. Megargee, "The Role of Inhibitor in the Assessment and Understanding of Violence," in *The Control of Aggression and Violence*, ed. Jerome Singer (New York: Academic Press, 1971), p. 130; Bandura, "Social Learning Perspective," p. 224.

164. Bandura, "Influences of Models Reinforcement Contingencies," p. 594; Owens and Straus, "Social Structure of Violence," p. 207.

165. Leyens, "Effects of Movie Violence," p. 346; Fromm, *Anatomy of Human Destructiveness*, p. 93.

166. Hartman, pp. 280-288; Goldstein, *Aggression and Crimes of Violence*; Charles Mueller, Robin Nelson, and Edward Donnerstein, "Facilitative Effects of Media Violence on Helping," *Psychological Reports* 40 (June 1977): 775-78; Arnold Buss et al., "Firing a Weapon and Aggression," *Journal of Personality and Social Psychology* 22 (June 1972): 296-302; Leonard Berkowitz and Anthony LePage, "Weapons as Aggression-Eliciting Stimuli," *Journal of Personality and Social Psychology* 7 (1967): 202-207; Monte Page and Rick Scheidt, "The Elusive Weapons Effect," *Journal of Personality and Social Psychology* 20 (December 1971): 304-318; Lenonard Berkowitz and Joseph Alioto, "The Meaning of an Observed Event as a Determinant of Its Aggressive Consequences," *Journal of Personality and Social Psychology* 28 (November 1973): 206-217; Edward Diener, "Effects of Altered Responsibility, Cognitive Set, and Modeling on Physical Aggression and Deindividuation," *Journal of Personality and Social Psychology* 31 (1975): 328-337; Glen S. Sanders and Robert Steven Baron, "Pain Cues and Uncertainty as Determinants of Aggression in a Situation Involving Repeated Instigation," *Journal of Personality and Social Psychology* 32 (September 1975): 495-502; Wade Silverman, "The Effects of Social Contact, Provocation, and Sex of Opponent upon Instrumental Aggression," *Journal of Experimental Research in Personality* 5 (December 1971): 310-316; Ervin Straub, "The Learning and Unlearning of Aggression," in Singer, *The Control of Aggression and Violence*, p. 111; Leonard White, "Erotica and Aggression: The Influence of Sexual Arousal, Positive Affect, and Negative Effect on Aggressive Behavior," *Journal of Personality and Social Psychology* 37 (April 1979): 591-601.

167. R. J. Sebastian, "Immediate and Delayed Effects of Victim Suffering on the Attacker's Aggression," *Journal of Research in Personality* 12 (September 1978): 312-28; Sanders and Baron. p. 501.

168. Straub, "Learning and Unlearning of Aggression;" Buss, *Psychology of Aggression*; Goldstein, *Aggression and Crime*.

169. D. J. West, "The Response to Violence," *Journal of Medical Ethics* 5 (1979): 128.

170. Michael R. Chatterton, "The Social Contexts of Violence," in *Violence in the Family*, ed. Marie Borland (Atlantic Highlands, N.J.: Humanities Press, 1976), pp. 25-33, 31.

171. Monica Blumenthal et al., *Justifying Violence* (Ann Arbor, Mich.: Braun-Brumfeld, 1972), p. 243.

172. Lundsgaarde, *Murder in Space City*, pp. 11, 186, 190-192.

173. David G. Gil. "Societal Violence and Violence in Families," in *Family Violence*, ed. John M. Eckelaar and Stanford N. Katz (Toronto: Butterworth and Co., 1978), p. 14.

174. Ibid, pp. 17, 20.

175. Bernard Bergen and Stanley Rosenberg. "Culture as Violence," *Humanitas* 12 (May 1976): 196, 197.

176. Marvin Wolfgang, "A Preface to Violence," *Annals of the American Academy of Political and Social Science* 364 (March 1966): 1-7, 3.

177. Toch, *Psychology of Crime and Criminal Justice*, p 167.

178. Robert K. Merton, "Social Structure and Anomie," *American Sociological Review* 3 (October 1938): 672-682.

179. Ibid., p. 681; Richard A. Cloward and Lloyd E. Ohlin, *Delinquency and Opportunity* (Glencoe, Ill.: Free Press, 1960), p. 78.

180. Cloward and Ohlin, *Delinquency and Opportunity*, pp. 97, 117.

181. J. P. Scott, "Agnostic Behavior: Function and Dysfunction in Social Conflict," *Journal of Social Issues* 33 (Winter 1977): 9-11.

182. Lester D. Jaffe, "Delinquency, Proneness, and Family Anomie," *Journal of Criminal Law, Criminology, and Police Science* 54 (June 1963): 147.

183. Bandura, "Influence of Models' Reinforcement Contingencies," p. 2; Claire Russell and W. M. J. Russell, "The Natural History of Violence," *Journal of Medical Ethics* 5 (1979): 110.

184. Paul Spector, "Population Density and Unemployment," *Criminology* 12 (February 1975): 400; Omar R. Galle, Walter R. Gove, and J. William McPherson, "Population Density and Pathology: What are the Relations for Man?" *Science* 176 (7 April 1972): 25.

185. Galle, Gove, and McPherson, "Population Density and Pathology," p. 26.

186. Spector, "Population Density and Unemployment," p. 40.

187. Dane Archer et al., "Cities and Homicide: A New Look at an Old Paradox," *Comparative Studies in Sociology* 1 (1978): 76, 87.

188. Harold M. Rose, "Lethal Aspects of Urban Violence: An Overview," in *Lethal Aspects of Urban Violence*, ed. Harold M. Rose (Lexington, Mass.: Lexington Books, 1979), pp. 5-7.

189. Lynn A. Curtis, *Criminal Violence* (Lexington, Mass.: D. C. Heath & Co., 1974), p. 159.

190. Marvin Wolfgang, *Crime and Race* (New York: Institute of Human Relations Press, 1964), p. 58.

191. Robert Liston, *Violence in America* (New York: Julian Messner, 1974), p. 151.

192. Robert Nash Parker and M. Dwayne Smith, "Deterrence, Poverty, and Type of Homicide," *American Journal of Sociology* 85 (November 1979): 622.

193. Spector, "Population Density and Unemployment," p. 399.

194. Curtis, *Criminal Violence*, pp. 150, 151.

195. Rose, "Lethal Aspects of Urban Violence," p. 8.

196. Edward Greene and Russell Wakefield, "Patterns of Middle and Upper Class Homicide," *Journal of Criminal Law and Criminology* 70 (Summer 1979): 175.

197. Elmer Luchterhand and Leonard Weller, "Effects of Class, Race, Sex, and Educational Status on Patterns of Aggression in Lower Class Youth," *Journal of Youth and Adolescence* 5 (March 1976): 63, 65.

198. Carolyn Balkwell et al., "On Black and White Family Patterns in America: Their Impact on the Expressive Aspect of Sex-Role Socialization," *Journal of Marriage and the Family* 40 (November 1978): 744.

199. Robert Coles, "Violence in Ghetto Children," *Children* 14 (May-June, 1967): 101-104. Judging from this chapter author's experience with hundreds of black adolescents, this author found them to be more verbally expressive in all emotions than white teenagers.

200. Daniel P. Moynihan, in Moynihan and the National Commission on the Causes and Prevention of Violence, "Toward a National Urban Policy," *Violent Crime* (New York: George Braziller, 1969), p. 10; Frank R. Scarpitti, "The Good Boy in a High Delinquency Area: Four Years Later," *American Sociological Review* 25 (August 1969): 556.

201. Wade W. Nobles, "Toward an Empirical and Theoretical Framework for Defining Black Families," *Journal of Marriage and the Family* 40 (November 1978): 680, 687.

202. Karen W. Bartz and Elaine S. Levine, "Childrearing by Black Parents: A Description and Comparison to Anglo and Chicano Parents," *Journal of Marriage and the Family* 40 (November 1978): 709-720, 714-15.

203. Rose, "Lethal Aspects of Urban Violence," p 7.

204. Cloward and Ohlin, *Delinquency and Opportunity*, pp. 20, 23, 27.

205. Marvin Wolfgang and Franco Ferracuti, *The Subculture of Violence* (London: Tavistock Publications, 1967), pp. 275, 282, 298.

206. John Hepburn, "Subcultures, Violence, and the Subculture of Violence: An Old Rut or a New Road," *Criminology* 9 (May 1971); 87-98: 93.

207. Maxine Letcher, "Black Women and Homicide," in *Lethal Aspects of Urban Violence*, ed. Harold M. Rose (Lexington, Mass.: Lexington Books, 1979), p. 89.

208. Richard Moran, "Criminal Homicide: External Restraint and Subculture of Violence," *Criminology* 8 (February 1971): 358, 362, 363, 367, 372.

209. William H. Webster, *Uniform Crime Reports* (Washington, D.C.: U.S. Department of Justice, 1978), p. 10.

210. Raymond Gastil, "Homicide and a Regional Culture of Violence," *American Sociological Review* 36 (June 1971): 412, 414.

211. William Doerner, "A Regional Analysis of Homicide Rates in the United States," *Criminology* 13 (May 1975): 90-101; Alvin Jacobsen, "Crime Trends in Southern and Non-Southern Cities: A Twenty-Year Perspective," *Social Forces* 54 (September 1975): 226-42; James O'Connor and Alan Lizotte, "The Southern Subculture of Violence: Thesis and Patterns of Gun Ownership," *Social Problems* 25 (April 1978): 420-29; Howard Erlanger, "Is There a Subculture of Violence in the South?" *Journal of Criminal Law and Criminology* 66 (December 1975): 483-90; William C. Bailey, "Some Further Evidence on Homicide and a Regional Culture of Violence," *Omega* 7 (1976): 145-70; Howard S. Erlanger, "The Empirical Status of the Subculture of Violence Thesis," *Social Problems* 22 (December 1974): 280-92.

212. Lynn A. Curtis, *Violence, Race, and Culture* (Lexington, Mass:, D. C. Heath & Co., 1975), p. 163.

213. Hepburn, "Subcultures, Violence, and the Subculture of Violence," p. 93; Erlanger, "Empirical Status," p. 289; Curtis, *Violence, Race, and Culture*, p. 24; Wolfgang and Ferracuti, *Subculture of Violence*, p. 259.

214. Stuart Palmer, *The Violent Society* (New Haven: College and University Press, 1970), pp. 16, 26, 30.

215. Ashley Montagu, Introduction in his *Learning Non-Aggression*, (New York: Oxford Press, 1978), p. 6.

216. Fromm, *Anatomy of Human Destructiveness*, pp. 194, 195, 196.

217. Colin Turnbull, "Politics of Non-Aggression," in *Learning Non-Aggression*, ed. Ashley Montagu (New York: Oxford Press 1978) p. 218; Jean L. Briggs, *Never in Anger* (Cambridge: Harvard University Press, 1970), p. 64; Fromm, p. 196.

218. Briggs, *Never in Anger*, p 154.

219. A. P. Elkin, *The Australian Aborigines* Natural History Library Edition (Garden City, N.Y.: Doubleday, 1964), p. 53; Joseph W. Eaton, "Controlled Acculturation: A Survival Technique of the Hitterites," *American Sociological Review* 17 (June 1952): 333; Margaret Mead, *Male and Female* (New York, William Morrow & Co., 1949) p. 65.

220. Sorenson, "Fore of New Guinea," p. 27; Levy, "Tahitian Gentleness," 228-29, 231; Turnbull, "Politics of Non-Aggression," p. 200; Briggs, *Never in Anger*, pp. 329, 345; Robert Knox Denton, "Notes on Childhood in a Nonviolent Context: The Semai Case," in Montagu, *Learning Non-Aggresion*, p. 128; Louis Jolyin West, "Discussion: Violence and the Family in Perspective," in Green, *Violence and the Family*, pp. 90-104.

221. Catherine H. Berndt, "In Aboriginal Australia," in Montagu, *Learning Non-Aggression*, p. 154.

222. Elkin, *Australian Aborigines*, pp. 53, 87, 130, 190, 226.

223. Ibid, p. 53; Berndt "In Aboriginal Australia," p. 150.

224. Berndt, "In Aboriginal Australia," p. 148; Elkin, *Australian Aborigines*, pp. 190, 192.

225. John Paddock, "Studies on Antiviolent and 'Normal' Communities," *Aggressive Behavior* 1 (1975): 217-33; John Paddock, "Values in an Antiviolent Community," *Humanitas* 12 (May 1976): 183-94.

226. Paddock, "Studies on Antiviolent and 'Normal' Communities," p. 225.

227. Paddock, "Values in an Antiviolent Community," p. 191.

228. Paddock, "Studies on Antiviolent and 'Normal' Communities," p. 229.

229. Leopold Bellak and Maxine Antell, "An Intercultural Study of Aggressive Behavior on Children's Playgrounds," *American Journal of Orthopsychiatry* 44 (July 1974): 504, 508.

230. Shirley A. McConahay and John B. McConahay, "Sexual Permissiveness, Sex-Role Rigidity, and Violence Across Cultures," *Journal of Social Issues* 33 (1977): 139, 140.

231. William Tulio Divale and Marvin Harris, "Population, Warfare, and the Male Supremacist Complex," *American Anthropologist* 78 (September 1976): 532, 533.

232. James W. Prescott, "Body Pleasure and the Origins of Violence," *The Futurist* 9 (April 1975): 66, 73.

233. Martin G. Allen, "A Cross-Cultural Study of Aggression and Crime," *Journal of Cross-Cultural Psychology* 3 (September 1972): 265.

234. Beatrice B. Whiting, "Sex Identity Conflict and Physical Violence: A Comparative Study, Part 2," *American Anthropologist* 67 (December 1965): 128, 130, 132, 135.

235. Ibid., pp. 131, 133, 136; Fran P. Hosken, "Female Circumcision in Africa," *Victimology* 2 (1977–78): 487.

236. Melvin Ember, "Warfare, Sex Ratio, and Polygyny," *Ethnology* 13 (April 1974): 202.

237. Allen G. Pastron, "Collective Defenses of Repression and Denial: Their Relationship to Violence among the Tarahumana Indians of Northern Mexico," *Ethos* 2 (Winter 1974): pp. 388, 391–393, 400.

238. William Eckhardt, "Anthropological Correlates of Primitive Militarism," *Peace Research* 5 (February 1973): 6.

239. Martin King Whyte, "Cross-Cultural Code Dealing with the Relative Status of Women," *Ethnology* 17 (April 1978): 214.

240. Lester, "Cross-Culture Study of Wife Abuse."

Family Well-Being

Susan Blanch Meister

"The family,
as a set of real human beings interacting
with one another,
transcends any model."

Abraham Kaplan

Conduct of Inquiry (New York: Chandler, 1964).

Family well-being is a construct that offers particular value and pertinence to nursing practice, theory, and research. Family well-being is a function of the fit between demands and resources, and dysfunctional fits are associated with decreased well-being and sometimes even violence. Currently, the empirical knowledge to define and measure family well-being is lacking. However, research in contributing disciplines substantiates the viability and importance of the concept. A representative subset of this research is presented in this chapter to describe "the family" as a convoy of relationships which is affected by the needs and abilities of its members, and contributes to defining and meeting both aggregate and individual needs. Results of extensive research in the well-being of individuals are also presented. The chapter closes with issues in family well-being which are pertinent to nursing care of violent families.

THE CONCEPT OF FAMILY WELL-BEING

Family well-being is a hybrid concept. "Family" has been the subject of decades of research and theory building, while "well-being" has a shorter history in scientific study. Traditional frameworks for describing families have used significantly different definitions of and perspectives on the family. For example, the developmental framework defines the family as an aggregate and studies the developmental issues that confront that aggregate: establishing a home, negotiating school entry of the oldest child, managing the changes caused by the departure of the youngest child from the home. On the other hand, the structure-function framework emphasizes the organization of the family and studies the family functions that are achieved and ascribed: reproduction of the species, socialization of children, provision of adequate living environments. The roles framework emphasizes roles that are associated with each position in the family and describes how those roles are defined, enacted, and changed: establishment of spouse roles, enlargement of spouse role complexes to include parenting, and adjustments of parenting roles in response to development of the children. The interactionist framework focuses on the communication patterns within the family and describes short- and long-term effects of various patterns: effect of open communicative styles in young children and later impacts when those children are adolescents, effects of ritualized and rigid communicative styles in similar time periods. Systems frameworks emphasize systems within and beyond the family, and describe the mutual effects of those systems: family purchasing patterns and the larger economy, educational requirements and costs, and childbearing choices by families.

Each of these distinct frameworks in family studies offer unique information about families. However, the very nature of a framework requires assumptions about the subject. In this instance each family framework applies assumptions about the nature and composition of the family. These assumptions are valuable assets in scientific study, but those same assumptions may not apply to all families in our current society or violent families in particular. More to the point, the assumptions may define "family" in ways that are irrelevant, wrong, or too narrow for application to nursing practice with families. For example, how well does the developmental framework fit the family with adult children returning to the home? Can structure-function theory be applied to the voluntarily childless family? Does role theory apply to single parent families? Could the interactionist principles be applied to families with two employed parents who are working separate shifts? Would systems theory contribute to understanding the needs of the "reformulated" family with two previously divorced parents? Any one of these families might experience difficulties that result in contact with nursing; any one of these families might experience violence. Practice would be hindered by a scientific base that does not address the type of family in which the problems occur.

If the broad range of current family types is to be captured in the science that supports practice, then new family frameworks are necessary. These frameworks would be shallow if they did not incorporate the wisdom and findings of more traditional approaches, but more comprehensive and flexible concepts are needed as well.

"Well-being" is a comprehensive and flexible concept of a variable commodity that is larger in scope than "health." If you ask someone, "How do you feel about your life as a whole?" you are asking them to evaluate their degree of well-being. Because this concept emphasizes strengths and resources as well as problems and needs, it is congruent with the perspective of nursing.

Well-being has both objective and perceived dimensions, that is, comparative (objective) and subjective (perceived) indexes of current status. The two dimensions do not necessarily match. For example, an aging grandmother may simultaneously think that she is fortunate to be living in her family's home (objective sense of well-being), and feel that she has been cruelly stripped of a meaningful, productive adult role (perceived well-being). The concept of well-being can be applied to families as well. For example, consider a family that has a relatively stable economic status while also experiencing tremendous daily stress in meeting demands for heat, food, and other necessities. The objective well-being of this family is more positive than the perceived well-being.

Several characteristics of the interactions between the family and its members make family well-being especially relevant to the discussion of family violence. First, although the family comprises a most intense and enduring segment of each member's environment, the members also comprise vital components of the family's environment. The members affect the nature of demands on and resources for the family, and vice versa. Second, because both the family and its members experience ongoing development, they have concurrent changes in needs and abilities.

Ongoing development of the family member is a more familiar concept: the member grows and changes with help, and hindrance, from the family. This chapter emphasizes the family's perspective as well: a family faces old and new demands, and it sometimes finds new resources for meeting those demands. When the family does well in achieving resource/demand fit, then it has a greater capacity to contribute to the members—who are also juggling personal resources and demands. Similarly, members achieving functional degrees of fit have greater capacities to contribute to family-level resources.

If the family is not able to "fit" resources to demands, then the family is less able to contribute to the efforts of its members as they face individual requirements to "fit" resources and demands. Over time, members who are struggling to meet demands become less able to contribute to the family's processes of coping with demands. A wealth of data associates poor fit with illness, and these findings apply to families as well as to family members. It is the *dysfunctional fit of resources and demands* that bears directly upon family violence.

The victim of family violence is an especially acute example of recurrent cycles of poor fit. The breadth of content in this volume speaks to the complexity of the problems, and solutions, associated with such cycles. This chapter addresses family well-being as a basic component of those problems and solutions. Because there has been little direct study of family well-being, the discussion draws upon a range of theory and research in social networks, family functioning, social support, life span development, and person-environment fit. These concepts are central to understanding and responding to family violence, as it has already been established that violence and aggression have both social and environmental components—and the family produces an intimate relationship between those components.[1] The work reviewed here defines a context from which the concept of family well-being may be derived, and issues in disruption of family well-being may be defined. Most important, the work reviewed here comprises a baseline from which nursing may prepare to assist the victim of family violence.

FAMILY AS A CONVOY OF RELATIONSHIPS

The Convoy

Although there are differences, the constructs of family and social network have a number of commonalities. Social network is the more general construct, and refers to a constellation of cohesive and regularly activated bonds.[2] In other words, social networks are actually aggregates of social bonds. Family, therefore, is a specific form of social network and defined by particular types of bonds. A great deal of research has been designed to identify which bonds define the family network and the answer seems to be "it depends on who you ask." For example, a study of entire families demonstrated significant interindividual differences and intraindividual stability in perceived family networks.[3] Although the network of one subject was notably different from the net-

Family Well-Being

work of another subject, each study subject was relatively consistent in defining his or her own network. One family in the study illustrates this pattern particularly well: the father consistently included his adult children and their spouses in his perceived network, the mother included the adult children and her daughters' husbands, and only the youngest adult child and his spouse included both parents in their networks. Given the importance and variance of individual perception in defining family networks, this chapter examines the literature on the general construct of social network as the background against which an individual situation may be considered.

The issue here is egocentric social networks, where the social bonds all include "Ego," or the person defining the network (Figure 3-1). It may also be important to know which of the network members share bonds, but that level of network connectedness differs from the egocentric level and is not the focus of this chapter. Rather, the discussion focuses on the bonds that include the person and define a perceived, person-specific network.

Egocentric social networks are important because they are enduring, indigenous, and nonrandom. The network accompanies the person throughout the life span, and there are changes in the quantity, quality, and nature of individual bonds. R. L. Kahn and T. Antonucci noted this enduring quality of social networks and proposed the "convoy" as the construct for social networks viewed as part of life experience.[4] The network evolves around the person, and its particular nature is a reflection of that interaction. In other words, the egocentric network is indigenous and person-specific. The membership of a particular network is certainly

——— = Egocentric bonds
— — — = Intranetwork bonds

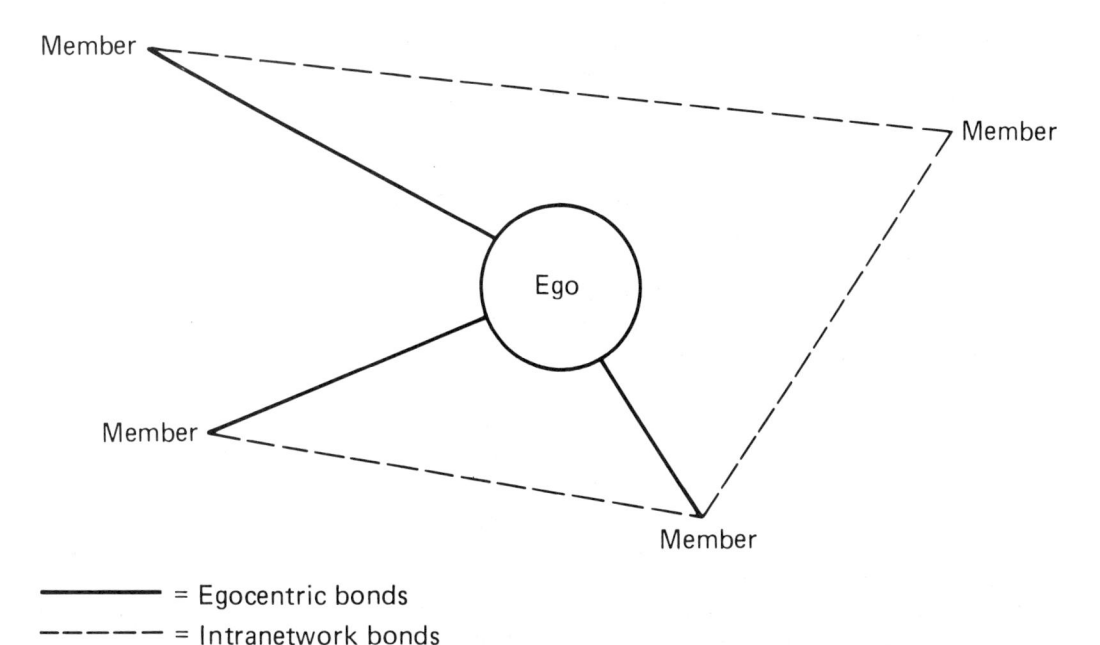

Figure 3-1: Egocentric versus Intranetwork Bonds

not random. For example, emotional bonds are a foundation of family networks and the perceived membership in affective networks varies sharply from what stereotypical and sanguinal traditions would predict: mothers are not always included; children are not equally close; and spouses are not always important in perceived affective networks.[5]

The family has been identified as a special case of social networks. A number of potent variables are associated with this special social network, the family. For example, the family develops a paradigm, or framework, of shared assumptions, constructs, fantasies, and expectations about the world. This paradigm provides a central organizing force for the family.[6] Stress disrupts the texture of family life and challenges the substance of the family paradigm. When families are dysfunctional in response to stress, the dysfunctional behavior does not reflect the full potential of the family; it simply constitutes the behaviors which are most available at that moment in time. Although dysfunctional behavior may be destructive or even violent, it is essential to recognize that there are likely to be other responses which the family can utilize with assistance.[7]

The family has a set of vulnerabilities which alter the effects of stress. Both family organization at the point of stress and the nature of the larger social environment have major impacts on the manner in which the stressor is perceived. More important, family organization and the environment may either threaten or support the family paradigm, which in turn has a major impact upon the types of responses available to the family.[8] This cycle of effects is apparent in violent families; violence stresses the family, and the family often responds to stress with violence.

Even a family with a well-developed organization and a helpful environment is affected by change, and the effects of normative family life changes are especially pertinent to the convoy construct. As the years pass, each member experiences a unique trajectory of life span development and these changes present new issues to the family. Normative changes are associated with developmental patterns, and members' developmental milestones introduce gains and losses for the family. The birth of the first grandchild, the youngest child's school entry, the employment and apartment living of an adult child are each examples of normative changes that produce loss to the family. Precipitous loss of members has a major impact on the family, but even normative loss is a powerful variable in family stress.[9]

Society is also changing as the years pass. Social changes are pervasive and in recent years they have altered the ideology regarding families. B. Laslett describes the expectations of families as an overwhelming burden.[10] She emphasizes the psychological importance of the family as an attribute that gives the ability to alleviate, as well as cause, tremendous pain for members. She questions the degree to which families can realistically and effectively cope with this social ideology. For example, how can families faced with economic stress and uncertainty also muster the stability to provide a safe, secure environment? When the environment becomes so unsafe as to include violence, is the primary cause the family or the social ideology?

Of course, social changes are not perfectly organized and consistent. J. R. Miller identified coherence of issues as another factor in the effects of social changes.[11] Social issues with regard to women, work, dispersion of family members, and psychological propinquity are complex, and the degree to which they are coherent is the degree to which families may be expected to be able to cope effectively with them. Even social issues which are apparently quite general in nature eventually affect families in a profound manner. For example, Ann Wolbert Burgess demonstrated the potent reverberation of the recent American fuel and energy shortages across a wide range of day-to-day aspects of family survival and described the associated and subsequent stress perceived by the families.[12]

Effects of Members on the Convoy

Each member of the family is involved in a trajectory of life span development. This development changes the needs and abilities of the person. The changes echo through the family group, causing changes in family needs and abilities.[13] There is interaction between both of these types of changes and the mutual abilities of families and members to contribute to each other.

Life span development changes do not necessarily occur smoothly or in an organized fashion. There is ample opportunity for changes to cause both conflict and concordance among the members of the family. It is also clear that life change events do not have uniform meanings or effects across individuals.[14]

Attachment is central to the familial bonds that endure throughout these life span changes. John Bowlby defines attachment as a strong disposition to seek proximity to and contact with the attachment figure and to do so especially in situations involving emergencies, fear, anxiety, or threat.[15] Attachment is a persisting attribute and provides a strong, pervasive sense of security. Bowlby also emphasizes that although the behaviors associated with attachment change over the life span, the relationship continues to offer a secure base for testing and exploring the environment.

D. Heard suggests that the degree to which attachment relationships are adaptive is the degree to which the members of the family will gain confidence and the ability to cope from their familial bonds.[16] Roles have an effect in this process. Each member holds a number of roles within the family and as those roles are evolved and adjusted, the aggregate nature of the family is affected.[17] For example, parenting is a major role shift which affects the majority of adults. Maternal role characteristics and experiences are significantly different from those associated with the paternal role.[18] C. Jones demonstrated that expectations of the role change, readiness for the parenting experience, and match of temperaments between father and infant were central to explaining success in paternal role transition.[19] These findings describe one process of adjusting the "fit" between person and environment.

Unusual events are equally viable factors in the effects of members upon their families. In the instance of hospitalization, the crisis of one member reverberates through the entire family system. K. A. Knafl reported that when a sibling is hospitalized, parental expectations of nonhospitalized siblings and their roles in adjustment were related to the preexisting family structure.[20] J. R. Bloom found the same type of pattern in the case of adjustment to breast cancer, during which the amount of contact with significant others and type of family cohesiveness were both predictive of coping.[21] A significant amount of variance in self-concept was explained by the coping variables, and so this study serves as an illustration of the relationship between family and member characteristics.

M. L. Velasco de Parra demonstrated the processual aspects of family changes in a study of renal transplant patients and their families.[22] Following the transplant, the families reflected major shifts in alliances and relational hierarchies. These results emphasize the cyclic, interrelated effects of change in one member and resultant changes in the family.

The composition of the family changes over time, in relation to life span development patterns. The composition also changes with respect to social patterns of behavior, and the interaction of cohort and life span development changes is particularly evident in our society. One-half of recent marriages will end in divorce, one out of six women are unmarried at age thirty, there has been a rise in cohabitation, and one-third of today's young adults will eventually divorce and remarry.[23] To what degree will other social standards even permit, much less assist, people exhibiting these new behavior patterns? How could these new family forms "fit" their environments—and what nursing assistance will be most useful?

been defined here as a convoy of relationships because of the importance of a life span view. This temporal dimension has several general implications for the outcomes of family functions. For example, family influences are different for each stage of development as well as each particular need or behavior of the members.[24] Therefore, time affects the relative impact of family functions for the individual because the importance of family influence varies across the life span. Erik Erikson's discussion of the eight ages of humans includes an example of the variability of family influence.[25] The generativity stage of later life requires a sense of guiding younger generations, while the identity stage of adolescence requires a sense of testing and establishing a unique self. Both stages can profit from, or be demolished by, family functions. It is equally important to note that the kinds of family functions that can contribute to each stage are different.

Time is also a factor in generational differences, which affect the outcomes of family functions. Parental influence on teens, stability of housing and energy sources, composition of the family, courtship and marriage mores, security and employment, and childrearing patterns each change over generations or cohort groups and carry real impact on the functioning of families.[26] Ethnicity is most certainly a viable factor which overlays the effects of member and cohort changes across time.

FAMILY CONTRIBUTIONS TO AGGREGATE AND INDIVIDUAL NEEDS

In theory, the family fulfills a number of functions that serve its own needs as well as those of its members. The family has

Family Functions

The primary outcome of family functions is to maximize coping and motivation. Members, at least potentially, gain psychological equilibrium as a result of family functioning, and that equilibrium is critical to engaging in effective coping responses.[27] The issue at hand is how does the family accomplish this formidable task? What are the mechanisms available to the family in terms of achieving this facilitation of successful coping by its members?

Research in family functioning measures the range of differences in family functions, but that research faces a number of conceptual and methodological problems. These problems are rooted in the fact that although one may interview every family member and strive to conceptualize all the information at the family level, the actual family is more than the sum of its parts.

Carolyn Sara Roberts and Suzanne L. Feetham measured two aspects of members' assessments of family functioning: what kind of family functioning each member perceived, and, what kind of functioning they believed "should be."[28] These assessments were applied to twenty-one examples of family functions, derived from three clusters of relationships (relationships between family and the broader social context, family and intrafamily systems, family and individual members). With a third question regarding how important each function seemed to the members, the researchers obtained a full measure of perceived family functioning. Their definition of family functioning provides the link between the perceptions of members and the aggregate family: family functioning includes the activities and relationships among and between persons and the environment which in combination enable the family to maintain itself as an open system. The Feetham Family Functioning Survey, both valid and reliable, provides a measure of discrepancy between expected and perceived family functioning. Reviewing degrees of discrepancy on each family function would provide a systematic method for identifying priorities for intervention. Functions with high discrepancies between expected and perceived are likely to be ones in which the family is limited in ability to contribute to either member or aggregate needs.

Perception has another, more basic, effect on outcomes of family functioning. The perceived nature of a relationship is associated with family contributions to the member. For example, Susan B. Meister found that an affective bond is not necessarily sufficient for providing assistance.[29] The 252 young adults in her study identified 4,544 network members. Network members were first classified in terms of affective, instrumental, and helping bonds, and then matched with the type of assistance offered over a four-month period of life change adjustment. Over one-third of the network members were reported as having an affective bond with the subject, yet offering *no* assistance during the adjustment period. This finding is important here because it highlights the errors which could result if affective family relationships were identified and then simply assumed to be functional or supportive.

Social Support

Much of what the family contributes to members can also be called social support. Defining social support has puzzled researchers for years, but we may estimate the definition as the provision of direct *aid*, expression of *affect*, and/or the *affirmation* of agreement or valuation of thoughts, feelings, or actions. Each of these forms of support describe what the family, or some of its members, might contribute to another member in need.

A review of the support literature confirms the existence and health effects of support. The theoretical value of social support lies in its dynamic effects within people's lives and its contribution to adjustment and well-being. Although researchers have employed a wide range of definitions of support, they have also had consistent success in showing effects of various forms of support. Most research has also used the more general construct of social network, rather than family, as the source of social support. Including this research in a discussion of family requires only two assumptions: (1) that the family is not wholly divorced from the egocentric social network, and (2) that holding a familial form of membership in the social network does not necessarily preclude the ability to offer social support. N. J. Pender and Susan B. Meister have demonstrated that these assumptions are defensible.[30]

Kahn and Antonucci propose a typology which is purposefully constructed for concordance with their concept of the convoy.[31] Recognizing that social support is important throughout the life span, they also note that the appropriate form and amount of support vary with age. Their typology is defined with an interest in exploring age, cohort, and individual differences in social support. Nursing and health care require the same kind of information and that concordance makes Kahn and Antonucci's typology particularly useful here (see Table 3–1).

The existence and viability of affective support has been demonstrated in several contexts: adjustment to job loss, prognosis and complication outcomes of pregnancy, hospitalization, and maintenance of mental health therapy.[32] In each instance, emotional support was associated with or predictive of an aspect of well-being.

Table 3–1 *Summary of Kahn and Antonucci's Typology*

Form of Social Support	Definition
Affect	The expression of liking, admiring, respecting, loving Ego
Affirmation	The expression of agreement or acknowledgment of the appropriateness or rightness of Ego's acts or statements
Aid	The provision of direct assistance, things, money, information, time, entitlement to Ego

Information and aid forms of support have also been empirically verified. J. S. House demonstrated their relationships to well-being in a series of work stress studies and B. H. Gottlieb produced them via a content analysis.[33] The combination of emotional and informational support has also been tested. L. D. Egbert et al. compared the recovery period of two groups of surgical patients. The experimental group received optimistic, enthusiastic, and reinforced preoperative teaching, and that group required less postoperative medication and length of hospitalization than did the control group.[34]

Affirmation has been demonstrated as a function of postpartum support groups. These volunteer groups were developed by the women who joined them and those women identified three principal elements of group support: an increased belief in their ability to parent, increased self-esteem and coping ability, and recognition of their postpartum feelings as normative.[35] These results suggest that affirmation may contain aspects of the other forms of support, that is, a statement of admiration is technically an expression of affect, but it contributes to increased self-esteem, which is associated with affirmation.

The arenas of work and home have been the context for many support studies. These two focuses of daily life involve many forms of support, induce and may meet needs for support, as well as define degrees of access to potential supporters.[36] Each arena includes some unique sources of support, but family members appear in each as well. The studies also demonstrated that some forms of support are situation (such as work or home) or relationship specific.

Family members are embedded in each of these studies of social support. The consistency of these results implicates familial bonds as support resources and emphasizes the specificity of relationships as a factor in support. For example, support which was sought out in relation to a particular concern was the most predictive of a sense of well-being at life change.[37] Patricia A. Brandt and Clarann Weinert, and B. L. Wilcox also found support to be associated with well-being; a sense of worth and social integration in the first study, psychological symptoms in the second.[38]

These findings are congruent with the basic elements of support. Support can buffer some stress effects, it can provide ongoing contributions to well-being, but it is neither a general panacea nor a completely independent factor in outcomes. There is disagreement about theoretical and methodological definitions of support mechanisms.[39] The majority of research demonstrates a modest and reliable association between social support and well-being, and the strength of that association mirrors the degree of stress in the person's situation.[40] Studies and theories of intrafamily abuse often emphasize lack of social networks among abusers, suggesting a particular vulnerability to stress in the instance of limited sources of social support.

Utilization and Help-Seeking

The simple existence of network sources of support does not assure that the support is actually received. In some instances, supporters spontaneously offer assistance, but support is most often effective when it is sought out.[41] The family may contribute to members either by making them more able to seek support or by making its own support more accessible.

The majority of adults who experience a problem will initially seek some form of help from their social network, but perception of the network is a critical factor in this process.[42] For example, some people are "nonutilizers," that is, they attempt to manage problems in an independent fashion. Nonutilizers are not a homogeneous group. Awareness that help is available permits some nonutilizers to handle problems independently because they perceive their networks as effective backup, while other nonutilizers choose that route because they view their networks as insufficient, unpredictable, or inaccessible.[43] Therefore, how the family is perceived is a potent precursor to how it is (or is not) utilized by a member.

The network also has an effect on utilization of other resources, such as the health care system. B. A. Hamburg and M. Killilea describe the egocentric network as including both a lay referral system and a lay treatment network.[44] The network is needed during stress because a stressful event constitutes a situation with anxiety, impaired informational processes, and needs for new or expanded assistance. The indigenous, enduring network affects both the nature of these stress components and the options available to resolve them.

J. McKinlay found that utilization of routine prenatal services was strongly related to the types of network differentiation.[45] The pregnant women described their networks in two ways: either as a relatively homogenous group or as a group with clear subsets. The women who were utilizing prenatal services also reported networks in which they clearly distinguished between friends and relatives. Nonutilizing women made less of an intranetwork discrimination and were more likely to seek advice and opinions from their social network than from the health care system. This pattern of network perceptions affecting access to other resources is of great importance to health care providers. Patients are part of their enduring environment; thus, the effects of that environment upon episodic utilization of health services are pertinent to both theory and practice.

Not all studies have reported these types of extranetwork effects. For example, F. D. Wolinsky found no significant relationships between physical symptoms, subjective psychological well-being, social role, and utilization of health services.[46] It is important to note that the variables were coded as 0 (no) or 1 (yes) dichotomies. When symptoms, stress, and health care utilization are measured over time and coded in a more substantive manner, utilization *is* sensitive to daily, short-term family processes.[47]

When the issue is whether or not to see a doctor, the perceptions of *both* the person with a symptom and the network are viable, interactive variables. E. Berkanovic and C. Telesky studied two groups of people with symptoms: those who thought a physician contact was important and those who did not.[48] In the first group, when the network members did not endorse seeing a physician, only 68 percent actually had a physician contact. In the second group, when most of the network members thought it was important to see a physician, 33 percent of the subjects actually contacted a physician. In this study, network opinion played an important but not independent role in seeking health care. These results are noted here as evidence of the active role of the person. Opinions and actions of network, or family, members impact upon the person's choices, but they do not dictate final outcomes.

L. McCallister and C. S. Fischer have also demonstrated the importance of perceived social bonds as discriminators in networks.[49] Their subjects first defined a "probable exchange network"; they used a set of assistance functions to identify the set of individuals who were likely to provide each function. Many functions were suggested, including helping out during illness, responding to emergencies, loaning money. Subjects then identified any people who were "important to keep in touch with," and most subjects added names to their networks. At least one-half of the total network membership was *only* elicited by the importance criterion (51 percent in the first study, 62 percent in the second). This result illustrates that networks must be viewed across all relevant components. Failure to tap an important subset of the network will result in failure to identify all network members. More important, some levels of connection between members and subject will be missed. This issue of accuracy in range is one of the most difficult to address, as well as one of the major sources of measurement error.[50]

Accuracy in range is further complicated when networks are viewed across the life span. The attachment literature stands as powerful evidence of intraindividual life span changes in both particular bonds and the general nature of desired bonds.[51] For example, the women interviewed by S. G. Candy, L. G. Troll, and S. G. Levy represented a cross section of the adult life span, and particular functions of friends varied with the age of the woman.[52] There is clearly a temporal dimension to social bonds and this dimension requires recognition in research, theory, and practice.

FAMILY WELL-BEING: DEFINITIONS AND ISSUES

Person-Environment Fit

J. R. P. French, W. Rodgers and S. Cobb developed the construct of person-environment fit and set it into the context of adjustment or adaptation.[53] Person-environment fit is a function of four factors:

E (objective):	The objective amount of environmental supplies that are available.
P (objective):	The objective amount of supplies that are necessary to meet current demands.
E (subjective):	The subjective amount of environmental supplies that are available.
P (subjective):	The subjective amount of supplies that are necessary to meet current demands.

The degree of balance between demand and supply defines the degree of "fit." French, Rodgers, and Cobb included both subjective and objective factors in their construct, and they emphasized that overall fit predicts outcome variables such as coping and strain. Because person-environment fit is a multidimensional construct, coping and strain are related to a number of demand/supply balances. French, Rodgers, and Cobb used the balance of relationships and privacy as an illustration: if one demand requires an increase in interpersonal contacts, then the supply of privacy must decrease. For example, when an infant is born, the family must strike a new balance of contact and privacy.

French, Rodgers, and Cobb drew attention to the multiplicity of demand/supply balance and suggested that the relative importance of each balance was critical to the overall degree of fit. In the affiliation and privacy example, if the person placed minimal importance on privacy, then the loss of a supply of privacy would have little impact on overall fit. On the other hand, if loss of privacy was important, then such a loss would define a new and unmet demand. Unmet demands decrease overall fit, and French, Rodgers, and Cobb cite such deprivations as part of the complex of motivations which precipitate the need for adjustment and adaptation. The magnitude, relative importance, immediacy, and duration of deprivations affect the type of responses people make in terms of achieving overall adjustments.

The objective and subjective components of overall fit are not necessarily related. In fact, French, Rodgers, and Cobb presented two primary mechanisms of adjustment: actually altering the discrepant fit, and, altering perceptions of the fit. These mechanisms include both useful and problematic coping strategies, although they differ in terms of objective or subjective emphasis.

Person-environment fit offers a comprehensive and specific description of human adjustment, coping, and strain. How might that description be quantified to obtain estimates of the relationships between fit, coping, and strain? The answer is far from complete, but measures of overall well-being and factors which predict it address a significant portion of the question.

Perceived Well-Being

F. M. Andrews et al. developed a measure of global perceived well-being and a set of specific perceived well-being measures.[54] The global well-being measure was the subject of extensive study. F. M. Andrews and S. B. Withey investigated sixty-eight global measures and demonstrated the importance of measures which tap general evaluations of life as a whole within a current time frame.[55] The measures which asked a subject to evaluate current well-being, using the full range of current experience, also clustered together regardless of wording or measurement scale. Andrews's "Life no. 3" is one of these measures and asks subjects how they feel about their "life as a whole."

This global measure was included in a test of the affective and cognitive components of global well-being measures.[56] It captured a fairly even representation of affective and cognitive dimensions and achieved a high degree of validity.

Specific perceived well-being measures request evaluations of particular domains of life. For example, subjects evaluate feelings about how much they are accomplishing in life (using a seven-point scale, "terrible" to "delighted"). Eleven such items, all measuring interactions between life domains and subjects' values were found to cluster into three dimensions.[57] Content, relationships, and psychological immediacy split the items into statistically and theoretically substantive groups.

Andrews and Withey pursued a larger test involving the prediction of global well-being from the specific well-being items.[58] Beginning with 123 items, they determined that a small subset formed a linear, additive, and highly predictive combination. Four major life domain indexes occur within that predictive subset: family index, efficacy index, fun index, and money index. These four life domain indexes account for 70 percent of the variance in global well-being.

Meister used perceived well-being as the outcome variable in a study of perceived social support and networks.[59] The results have particular meaning to nursing because support and network variables accounted for more variance in the efficacy life domain than in the global well-being measure. The subscale of efficacy asks the subjects in estimate how they feel about: themselves, what they are accomplishing in life, and how they handle problems. These results emphasize the focal effects of support and selected network members on the precise individual characteristic of greatest importance to nursing; the basis for self-care. J. S. Norbeck, also a nurse, has similarly underscored the importance of social support to nursing theory and practice, and there has been a recent increase in nursing research in this arena.[60]

We have now come full circle. The discussion began with the interactive nature of family and family members, worked through an overview of the convoy and member's life span development, examined social support as a function of families, and set those parameters into the larger theory of person-environment fit, as evidenced by perceived well-being. We now note that the family makes a direct contribution to well-being, and the next step is to recall that the well-being of the family determines its ability to make such a contribution.

The Promise of the Construct of Family Well-Being

Previous research has demonstrated the utility of well-being as a construct which can quantify the more general idea of person-environment fit. Because "fit" is a multivariate function of subjective and objective components of the person and the environment, it would be nearly impossible to measure each factor which contributes to "fit." Rather, research designs are planned to incorporate some of the most salient factors, and well-being is used as a measure which taps a large segment of the degree of "fit" achieved by an individual. This approach has been fruitful in terms of individuals, and this chapter has been developed to posit the promise of using the same approach in terms of families.

Family well-being, as a substantive indicator of family-environment fit, would answer a number of questions that are crucial to nursing practice with families in general. It is presented here because of its potential role in developing nursing responses to family violence.

Practice hinges upon the identification of not only the problems, demands, and needs of the person, but also the available resources, strengths, and options. Family well-being is an indicator of the types of help and hindrance that are forthcoming for the person. As such, family well-being is a major factor in the adaptive capabilities of the person and constitutes a pressing issue in nursing assessments.

The practice setting and role of the nurse will affect the interventions which are developed from the assessment data. In most instances, interventions will focus on the person and use knowledge of the family's well-being as a guideline. Some nurses will be in positions to develop family-based interventions as well, and family well-being measures will be of particular value to them.

Nursing research can intensify the practice value of family well-being measures. We need two particular types of information. First, what are the interactive effects of family and member well-being in an enduring context? These effects may well vary in terms of normative and nonnormative changes, and both types of change are viable factors in nursing practice. Second, what are the predictors of family-environment and person-environment fits? The relative predictive powers of the context, time, and developmental stage are not known, but they will define the relative priorities of the context, time, and developmental stage in nursing practice with families.

LINKS BETWEEN THE CONSTRUCT OF FAMILY WELL-BEING AND VIOLENCE

There are three links between family well-being and family violence which are particularly pertinent and promising to nursing: the role of deprivation, the contextual meaning of change, and potential strategies for intervention in social networks. Each of these links is based upon current knowledge of an aspect of family well-being and may explain major factors in family violence.

French, Rodgers, and Cobb identified deprivation as a powerful source of motivation to adjust person-environment fit.[61] Some deprivations are predictable aspects of the family life cycle, and nursing research has examined the effects of instituting, expanding, and contracting the family.[62] Those studies emphasized the range of individual differences which result from attempts to adjust to change. Failed or torturous attempts at adjustment, whether to normative or unusual episodes of poor "fit," may well contribute to family violence. Because deprivation is at the root of attempts to adapt, particular deprivations may predict adaptive failures among certain people. If so, those deprivations could serve as cardinal warning signs of the potential for family violence.

The predictive value of the deprivations would be associated with specific characteristics of individuals, which brings us to the second link between family well-being and violence. Change is always an active factor in human experience, but some changes are more threatening than others. D. A. Hamburg, G. V. Coelho, and J. E. Adams emphasized individual differences in perceived threats and identified the importance of coherence between skills acquired from earlier socialization and skills demanded by the current environment.[63] In other words, if the environment is relatively stable, then the adaptive skills learned early in life are likely to be useful during later years as well. Is violence associated with lack of coherence? L. Rubin painted a disturbingly grim picture of the struggles and slim hopes of working-class families today, and much of her data defines precisely the lack of coherence described by Coelho, Hamburg, and Adams.[64] The potency of coherence between skills and demands also reflects the enduring role of the family, as early socializer and later environment, in creating situations which can result in adaptive or violent outcomes.

Intervention strategies are the third link between family well-being and violence. The family, as a social network, is the seat of attachments that promotes or inhibits mastery of life experience.[65] Families can, and indeed must, change over time. The nature of this change defines both family well-being and the degree to which the family can contribute to its members. Intervention to promote positive changes is possible. L. C. Ford, A. L. Whall, S. R. Miller and P. Winstead-Frye have each developed a framework for nursing interventions with families, and each addresses several aspects of health-promoting interventions.[66] Hamburg and Killilea have similarly emphasized the need to develop interventions which build upon inherent resources, such as the family.[67] They also raise a pivotal issue: which *member*-focused interventions are best accomplished by the family, and which are most effectively instituted by health care professionals? This issue takes on particular urgency when it is applied to violent families. The strengths and inherent resources of these families are essentially undefined in extant research and theory.

The issue of splitting contributions to member well-being between two potential resources presents the second step in developing the construct of family well-being. Once we can estimate such well-being, we are able to identify pathways to effective facilitation of the family as well as the parameters of a nursing role with the members. When the enduring family network has achieved a healthy level of well-being, that network is often a wise source of intervention for the members. The nursing role must expand significantly in the instance of decreased or fragile family well-being, which is the focus of the remainder of this volume.

The profession of nursing can respond to these needy families by continuing basic and applied research, while voicing political and professional endorsements of multiple, diverse supports for families. Each nurse can respond by continuing to seek fuller knowledge of these families and stretching to develop a more complete perspective on how to best meet their needs.

Summary

Although traditional family frameworks have produced a broad and useful body of knowledge, nursing requires a more comprehensive and flexible conceptualization of families. Family forms are more widely variant in our society, and practice is hindered by a scientific base that does not address the type of family in which health problems happen to occur. Well-being is a concept with great promise for nursing theory, research, and practice with families.

Well-being is of particular value because it is an index of family-environment, or person-environment, fit. The degree of fit between supplies and demands affects both the family and its members. When the family does well in achieving fit, then it has a greater capacity to contribute to the members—who are also juggling personal resources and demands. The same principle determines the degree to which members are able to contribute to the family. Dysfunctional fit of resources and demands (decreased family well-being and member well-being) bears directly upon family violence.

The family is a specific form of social network (convoy) and its membership is a function of the bonds perceived by the members. Across the life span, developmental experiences affect both the members and the family. These changes result in both conflict and concordance within the family. Members are faced with normative and nonnormative personal changes, and their roles and well-being are affected. Social mores affect life span patterns, including familial ones. Each member-based change affects other members of the family as well as the aggregate nature of the convoy.

Family functions best serve the members when they contribute to the psychological equilibrium essential to coping. Family assistance may take the form of social support, which is not a general panacea, but rather relates to well-being in a number of situation specific and person specific manners. While the nature of family functioning and support also affect member utilization of other resources, neither family nor member effects are necessarily independent predictors of outcomes.

Practice hinges upon the identification of not only the problems, demands, and needs of the person, but the available resources, strengths, and options as well. Family well-being is an indicator of the types of help and hindrance that are forthcoming for the person. As such, family well-being is a major factor in the adaptive capabilities of the person, and it presents a pressing issue in nursing assessments of families in general, as well as nursing responses to family violence.

Research findings, the practice setting, and role of the nurse will affect the interventions which are developed from the assessment data. In most instances, interventions focus on the person and would use knowledge of the family well-being as a guideline. Some nurses will be in positions to develop family-based interventions as well, and family well-being measures would be of particular value to them.

Nursing research can intensify the practice value of family well-being measures. The degree of family well-being is a factor in determining pathways to effective facilitation of the family as well as the members. The family with a healthy level of well-being is often a potent source of intervention for the members, while decreased family well-being may indicate a greater need for nursing intervention. The vulnerabilities and needs of these fragile families are all the more compelling when viewed in light of the strength embedded in healthier levels of family well-being.

Chapter 3

1. D. A. Hamburg and M. B. Trudeau, "Behavioral Aspects of Aggression: An Overview," in *Biobehavioral Aspects of Aggression*, ed. D. A. Hamburg and M. B. Trudeau (New York: Alan R. Liss, 1981).

2. N. Friedkin, "A Test of Structural Features of Granovetter's Strength of Weak Ties Theory," *Social Networks* 2, (1980): 411–422.

3. S. B. Meister, "Measurement of Perceived Affective Networks Defined by Whole Families: Reliability and Validity" (unpublished research report, University of Michigan, 1980).

4. R. L. Kahn, and T. Antonucci, "Convoys over the Life Course: Attachment, Roles, and Social Support," in *Life-span: Development and Behavior*, ed. P. B. Baltes and O. Brim, vol. 3 (Boston: Lexington Press, 1980).

5. Meister, "Measurement of Perceived Affective Networks."

6. D. Reiss, *The Family's Construction of Reality* (Cambridge: Harvard University Press, 1981). M. E. Oliveri and D. Reiss "A Theory Based Empirical Classification of Family Problem-Solving Behavior," *Family Process* 20 (1981): 409–18.

7. S. Minuchin and H. C. Fishman, *Family Therapy Techniques* (Cambridge: Harvard University Press, 1981).

8. D. Reiss, *Family's Construction of Reality*.

9. M. P. Andrews, M. M. Bubolz, and B. Paolucci, "An Ecological Approach to the Study of the Family," *Marriage and Family Review* 3 (1980): 29–49. E. M. Duvall, *Marriage and Family Development*, 5th ed. (Philadelphia: J. B. Lippincott, 1977), R. B. Taylor, R. L. Michielutte, and A. Herndon. "Family Life Events: A Study of 198 Families" *Family Practice Research Journal* 1 (1981): 68–74.

10. B. Laslett, "The Significance of Family Membership," in *Changing Images of the Family*, ed. V. Tufte and B. Myerhoff (New Haven: Yale University Press, 1979).

11. J. R. Miller, "Family Support of the Elderly," *Family and Community Health* 3 (1981): 39–49.

12. A. W. Burgess, "Energy Related Stress and Families' Coping Response." (paper presented at the annual meeting of the American Academy of Nursing, 1980).

13. E. M. Duvall, *Marriage and Family Development;* D. P. Hymovich and R. W. Chamberlain, *Child and Family Development: Implications for Primary Health Care* (New York: McGraw-Hill, 1980).

14. A. H. MacFarlane, G. R. Norman, D. L. Streiner, R. Roy, and D. J. Scott, "A Longitudinal Study of the Influence of the Psychological Environment on Health Status: A Preliminary Report," *Journal of Health and Social Behavior* 21 (1980): 124–33.

15. J. Bowlby, "Attachment and Loss: Retrospect and Prospect," *American Journal of Orthopsychiatry*, 52, (1982): 664–78.

16. D. Heard, "Family Systems and the Attachment Dynamic," *Journal of Family Therapy* 4 (1982): 99–116.

17. P. Robischon and D. Scott, "Role Theory and its Application in Family Nursing," in *Family-Centered Nursing: A Sociological Framework*, ed. A. Reinhardt and M. Quinn (St. Louis: Mosby, 1973).

18. W. K. Wilson and L. Cronenwett, "Nursing Care for the Emerging Family: Promoting Paternal Behavior," *Research in Nursing and Health* 4 (1981): 201-211. Bowlby, "Attachment and Loss."

19. C. Jones, "Father To Infant Attachment: Effects of Early Contact and Characteristics of the Infant," *Research in Nursing and Health* 4 (March 1981): 183-192.

20. K. A. Knafl, "Parent's View of the Response of Siblings to a Pediatric Hospitalization." *Research in Nursing and Health* 5 (1982): 13-20.

21. J. R. Bloom, "Social Support, Accommodation to Stress, and Adjustment to Breast Cancer," *Social Science and Medicine* 16 (1982): 1329-38.

22. M. L. Velasco de Parra, "Changes in Family Structure after a Renal Transplant," *Family Process* 21 (1982): 195-202.

23. A. J. Cherlin, *Marriage, Divorce, Remarriage* (Cambridge: Harvard University Press, 1981).

24. B. Hamburg and A. J. Solnit, "Workshop on Family and Social Environment," in *Adolescent Behavior and Health: A Conference Summary* (Institute of Medicine, National Academy of Sciences, Washington D.C., 1978).

25. E. H. Erikson, *Childhood and Society*, 2d ed. (New York: W. W. Norton, 1963).

26. U. S. Congress, *Editorial Research Reports on the Changing American Family* (Washington, D.C.: Congressional Quarterly, 1979).

27. D. Mechanic "Social Structure and Personal Adaptation: Some Neglected Dimensions," in *Coping and Adaptation*, ed. G. V. Coelho, D. A. Hamburg, and J. E. Adams (New York: Basic Books, 1974).

28. C. Roberts and S. L. Feetham, "Assessing Family Functioning Across Three Areas of Relationships," *Nursing Research* 31 (1982) 231-35.

29. S. B. Meister, "Perceived Social Support Subnetworks and Well-Being at Life Change (Ph.D. diss., University of Michigan, 1982).

30. N. J. Pender, *Health Promotion in Nursing Practice* (Norwalk, Conn.: Appleton-Century-Crofts, 1982), Meister, "Perceived Social Support Subnetworks."

31. Kahn and Antonucci, "Convoys over the Life Course."

32. S. Cobb, "Social Support as a Moderator of Life Stress," *Psychosomatic Medicine* 38 (1976) 300-314; S. Gore, "The Influence of Social Support in Ameliorating the Consequences of Job Loss" (Ph.D. diss. University of Pennsylvania, 1973); G. deAraujo et al., "Life Change, Coping Ability and Chronic Intensive Asthma," *Journal of Psychosomatic Medicine* 17 (1973): 359-63.; F. Baekland and L. Lundwell "Dropping out of Treatment: A Critical Review," *Psychological Bulletin*, 82 (1975): 738-83; S. Cobb "Social Support and Health through the Life Course," in *Aging from Birth to Death: Interdisciplinary Perspectives*, ed. M. W. Riley (Washington D.C.: American Association for the Advancement of Science, 1979).

33. J. S. House, *Work Stress and Social Support* (Reading, Mass.: Addison-Wesley, 1981); B. H. Gottlieb, "The Development and Application of a Classification Scheme of Informal Helping Behaviors," *Canadian Journal of Science* 10, (1978): 105-115.

34. L. D. Egbert, G. E. Battit, C. E. Welch, and M. K. Bartlett, "Reduction of Post-Operative Pain by Encouragement and Instruction of Patients," *New England Journal of Medicine* 270 (1964): 825-27.

35. L. R. Cronenwett, "Elements and Outcomes of a Postpartum Support Group Program," *Research in Nursing and Health* 3 (1980): 33-41.

36. E. Bott, *Family and Social Networks*, 2d ed. (New York: Free Press, 1971); House, *Work Stress and Social Support*; R. L. Kahn, "Aging and Social Support," in Riley, *Aging from Birth to Death*; Kahn and Antonucci, "Convoys over the Life Course;" F. E. Katz, "Occupational Contact Networks," *Social Forces* 37 (1958):

52-55; B. Raphael, "Preventive Intervention with the Recently Bereaved," *Archives of General Psychiatry,* 34, (December 1977) 1450-1454; R. C. Stephens, "Aging, Social Support Systems and Social Policy," *Journal of Gerontological Social Work* 1 (1978): 33-45.

37. Meister, "Perceived Social Support Subnetworks."

38. P. A. Brandt, and C. Weinert, "The PRQ—a Social Support Measure," *Nursing Research* 30 (1981): 277-80; B. L. Wilcox, "Social Support, Life Stress, and Psychological Adjustment: A Test of the Buffering Hypothesis," *American Journal of Community Psychology* 9, (1981): 371-85.

39. J. M. LaRocco, J. S. House, and J. R. P. French "Social Support, Occupational Stress, and Health," *Journal of Health and Social Behavior* 21 (1980): 202-18; C. Schaefer, "Sharing up the 'Buffer' of Social Support," *Journal of Health and Social Behavior* 23 (1982): 96-98; J. S. House, J. M. LaRocco, and J. R. P. French "Response to Schaefer," *Journal of Health and Social Behavior* 23 (1982): 98-101; P. A. Thoits, "Conceptual, Methodological, and Theoretical Problems in Studying Social Support as a Buffer against Life Stress," *Journal of Health and Social Behavior* 23 (1982): 145-59.

40. K. B. Nuckolls, J. Cassel, and B. H. Kaplan, "Psychosocial Assets, Life Crisis, and the Prognosis of Pregnancy," *American Journal of Epidemiology* 95 (1972): 431-41; R. J. Turner, "Social Support as a Contingency in Psychological Well-Being," *Journal of Health and Social Behavior* 22 (1981): 357-67; Meister, "Perceived Social Support Subnetworks."

41. Meister, "Perceived Social Support Subnetworks."

42. N. Gourash, "Help-Seeking: A Review of the Literature," *American Journal of Community Psychology* 6 (1978): 413-23.

43. B. B. Brown, "Social and Psychological Correlates of Help-Seeking Behavior among Urban Adults," *American Journal of Community Psychology* 6 (1978): 425-39.

44. B. A. Hamburg and M. Killilea, "Relation of Social Support, Stress, Illness, and Use of Health Services," in *Healthy People: The Surgeon General's Report on Health Promotion and Disease Prevention: Background Papers,* Department of Health, Education, and Welfare Public Health Service publication no. 79-55071A; Institute of Medicine, National Academy of Sciences, 1979.

45. J. McKinlay, "Social Networks, Lay Consultants, and Help-Seeking Behavior," *Social Forces* 51 (1973): 275-92.

46. F. D. Wolinsky, "Assessing the Effects of the Physical, Psychological, and Social Dimensions of Health on the Use of Health Services" *Sociological Quarterly* 23 (1982): 191-206.

47. S. L. Gortmaker, J. Eckenrode, and S. Gore, "Stress and the Utilization of Health Services: A Time Series and Cross-Sectional Analysis," *Journal of Health and Social Behavior* 23 (1982): 25-38.

48. E. Berkanovic and C. Telesky, "Social Networks, Beliefs, and the Decision to Seek Medical Care: An Analysis of Congruent and Incongruent Patterns," *Medical Care* 20 (1982): 1018-26.

49. L. McCallister and C. S. Fischer, *Studying Egocentric Networks by Mass Survey,* Working Paper no. 284 (Berkeley: Institute of Urban and Regional Development, University of California, 1978a); L. McCallister and C. S. Fischer, "A Procedure for Surveying Personal Networks," *Sociological Methods and Research* 7 (1978b): 131-48.

50. P. W. Holland and S. Leinhardt, "A Method for Detecting Structure in Sociometric Data," *American Journal of Sociology* 70 (1970): 492-513.

51. Kahn and Antonucci, "Convoys over the Life Course."

52. S. G. Candy, L. G. Troll, and S. G. Levy, "A Developmental Exploration of Friendship Functions in Women," *Psychology of Women Quarterly* 5 (Spring 1981): 456-472.

53. J. R. P. French, W. Rodgers, and S. Cobb, "Adjustment as Person-Environment Fit," in *Coping and Adaption,* ed. G. V. Coelho and D. A. Hamburg (New York: Basic Books, 1974).

54. F. M. Andrews and R. C. Messenger, *Multivariate Nominal Scale Analysis* (Ann Arbor: Institute for Social Research, 1973); F. M. Andrews and S. B. Withey, "Developing Measures of Perceived Life Quality: Results from Several National Surveys," *Social Indicators Research* 1 (1974): 1–26; F. M. Andrews and S. B. Withey, *Social Indicators of Well-Being* (New York: Plenum Press, 1976); F. M. Andrews and A. C. McKennell, *Measures of Self-Reported Well-Being: Their Affective, Cognitive, and Other Components* (Ann Arbor: Institute for Social Research, 1978); F. M. Andrews, and R. F. Inglehart, "The Structure of Subjective Well-being in Nine Western Societies," *Social Indicators Research* 6 (1979): 73–90.

55. Andrews and Withey, "Developing Measures."

56. Andrews and McKennell, *Measures of Self-Reported Well-being*.

57. Andrews and Inglehart, "Structure of Subjective Well-being."

58. Andrews and Withey, "Developing Measures."

59. Meister, "Perceived Social Support Subnetworks."

60. J. S. Norbeck "Social Support: A Model for Clinical Research and Application," *Advances in Nursing Science* 3 (1981): 43–60; J. S. Norbeck, A. M. Lindsay, and V. L. Carrieri, "The Development of an Instrument to Measure Social Support," *Nursing Research* 30 (1981): 264–69.

61. French, Rodgers, and Cobb, "Adjustment as Person-Environment Fit."

62. K. A. Knafl and H. K. Grace, *Families across the Lifecycle: Studies for Nursing* (Boston: Little, Brown. 1978).

63. D. A. Hamburg, G. V. Coelho, and J. E. Adams, "Coping and Adaptation: Steps towards a Synthesis of Biological and Social Perspectives," in Coelho, Hamburg, and Adams, *Coping and Adaptation*.

64. L. Rubin, *Worlds of Pain* (New York: Basic Books, 1976).

65. "Changes in Human Societies, Families, Social Support, and Health," in *Health and Behavior: Frontiers of Research in the Biobehavioral Sciences*, ed. David A. Hamburg, Glenn R. Elliott, and Delores L. Parron (Washington, D.C.: National Academy Press, 1982).

66. L. C. Ford, "The Development of Family Nursing," in *Family Health Care*, ed. D. P. Hyovich and M. U. Bernard, vol. 2, 2d. ed. (New York: McGraw-Hill, 1979); A. L. Whall, "Family Systems Theory: Relationship to Nursing Conceptual Models," in *Nursing Models and Their Psychiatric Mental Health Applications*, ed. J. J. Fitzpatrick, A. L. Whall, R. L. Johnston, and J. A. Floyd (Bowie, Md.: Prentice-Hall, 1982); S. R. Miller and P. Winstead-Frye, *Family Systems Theory in Nursing Practice* (Reston, Va: Reston ing Co., 1982).

67. Hamburg and Killilea, "Relation of Social Support, Stress, Illness, Services."

Abuse of Female Partners

Jacquelyn Campbell, MS, RN

"Every 12 Seconds"

every 12 seconds
a woman is beat
fast comes the fist
the gun to her head
knife at her throat
boot in the ass
bicycle chain
bites her flesh
keeps her in place
smashes her face
every 12 seconds
a woman in pain
out on the streets
in the dark
in the rain
running with children
from a dangerous man

Susan Venters

Reprinted from *Every Twelve Seconds*, compiled by Susan Venters (Hillsboro, Oregon: Shelter, 1981) by permission of the author.

Abuse of female partners has recently begun to attract widespread attention in the literature as a significant societal problem. The theoretical formulations which have been advanced to explain the phenomenon are related to coexisting theories of violence and family functioning. This chapter uses results of research in the area of wife abuse to suggest a theoretical base for nursing research and practice with battered women. Abuse of female partners is examined as a significant health problem of necessary concern to nursing. The historical roots and traditional and contemporary theoretical approaches to the phenomenon are analyzed, and the concept of machismo is described as a theoretical construct providing gender-related insight into the abuse of women. Finally, the explanatory frameworks which suggest the reasons for the continuation of battering relationships are critically examined.

THE PARAMETERS OF ABUSE OF FEMALE PARTNERS

Significance as a Health Problem

Abuse of female partners is a significant and complex health problem. J. J. Gayford's definition of wife abuse as "severe, deliberate and repeated demonstrable physical violence" inflicted on a woman by a man with whom she has or has had an intimate relationship has been accepted for the purposes of this article.[1] It is thus a pattern, not a single incident, and the man and woman are not necessarily married. Therefore, the phrase "abuse of female partners" is felt to most accurately reflect the pattern, although wife abuse and female battering will also be used.

To give some indication of the physical problems that have resulted from this abuse, R. Emerson Dobash and Russell Dobash, in their interviews of 109 battered women, found that 100 of them had injuries more extensive than bruises (such as broken bones, head injuries leading to unconsciousness, internal injuries, miscarriages) and that 80 percent had visited their doctor on at least one occasion because of physical problems from battering.[2] In a review of records of 481 women who sought treatment in a hospital emergency room for any reason during one month, Evan Stark and her associates found 10 percent who had definitely been battered at least once, 15 percent who had trauma histories pointing to husband assault, and another 16 percent with injuries suggesting abuse.[3] Virginia Koch Drake, in her pilot nursing research study, found that in the cases of twelve abused women interviewed, there was a history of eleven women battered while pregnant, fourteen fractures, seven multiple contusions, seven head and facial lacerations, seven incidences of hair being pulled out, five burn injuries, five spontaneous abortions within ten days of a battering incident, four head injuries, and three dislocated jaws.[4] Physical problems must also include the stress-related physical symptoms frequently reported by abused women.

In examining abuse of female partners as a serious health problem, the emotional effects on the women, not only of the violence itself but also of the psychological abuse typically heaped upon these women, must also be considered. Some authors have included emotional or psychological violence in their formal definitions, and several accept the woman defining herself as abused, no matter what consequences occurred.[5] Forms of psychological abuse certainly exist, which would be considered potential precursors to physical violence and therefore in need of nursing intervention, but this analysis will be limited to wife abuse resulting in physical injury. Emotional abuse will be considered as a sign of family dysfunction and examined as such in Chapter 8.

Wife Abuse Not Spouse Abuse

Another conceptual problem to be addressed is the deliberate choice of the term abuse of female partners or more loosely, wife abuse, in this chapter, rather than spouse abuse. Although it is true that husband battering does occur, the preponderance of evidence suggests that the incidence is so low that its significance as a health problem can be considered negligible. This is somewhat controversial, since the respected author, Suzanne Steinmetz, has concluded that husband abuse is close to as prevalent as wife abuse, the major difference being the husband's ability to do more damage because of his greater physical strength. She bases her conclusions on a study of fifty-seven families, urban and suburban, representing various economic statuses, ethnic groups, and geographic locations. The survey revealed that the husband and wife were approximately equal in the type and frequency of violence that they used against each other during conflicts throughout the duration of the marriage. The extremely small sample size limits generalizations (as Steinmetz admits), and may have not been picked up any cases of actual battering at all! In fact, only one person (a wife) reported using hitting with hands on an "almost always" basis; the rest of the spouses who used various means of physical force used them on a "hardly ever" or "sometimes" basis. Steinmetz is therefore only describing general violence within families, not abuse.[6]

Other data are used to support Steinmetz's proposition. She cites the M. A. Straus, R. G. Gelles, and S. K. Steinmetz national survey of 2,143 couples as also showing an equal number of husbands and wives who ever used violence in their marriage. She admits, however, that this same survey showed only 0.5 percent of the husbands, in comparison to 7 percent of the wives, experiencing severe enough violence to be considered battering. This translates to 150 abused wives versus 11 abused husbands. Such data are explained by Steinmetz in terms of the husband being more ashamed of admitting abuse and the wive's lesser ability to do damage.[7] It is difficult to say with certainty who is more reticent about their abuse, husbands or wives, although both are undoubtedly ashamed. In a study by Elaine Hilberman and Kit Munson, fifty-six of the sixty battered women were identified as such only because they were asked directly about it.[8] Murray A. Straus, after a careful analysis of the shame and guilt involved in family violence concludes: "Under-reporting of violence is greater for violence by husbands than it is for violence by wives."[9]

Steinmetz also uses R. G. Gelles's study of eighty (nonrandomly selected) families as support for her contentions about husband abuse. In this sample, 49 percent of the husbands had used violence against their spouse at least once in comparison to 32 percent of the wives. These percentages are fairly close, but Steinmetz fails to mention that 25 percent of these men used physical force on a regular basis versus only 11 percent of the wives.[10] As pointed out by Dobash and Dobash, Gelles's data also show husbands using more severe forms of violence, a wider range of techniques, and more use of threats of force than the wives.[11]

Most of the data on wife abuse tends to disprove Steinmetz's contention. George Levinger's survey of 600 couples applying for divorce in Cleveland revealed 36.8 percent of the wives in contrast with only 3.3 percent of the husbands claiming that their partner had hurt them physically.[12] Of 1,032 cases of intrafamily violence processed through the Edinburgh and Glasgow courts in 1974, 73.5 percent of the offenders were husbands who had attacked their wives, while only 1.1 percent were husband-assaulting women.[13] Dobash and Dobash also cite a survey of police responses to family disputes in 1974-75 in which 84 percent involved assault and 94 percent of those attacks were against wives.[14] Gayford maintains that "husbands may be subjected to marital violence, but it is extremely uncommon for them to be subjected to torture." Torture is defined by Gayford as the "premeditated infliction of physical injury performed in a sadistic setting."[15] This type of beating was reported by 15 of her sample of 100 abused wives and was also noted by Dobash and Dobash, and Lenore E. Walker.[16]

Another problem with Steinmetz's conclusions and other studies on general violence between husbands and wives is that they do not reflect who struck first. If as many married women hit, push, or throw things at their spouse as are victims of the same, it may only be indicative of retaliation for prior acts of violence. Hilberman and Munson found in their study that

> The few women who resorted to counter-violence did so as an act of desperation when there was no other option.... This is in contrast to the minimal provocation which precipitated violence by the husbands.[17]

The majority of the women in the Dobash sample of battered wives said they never (33 percent) or seldom (42 percent) attempted to use force against their husbands. The remaining 24 percent did so on at least a few occasions, but never in the magnitude or frequency of their husbands.[18]

Steinmetz also uses the statistics on homicide to support her position.

> Thus it appears that men and women might have equal potential toward violent marital interaction, initiate similar acts of violence, and, when differences of physical strength are equalized by weapons, commit similar amounts of spousal homicide.[19]

It is true that most studies of interspousal homicide in the United States show close to equal percentages of husbands and wives killing each other.[20] However, these authors talk in percentages and not in actual numbers which better indicate the magnitude of difference. For instance, the 1981 Federal Bureau of Investigation figures on homicide show 3.8 percent of the total victims as husbands compared with 4.8 percent being wives.[21] In actual numbers, we are talking about 761 husbands and 962 wives. Steinmetz mainly uses the figures from Martin Wolfgang's study of homicide in Philadelphia in this regard. His research does show approximately equal numbers of husbands and wives killing each other; however, Steinmetz fails to indicate a part of his data which changes the picture importantly. Wolfgang found a significantly greater number of husbands first using a weapon or striking a blow ("victim precipitation") in interspousal homicide situations. He also noted that husbands were significantly more likely to use "severe violence" (using more than five separate acts of physical attack to kill) than wives and were almost alone in beating a spouse to death.[22] This suggests more intent to kill and less of an element of self-defense when husbands murder wives.

Dobash and Dobash note that in the United States, women are motivated by self-defense when they kill 70 percent more often than men.[23] The courts are becoming increasingly likely to rule self-defense in cases where an abused wife kills her husband.[24] The general rule is that before people can legally defend themselves, they must "retreat to the wall or take all available escape routes known" unless they are in their own living quarters. It is beginning to be recognized that the woman has a right to be in her own home and has difficulty escaping the battering situation. The other legal self-defense criteria is "immediate threat of great bodily harm or death."[25] Judges and juries have set precedents in Illinois, South Dakota, and New York by allowing a long record of brutality against the wife to constitute an acceptable threat of great danger even though there was no immediately preceding use of great force or weapon.[26] One would assume that future statistics will find an even greater proportion of wives being found innocent in the eyes of the law for killing a battering husband than is presently true. Walker's sample of 120 abused wives contained 4 who had killed their husbands after severe and long-standing repetitive abuse, and "many" others who had lashed back with knives and other lethal weapons. In each case the woman said, "she only wanted to stop him from hurting her more."[27]

It is undoubtedly true that there are husbands who are abused by wives. It is also a fact that some couples are equally assaultive toward each other. However, in the opinion of most of the experts on battering, the kind of repetitive (weekly and sometimes daily), prolonged (forty-five minutes to occasionally more than five hours), serious assault involving severe injury and including sexual mutilation, done with minimal provocation, intent, and in the interest of coercive control, that constitutes actual abuse, is almost exclusively reserved for women.[28] This wife abuse does much to explain the nearly (but not totally) equal numbers of wives killing husbands and cannot be explained in terms of physical strength alone.

Wife Abuse and Homicide of Women

One of the most frightening aspects of wife abuse as a health problem is its connection with homicide of women. The most recent national homicide statistics, compiled by the FBI, indicate that of 538 women murdered in 1981, approximately 29 percent were killed by their husbands (including common law) or boyfriends.[29] This percentage does not include any women killed by estranged husbands and boyfriends, which was found to be a significant category in other research conducted on the problem. Data collection by close inspection of police records also revealed that some of the cases officially reported under the "friend" or "other family" category were actually also intimate male-female relationship members. Therefore, it can be stated with confidence that at least one-third of the women homicide victims in the United States in 1981 were killed by an actual or estranged husband or boyfriend. The data from research conducted by this author suggests that wife abuse was a significant factor in these homicides.

The connection between wife abuse and homicide has been noted in other research efforts. The most direct relationship was found in a study by Margaret Gregory who learned that the majority of husbands who killed their wives in England and Wales, between 1957 and 1968, had previously assaulted them.[30] Del Martin cites a Kansas City Police Department study indicating that 40 percent of the homicides in that city were spouse killing spouse.[31] Another study of homicide in England and Wales, this one covering 1976-71, shows that 58 percent of the female victims were married to or sexually intimate with their killers.[32] P. D. Scott, in a study of forty men who murdered their wives, found that twenty of them had battered their spouse previously.[33] In Atlanta in 1972, 31 percent of the 255 total homicides listed "domestic quarrels" as a factor in causation.[34] Most of the major scholars who have written about wife abuse agree that the potential for battering to escalate to homicide is a very real danger. As Walker states, "Thus, homicide between man and woman is not a 'crime of passion' but rather the end result of unchecked, long-standing violence."[35]

A nursing research study was conducted by this author in 1980 which used a retrospective analysis of the police files of murdered women and women who perpetrated homicide in Dayton, Ohio, a midwestern city of approximately 200,000 individuals.[36] The findings of this study cannot be generalized, but they follow in the tradition of at least nine major epidemiological research efforts which have looked at homicide in various urban areas to identify possible factors affecting inner city homicide. The most significant finding of the study was that between 1975 and 1979, 71.9 percent of the intersex killing between husband and wives, boyfriends and girlfriends or estranged same, involved a prior history of wife abuse. Of the twenty-eight women who were killed by a man in an intimate relationship, eighteen (64.3 percent) had been abused by that man. In these cases, the battering was reported by family members or friends and neighbors to the police when they were interviewed after the crime. Unless the police asked, the information was usually not offered, and the police frequently did not inquire nor did they always interview for the record someone who might have known of abuse. Thus the 64.3 percent figure may well be an underestimate.

Other findings from the Dayton study that are pertinent include that only 7.1 percent (2 cases) of the men who killed a woman with whom they were having or had had an intimate relationship, acted in self-defense, while of the twenty-nine men who were killed by a woman in the same type of relationship, twenty-three precipitated the murder by showing a weapon or striking a blow and usually the blows were repeated. In only two of these cases of intersex killings did the man and the woman have a history of being equally violent toward each other, and in no case was there indication of husband abuse.[37]

Battered wives themselves are certainly acutely aware that they are in danger of being killed.[38] They frequently give this as the reason for staying in the abusive relationship, but this has not always been treated as a realistic fear.[39] The Dayton data show that 30 percent of the female homicide victims from 1974 to 1979 who were killed by a husband or boyfriend, had divorced, separated from, or broken up with that man. Several other cases were the result of the female partner trying or threatening to break off the relationship.[40] Richard Makman theorizes that violent husbands are often dependent on control of their wives for continued self-esteem and that actual or threatened loss of the spouse by separation or divorce may lead to "paranoia," increasing the danger of further violence and murder.[41] Margaret Elbow asserts, "The abusive husband in formal or common law marriages is strongly opposed to his wife's terminating the relationship to the extent of threatening to kill her, and in some instances, carrying out the threat."[42]

Scope of the Problem

In trying to determine the incidence of abuse of female partners, virtually all authors have relied upon physical abuse as the criterion for estimation. Incidence estimates of severe and repeated battering range from 10 to 50 percent of the approximately 47.5 million married couples in the United States.[43] The wide variation is accounted for by various means of extrapolation from a number of different studies using different populations, the impreciseness of police data on assaults and family disturbance calls, and the lack of reporting of wife abuse to authorities (estimated at only 1 of each 270 cases).[44] Perhaps the most systematic and accurate indication of the amount of violence against wives is from the only national, representative sample survey of family violence done by Straus, Gelles, and Steinmetz in 1976. This survey showed 16 out of every 100 couples having violent confrontations during the course of a year and 4 of each 100 wives being seriously beaten within the same time period.[45] This translates into at least 1.8 million abused wives per year in this country alone. Other estimates cite 3 to 4 million battered women per year and FBI statistics indicate a higher rate of incidence than is true for rape.[46] Estimates from other nations indicate equally widespread and serious incidence.[47] To bring the numbers closer to home, a nurse should keep in mind that it is likely that approximately one in every twenty-five adult women, who live with a man, *encountered in any health care setting* may be a victim of abuse by her husband or lover.

Interface of Wife Abuse and Nursing

In the study of 481 females entering a hospital emergency room cited earlier, only 13 of the 197 probable battered women identified were recognized as such by the attending physician.[48] Drake quotes an abused woman as saying about nurses and doctors "I just wish somebody would of come right out and asked me. I always hope they'll do that."[49] Many battered women have recounted to this author that they felt the hospital was cold and impersonal, that their perception was that no one there really cared if they had been beaten or not. Other women have said that they were embarrassed or afraid because their spouse was present, or they thought the medical personnel would tell him.

In a random sample of twenty-six female psychiatric inpatients, 61 percent were identified as battered.[50] The sample is, of course, too small for generalizable conclusions, but the findings do suggest that mental health nurses need to be aware of and able to intervene with battered women more than is commonly thought. The same nursing study indicated that of the fourteen abused women, eight had reported the abuse to at least one health professional, and only four had received a clearly helpful response from one of the health professionals talked to. Other sources have also spoken of the generally detrimental role the health care system has played in the past with battered women. They are frequently (71 of 100 abused wives in one study) prescribed tranquilizers or antidepressants.[51] This insinuates that the woman is mentally ill and may mask her discomfort and encourage her to remain in the battering situation. Furthermore, it treats the symptoms, not the problem and certainly not the cause, the spouse.

The widespread incidence of battering during pregnancy suggests another important arena where wife abuse can be identified and attended to by nursing. Prenatal clinics, private obstetrical offices, childbirth education classes, and inpatient postpartum floors are all places where nurses practice and can be alert for wife battering. Drake's study found 100 percent of her sample (twelve) who had ever been pregnant to have been beaten while in that condition.[52] One-half of Flynn's sample of thirty-three wife abuse victims had been battered while carrying a child.[53] Walker found that most of the women she interviewed reported more severe and more frequent violence during pregnancy.[54] Extrapolating from previous incidence statistics, we can estimate that one in every fifty pregnant women is being beaten. This is a more common occurrence than placenta previa or diabetes in pregnancy. Are questions about abuse included in routine prenatal histories? Is wife battering mentioned in maternal-child health nursing texts?

In community health nursing, nurses are in clients' homes and dealing with families on a regular basis. In such settings wife abuse may easily come to light if the professional nurse is alert to the possibility and gently asks the right questions. Most battered women seem anxious to tell if asked empathetically and in a safe and private situation. Fortunately, more and more nurses are becoming aware of the problem and becoming active in both identifying and providing services for battered women in their regular work settings and are becoming involved in providing health services and group and/or parenting sessions in battered women's shelters. More of this nursing activity is indicated and needed and well within the scope of nursing.

HISTORICAL PERSPECTIVE

Dobash and Dobash place wife abuse in its historical context as a form of behavior which has existed for centuries as an acceptable, and, indeed, a desirable part of a patriarchal family system within a patriarchal society, and much of the ideology and many of the institutional arrangements which supported the patriarchy through the subordination, domination and control of women are still reflected in our culture and our social institutions.[55]

At least three excellent and comprehensive historical studies of the history of wife abuse have been done: Terry Davidson's "Wifebeating: A Recurring Phenomenon Throughout History," Margaret May's "Violence in the Family: An Historical Perspective," and the Dobash and Dobash research reported in their book, *Violence Against Wives*.[56] From these secondary sources, a brief summary of historical precedent is presented to convey its magnitude.

The Bible provides our earliest prescription for physical punishment of wives. Deuteronomy 22:13–21 gives a law condemning brides to death by stoning if unable to prove virginity.[57] In early Rome, husbands and fathers could legally beat or put women to death for many reasons, but especially for adultery or suspected infidelity, reflecting "not so much thwarted love but loss of control and damage to a possession."[58] Jesus was more egalitarian in his thinking, but the sexist statements of Saint Paul set the tone for the Christian Church. Constantine, the emperor and religious leader of the Byzantium branch of Christianity, set the example for treatment of wives by putting his own young wife to death by scalding.[59] By medieval times, the widespread nature of wifebeating had been documented in several ways. It was written in Spanish law that a woman who committed adultery could be killed with impunity. In France, female sexual infidelity was punishable by beating, as was disobedience. Italian men punished unfaithful women with severe flogging and exile for three years.[60] A medieval theological manual refers to the necessity of men beating their wives "for correction" according to church doctrine. A Catholic abbé decried the common cruelty to and murder of the wives of prominent Christian men.[61]

Dobash and Dobash explain that the medieval "age of chivalry" was actually an attitude based on the ideal of female chastity before marriage and fidelity afterwards which were important aspects of male property rights and outward signs of the master maintaining control. This glorification of women as asexual, weak adornments actually contributed to their subjugation and was associated with the use of male force in rescues and tournaments. The close of the Middle Ages saw the rise of the nuclear family along with the development of modern states and the beginning of capitalism, all of which eroded the position of women and strengthened the authority of men. In sixteenth-century England there was a campaign in support of the nuclear family and loyalty to husband and the king who was trying to consolidate his power. Allegiance to fathers and husbands was equated to loyalty to the king and God.[62]

The Effects of Capitalism and Protestantism

Capitalism and Protestantism rose together. The basic unit of production moved outside of the family, and for the first time wages were paid for work on a regular basis. Wives became separated from production and exchange. Because domestic work received no wages, it became devalued. The Protestant religion idealized marriage and equated wifely obedience with moral duty. The head of the household gained much of the power which used to belong to priests.[63] Martin Luther is considered less misogynistic than most of the men of his time, but even he equated female anatomy with the woman's role and admitted to boxing his wife's ear when she got "saucy."[64] John Knox insisted that the "natural" subordination of women was ordained by God. Wifebeating was discouraged by the Protestant theologians, but the husbands' right to do so was acknowledged and the practice was widespread.[65] As May explains, "children, property, earnings and even the wife's conscience belonged to the husband."[66] During the seventeenth, eighteenth, and nineteenth centuries in the Western world, there was little objection to the husband using force as long as it did not exceed certain limits. The wife could be beaten if she "caused jealousy, was lazy, unwilling to work in the fields, became drunk, spent too much money or neglected the house."[67] However, in direct conflict it was the prevailing perception that women's position was privileged and protected.

While the Reformation set the tone in the rest of Europe, Napoleon influenced France, Holland, Italy, and parts of Switzerland and Germany. He thought of wives as "fickle, defenseless, mindless beings, tending toward Eve-like evil" and deserving of punishment for such misdeeds as "causing" bankruptcy or criminality in her husband.[68] He is quoted as saying to the Council of State:

> The husband must possess the absolute power and right to say to his wife: "Madam, you shall not go out, you shall not go to the theatre, you shall not receive such and such a person; for the children you bear shall be mine."[69]

The common saying of the times was, "Women, like walnut trees, should be beaten every day."[70] German husbands had a duty to beat their wives for misdemeanors during this period; they were subject to fine if they did not. In France, King Humbert IV declared, "Every inhabitant of Villefranche has the right to beat his wife, providing death does not ensue."[71]

British common law in the eighteenth century also established the legal right of a man to use force with his wife to insure that she fulfilled her wifely obligations, "the consummation of marriage, cohabitation, conjugal rights, sexual fidelity and general obedience and respect for his wishes."[72] John Stuart Mill petitioned Parliament to end the brutal treatment of British wives in 1869. The changes in law that resulted were directed not toward eliminating the practice of wifebeating but toward limiting the amount of damage that was being done. The nineteenth century in England was also marked by more toleration for conjugal violence in the lower classes while more chivalry was expected by the upper classes.[73]

Historical Influence Today

In our own country, founded on the rights of *men*, not of women, John Adams rejected his wife's plea for better treatment of women in the new government. Sir William Blackstone's interpretation of English law which upheld the husband's right to employ moderate chastisement in response to improper wifely behavior, was used as a model for American law. In 1824 the state of Mississippi legalized wifebeating, and in 1886 a proposed law to punish battering husbands was defeated in Pennsylvania. North Carolina passed the first law against wifebeating, but the court pronounced that it did not intend to hear cases unless there was permanent damage or danger to life.[74] As late as 1915, a London police magistrate reaffirmed that wives could be beaten at home legally as long as the stick used was no bigger than the man's thumb ("the rule of thumb" from a 1782 judge's proclamation).[75] "The law has been condoning violence to wives for centuries."[76] The influences of the history of wifebeating are with us today, not only in the behavior of husbands but also in the attitudes of the courts, police, and society toward them. The conclusion of Dobash and Dobash is an appropriate summary.

> The ideologies and institutions that made such treatment both possible and justifiable have survived, albeit somewhat altered from century to century, and have been woven into the fabric of our culture and are thriving today.[77]

THEORETICAL FRAMEWORKS

Wife abuse was barely recognized, let alone carefully studied, until the 1970s. Most of the literature that has since been produced is descriptive and has relied on clinical samples of abused women, identified through shelter residence, self-report, or from mental health facilities or emergency rooms. Thus the findings suffer from a lack of generalizability and frequently an impreciseness in definitions of variables and measurement. One of the main purposes of the early research has been to show how widespread the problem is and to explode the myth that wifebeating is confined to a few pathologically exceptional men. This goal has been admirably carried out, and the descriptive studies have been helpful in identifying associated variables. However, few studies have employed statistically sophisticated analysis or nonabused control groups, and little has been done to formulate or empirically test actual explanatory theories of wife abuse. Therefore, it can be said that theoretical frameworks are beginning to be advanced toward delineating the causes of wife battering, and some of the descriptive data can be used as support or to question these frameworks, but causation is far from well identified, let alone proven.

The literature on the causes of wife abuse reflect the perspective of the various authors addressing the problem. As with the literature on violence in general, there are viewpoints that emphasize the psychological, sociological, and biological determinants, and there is also a feminist body of literature that emphasizes the patriarchal roots of this practice which so endangers women. The literature also reflects many serious and commendable attempts to integrate these causes and resist the temptation to rely on simplistic, single-cause formulations.

Theories of Causation

Traditional Psychiatric Viewpoints

The early literature on wife abuse was generally from the psychiatric field and tended to focus on the individual pathology of the abuser and especially his victim. For example, in 1964, a group of psychiatrists, drawing from twelve case studies from private practice, concluded, "We see the husband's aggressive behavior as freeing masochistic needs of the wife and to be necessary for the wife's (and the couple's) equilibrium."[78] This kind of study generally used small samples, often drawn from already diagnosed mentally ill populations, and are biased by adherence to the Freudian conceptualization that all women have masochistic tendencies. In contrast, the main body of literature, written from 1970 on, concludes that wife abusers are no more likely to be diagnosed as mentally ill than the rest of the population, and it dismisses female masochism as a myth.[79]

In spite of this overwhelming rejection of masochism as a causative factor in wife abuse, some vestiges of the theory remain even in recent literature. Natalie Shainess, in a 1979 issue of the *American Journal of Psychotherapy*, redefines masochists as women who do not enjoy suffering, but do employ an "all pervasive cognitive style" of submission and self-destruction which makes them more vulnerable to violence.[80] In contrast, this author joins the preponderance of experts on wife abuse in condemning the myth of masochism for causing much of society, many members of the helping professions, and more devastatingly, the abused women themselves, to feel that battered wives ask for and are to be blamed for their victimization.[81]

Another vestige of the masochism myth can be detected when authors overemphasize the role of the wife in provoking her abuse. On the basis of twenty-three cases of men in custody for murdering or assaulting their wives, M. Faulk concludes that nine of the wives were so "demanding" that the husband finally "exploded" and attacked her, implying that *her* behavior was the problem.[82] Morally it is impossible to justify murdering, attempting to murder, or doing grievous bodily harm to someone because of excessive verbal demands. As Walker states, "By perpetuating the belief that it is rational to blame the victim for her abuse, we ultimately excuse men for the crime."[83] The sentences that Faulk's offenders received reflects this mechanism. Five were placed on probation (including two who had killed their wives and had not pleaded self-defense) because their lack of previous offenses and the circumstances of the cases led the "court to a sympathetic approach."[84]

A separate viewpoint of psychiatric literature is represented by George R. Bach and Peter Wyden who maintain that fighting between married couples is necessary for true intimacy. They prefer verbal conflict and advocate rules to keep the fights fair but assert, "We believe that the exchange of spanks, blows and slaps between consenting adults is more civilized than the camouflaged or silent hostilities of ostensibly well-behaved fight-evaders. . . ."[85] In contrast to this view, there is substantial evidence from studies of abused wives showing that physical attack is often preceded by verbal arguments, that spouses who use screaming also tend to use violent means of conflict resolution, that as the level of verbal aggression increases, the level of physical aggression increases even more rapidly, and that physical abuse, once begun, escalates over time.[86] Bach and Wyden are operating from a catharsis belief which the wife abuse literature has tended to disprove adding to the weight of evidence against it from other studies reviewed in Chapter 2.[87]

The Role of Alcohol

Alcohol is a factor which has consistently been noted in connection with wife abuse, but which has not been proven as an actual cause. In the major studies of battered women, the percentages reporting association between husbands drinking and abuse varies from 25 to 85 percent, with a variety of figures in between.[88] The methods of gathering and reporting the data also vary considerably. Many questions remain unanswered. Is the husband always drunk when he is abusive? Conversely, is he always abusive when drunk? Is alcohol or drug abuse a major problem in his life, or is it only connected to wife abuse? Is the husband intoxicated or only had a few drinks? Until more of these questions are answered, the extent of the role of alcohol in wife abuse is difficult to more precisely identify.

Forty-five of a group of 100 wives of diagnosed alcoholics reported being beaten by their husbands in one research study.[89] This is a higher percentage of abusive behavior than is estimated to occur in the normal population. At the same time it suggests that more than one-half of alcoholic husbands do not batter their wives. John A. Byles found that violence was more than twice as likely to occur in families with alcohol problems than in those without alcohol problems in a survey of disintegrating families.[90] Gelles notes that although 48 percent of his battering husbands had problems with alcohol and most of their wives felt that no violence would have occurred without intoxication, drinking did not necessarily lead to violence in his sample, and the violent men were not necessarily drunk.[91] The preponderance of evidence tends to reveal some degree of correlation, not causation.

In an effort to unravel the connection, Morton Bard and Joseph Zacker studied 1,388 occasions of family disturbance involving a police visit. The police officers, who had received special training in observational and data recording skills for family crises, perceived alcohol to be the primary cause of the dispute in only 14 percent of the cases. The complainant had been using alcohol in 26 percent of the cases and the other party in 30 percent of the cases. These authors also conclude from their study and a review of others that alcohol cannot be said to *cause* violence in family disputes.[92]

However, there is still a strong connection to be explained. Such researchers as Gayford and Bard and Zacker use the so-called disinhibiting effect on violent behaviors as an explanation.[93] Bonnie Carlson also sees alcohol as a disinhibitor, but in addition regards its abuse as a symptom of structural stress and frustration which she feels is the main cause of wife abuse.[94] Gelles advances an interesting analysis of the relationship of alcohol. He notes that alcohol can provide an "excuse in advance," since alcoholism is regarded as an illness in our society, and behavior under the influence is seen as uncharacteristic and uncontrollable.[95] Walker found that for the problem drinkers described by her sample of battered women, "Drinking seemed to give them a sense of power" which was then demonstrated by violence.[96] Joanne Downey and Jane Howell conclude that battering men may drink *in order to* carry out violence.[97] In conclusion, a correlation between alcohol abuse and wife battering has been established similar to the connections between alcohol and violence in general described in Chapter 2. Alcohol as a cause of wife abuse has neither been claimed nor shown, and explanations for the connection vary considerably.

Socialization for Abuse

The majority of researchers in the field of wife abuse operate from a sociological perspective. They tend to emphasize social learning and/or situational stress or frustration factors as the main causes of wife abuse. However, most of these authors recognize the interrelationship of factors which lead to the battered wife phenomenon. Straus and his associates, Steinmetz and Gelles, have written extensively from this viewpoint. Straus has developed a multifactoral system which recognizes the societal background of a high level of violence in our culture, sexist organization of the society and its family system, and cultural norms legitimizing violence between family members.[98] With this background of societal influences, he points out that the family is inherently at high risk for violent interaction because of the great number of hours family members spend interacting; the broad range of activities over which a conflict can occur; the intensity of emotional involvement of the members; the involuntary nature of membership; the impingement of family members on each other's personal space, time, tastes, and life-styles; and the assumption of family members that they have the right to try to change each other's behavior. Within these societal and family contexts, these authors believe that people can be socialized to use violence for conflict resolution. Children learn this by observing parental violence, experiencing physical punishment, seeing their parents tolerate sibling fighting, and, if boys, being taught to value violence. This socialization teaches the association of love with violence and justifies the use of physical force as a morally correct means of solving disputes.

Abusive Behavior Learned in Childhood. There is much evidence to support the idea that abuse of women is behavior learned in childhood. In the Roy sample of violent husbands, 81.1 percent were reported to have been victims of child abuse or had parents who used violence on each other.[99] Steinmetz found, in a study of fifty-seven families, that all patterns of conflict resolution repeat themselves for at least three generations with a consistent degree of violence.[100] Other samples show variations from 27 percent (experiencing actual child abuse only) to 51 and 59 percent of abusive men having witnessed or experienced violence in their home as a child.[101] Again we are dealing with descriptive statistics of specific populations with these studies, but research done by Joseph C. Carroll used a control group of nonviolent individuals and is therefore somewhat more conclusive. His results showed a significantly higher incidence of physical punishment (36.6 percent) used in the childhood of those violent toward a spouse than those who were not (14.5 percent had experienced physical punishment).[102] Steinmetz summarizes this causative factor as follows: "Those who have witnessed or experienced family violence as a child, tend to approve of the use of violence and use violence themselves to resolve family conflicts."[103]

Another aspect of learning which is suspected to promote wife abuse is the influence of television. The most attractive men on television illustrate the compulsive masculinity syndrome, dominate their heterosexual relationships, and use violence without sanctions. Most television husbands control absolutely their families, and some programs teach the appropriateness of verbal abuse. Aggression is shown as an effective way to achieve power and success and maintain control. Lucien Beaulieu feels that this "important, insidious and pervasive impact" of television which fosters "norms, values and attitudes which favor violence" is an important factor in family violence.[104]

Gender Differences in Learning. Some authors have also linked learning theory to the woman's role as victim. Gelles theorizes that the more frequently a woman was hit by her parents, the more vulnerable she is to being a victim of marital violence.[105] The mechanism supposedly working here is that a woman learns to be a victim by prior conditioning.[106] Unfortunately, this theorizing echoes the old masochism myth in a slightly different form; because women have learned to be victims, they somehow precipitate and then accept their further victimization.

Actually the data tend not to support this theory nearly as strongly as the learning influence on male behavior. In Roy's sample, only 33.3 percent of the abused wives observed or experienced violence as a child.[107] Walker found that only a small number of her sample of battered women were beaten as children.[108] In Gayford's study, 23 percent came from homes where violence was a regular occurrence.[109] Carroll, using a control group of nonviolent couples, was surprised to note that, "In fact, daughters who received less physical punishment from their fathers were *more* likely to report that violence was a problem" (in their own conjugal relationship) than those subjected to a high amount of punishment.[110] Only 29 percent of the abused wives studied by Dobash and Dobash reported any violence at all in their childhood homes.[111] In all these studies the level of childhood violence was significantly higher for the abusers than for the victims.

Mildred Daley Pagelow separated out two distinct forms of experience with violence in the family of origin in her study of 307 abused women and their reports of spouses: (1) "being a victim of parental physical abuse and (2) observing one parent being physically violent with the other."[112] Only about one-fourth of the women saw their mothers being beaten by their fathers while more than one-half of their batterers had observed such. The men were also significantly "more frequently and severely physically punished" than the women (19 percent of the women severely victimized versus 48 percent of their spouses). In a study done by Barbara Star, using a control group of nonabused women (albeit small), 35 percent of the battered women came from homes where they experienced or witnessed violence, while 50 percent of the control group had.[113] Again the picture for the violent husbands was clearly the opposite; 55 percent observed beatings or had been abused, while only 17 percent of the nonviolent men came from that sort of background. The preponderance of evidence thus seems to indicate that social learning theory holds explanatory value for the behavior of abusive men, but cannot be said to be operating in teaching women to be victims of abuse.

Family Stress

The social scientists writing about wife abuse also emphasize the situational and societal stressors as causative factors in wife abuse. As Steinmetz points out, the family has to absorb emotional tension from external as well as internal sources.[114] This approach echoes the frustration leading to aggression theory on general violence. This is theorized to be especially important in the family since, "In general, people tend to take out their frustration on those to whom they are closest."[115] Central to this argument is the idea that poverty or low social status will create excessive stress in the family. As Carlson states this case, "Sources of family violence are complex structural circumstances creating environmental stresses that are distributed unevenly across the social structure." Her sample of 101 cases of abusive families included 29 percent unemployed males and 37 percent making less than $9,000 a year. Only 7.6 percent of the battering husbands were professionals.[116] Gayford found a 33 percent unemployment rate in his abusing husbands and a majority in the lowest social classes. He concludes from his research that wifebeaters have a low frustration tolerance, have seen crises solved with aggression and violence, and when they are faced with extra frustration from outside the home and experience stress inside the home, violence may result, especially if inhibitions are lowered by alcohol.[117]

Scott also finds the majority of wife batterers in the lower social classes and feels that wife abuse is a function of failure of adaptation of societal stresses.[118] In another study, unemployment was a factor for two-thirds of the men and "educational, economic and social deprivation found to be the norm".[119] A survey of petitioners for English divorce citing repeated physical beatings revealed an overrepresentation of abusers in the category of unskilled workers.[120] Middle-class divorce applicants in Greater Cleveland were found to be less likely to cite physical abuse as a reason than lower-class applicants.[121] From a national survey of 72,000 representative households, Deirdre Gaquin found that spousal abuse was more likely to occur in homes with incomes below $7,500 per year, but did not find any difference between black and white respondents.[122]

Other data tends to contradict these findings. John Flynn found no relationship to socioeconomic status in his review of police records on familial assaults, but he did find the majority of his families to be under stress of some kind.[123] Montgomery County, Maryland, one of the nation's richest suburbs, reports a high incidence of verified assaults on wives.[124] During the same period in 1974, Norwalk, Connecticut, a middle-class community, and Harlem, New York, had an approximately equal incidence (per 100,000 population) of wife abuse reported to police.[125] Jean Renvoize, along with many other authors, asserts that battering is spread throughout the socioeconomic strata.[126] She acknowledges that the major studies do not reflect this, but reasons that it is because middle- and upper-class victims are less likely to report its occurrence to police, resort to wife abuse shelters which provide most of the samples studied, or utilize other social service agencies.[127] The other problem with citing poverty and/or unemployment as the main stressor leading to wife abuse is that it fails to account for the preponderance of males who are doing the battering when the wife in such a situation would be equally frustrated or stressed.

The theory is better supported and made more explanatory when linked to the male prescribed role in society and when data cover in more detail the couples' employment and education status. Langley and Levy express this formulation when they state, "Many wifebeaters regard themselves as inadequate in some aspect of the prescribed male role in our society."[128] Another way of describing the same mechanism is to talk about the husband using violence to compensate for his lack of resources (financial, educational, occupational) needed to maintain his assumed dominant role in the family and in the culture. John O'Brien's study of 150 middle- and working-class applicants for divorce showed that more of the abusing husbands were underachievers in their work role in terms of education or satisfaction with their job than those who were nonviolent.[129] Gelles found a higher level of abuse when the wife's job was of higher status than the husband's, where the husband's occupational status was lower than the neighbors', and when unemployment was a threat in the man's job.[130] Suzanne Prescott and Carolyn Letko also found low job satisfaction related to severer forms of violence against wives.[131] Carlson's sample contained twenty-six (of fifty-eight) couples where the wife had more education than the husband, while only seventeen couples showed the opposite pattern.[132] This is a very different relationship from the one ordinarily found in married couples. Thus, there are considerable data to support this reworking of the basic premise of stress, lack of resources, or frustration as causative of wife abuse.

Other stressors that have been identified in at least one study as being linked to wife abuse are fewer verbal skills on the part of the husband, social isolation of the family resulting in decreased social support, pregnancy and other family developmental crises, differing religions or lack of family religion, and health problems.[133] Straus, Gelles, and Steinmetz found that high scores on a checklist of characteristics including such stressors as poverty, unemployment, worry about financial security, two or more children, a high score on a Stress Index, non-white racial group membership, and few support systems were predictive of spouse abuse.[134] When social scientists link stress to social learning theory and the norms and values regarding violence and marital relationships in our culture, they have identified an important group of factors predisposing toward wife abuse. However, the statistical relationships have been relatively small, and the many methodological and sample problems have prevented identification of actual causation. The other main criticism of this viewpoint is in its lack of parsimony and in terms of emphasis, not faulty reasoning. Although such researchers as Steinmetz and Straus mention "the male dominance and machismo values and norms which form a subtle but powerful part of our sexual and family system," they fail to see this as perhaps the underlying causative factor.[135]

Cultural Support for Wife Abuse

There is widespread cultural support for wife abuse. In a national, representative 1968 poll of 1,176 American adults, one-fifth approved of "slapping one's spouse on appropriate occasions."[136] Sixty-two percent of a primarily male sample of college students and middle-class businessmen felt that violence would sometimes be appropriate if the spouse was involved in extramarital sex.[137] Of Straus's national sample of married people, 27.6 percent thought that slapping a spouse was either necessary, normal, or good.[138] However, the authors warn that consistency between attitudes and behavior cannot be taken for granted according to their research.

More specific and behavioral but less generalizable evidence for the presence of societal attitudes supporting wife abuse is shown by two laboratory studies. In one such study done by Straus, student subjects were given a description of an assault of a woman by a man which resulted in her losing consciousness. If the subjects were told the couple was married, they suggested a significantly less severe punishment for the man than if they were described as "going together."[139] Another laboratory study, involving a staged physical attack on a female by a male, resulted in 65 percent of the subjects intervening when they had been led to believe the pair were strangers versus only a 19 percent intervention rate when they thought the couple was married. Those authors concluded: "If bystanders and, one would guess, society do not regard wife beating seriously, this act cannot be controlled."[140] In real life twenty-one of Bruce J. Rounsaville's sample of thirty-one battered women (68 percent) had been beaten in public, but only one received any help from strangers.[141]

Wife abuse can also be viewed in the context of behavior which is thought to be appropriate for the male sex in general. The National Commission on the Causes of Violence found that proving masculinity in our culture may require "frequent rehearsals of toughness" and the exploitation of women.[142] As Robert Whitehurst states, "When all other sources of masculine identity fail, men can always rely on being 'tough' as a sign of manhood."[143] Renvoize mentions the mining communities of England and Wales where physical strength is important to men and "roughing up" wives considered normal.[144] Dobash and Dobash note that men who assault their wives are living up to cultural prescriptions that are "cherished in Western society, aggressiveness, male dominance and female subordination."[145]

David Lester's cross-cultural study of wife abuse found that wifebeating was significantly more common in societies where the status of women was rated as inferior.[146] In a similar study of primitive societies, Wilfred T. Masumura found wife abuse significantly correlated with other forms of violence, such as warfare, personal crime, and feuding.[147] Carroll has argued that "the elements of a culture tend to be interdependent," that norms of male dominance (as in the Mexican-American culture) and prescriptions against challenging that dominance are consistent with high rates of battering, and equality and conflict resolution on the basis of discussion support nonviolence between spouses (as in the Jewish-American culture).[148] These "informal and ideological controls" can become so deeply embedded as to appear natural.[149] In a questionnaire survey of attribution of blame for wifebeating in a written vignette, 23.7 percent of 338 respondents said the wife was equally to blame for unprovoked or after a "heated verbal argument" violence against her, and 3.3 percent said she was predominantly or totally to blame.[150] Surely a violent attack on a woman by a stranger, even after an argument, would not be blamed at all on her by impartial observers! Within the context of marriage, there definitely seems to be overt as well as covert cultural support for violence against women.

Wife Abuse Within the Context of Violence Against Women

It is important to view wife abuse in a wider perspective. A crucial part of the cultural support for beating women comes from the historical and present context of various forms of violence against women that operate to help maintain the patriarchy of most societies. Patriarchy can be defined as "any kind of group organization in which males hold dominant power and determine what part females shall and shall not play, and in which capabilities assigned to women are relegated generally to the mystical and aesthetic and excluded from the practical and political realms."[151] As Margarete Sandelowski asserts, "women are immobilized by and imprisoned within the fear of violence."[152] Single acts of wife abuse do not keep our society sexist, but when the acts are multiplied and coupled with the frightening incidence of rape, homicide of women, and genital mutilation and joined with the historical precedents of suttee, witchburning, footbinding, mutilating surgery, and female infanticide, patriarchy's power can be seen to be based ultimately upon violence.

Historical Forms of Violence Against Women. Briefly examining the historical phenomena of types of violence against women, witchburning is the earliest well-documented form. "Tens of thousands of female peasant lay healers and midwives were burned as witches" in Europe and America from the 1500s to the 1700s.[153] Close examination of this occurrence by feminists has revealed that their main crime was a lack of submission to the stereotyped role of the subservient medieval woman. During the same time period, the practice of suttee or inclusion of the widow and concubines in the male's funeral pyre, was being carried out in India. The women were often drugged or coerced. Even when she was not forced, the widow knew that her alternatives were prostitution or a life of servitude and starvation with her husband's relatives, since culture prescribed that she was somehow to blame for the man's death, if not during her present life, then in her past ones. The Chinese custom of footbinding was forced by male insistence that women were not attractive unless their feet were tiny stumps caused by years of excruciatingly painful binding. As a result, women were forced absolutely to be totally dependent on men, since they could take only a few tottering steps without assistance. Western medicine in the late nineteenth century used the surgical procedures of clitoridectomy, oophorectomy, and hysterectomy to cure masturbation, insanity, deviation from the "proper" female role, heightened sexual appetites, and rebellion against husband or father.[154] Radical feminists would argue that the medical practices of superfluous hysterectomies, unnecessarily mutilating surgery for breast cancer, the use of the Dalkon Shield and Diethylstilbestrol (DES), and the coercive sterilization of poor women have continued the practice of violence against women by male-dominated medicine yet today.[155]

Contemporary Forms of Violence Against Women. Female infanticide, homicide of women, and genital mutilation are three forms of violence directed at females that are rooted in history and con-

Abuse of Female Partners

tinuing today. They are found in their most virulent forms in societies that most rigidly adhere to male dominance. Marie-louise Janssen-Jurreit points out that because of the higher life expectancy of females, the proportion of women should be higher in relation to men; however, world statistics show only a 49.78 female-to-male ratio.[156] That proportion is lowest in Arab and Islamic countries. Western countries show a higher male infant mortality rate, while Arab and Islamic nations, as well as India, have a significantly higher female infant mortality rate. The statistics seem to indicate "negligent care of female newborns" at the very least. India and the Arabic and Islamic nations also practice the killing of adult women with frightening regularity. Without punishment, men can kill wives and daughters for "public embarrassment," especially "habitual disobedience" and for having illegitimate children in contemporary India.[157] In rural Arabic villages a woman who has had sex before marriage is such a stigma to the family that they are obligated to kill her, even if she has been raped.[158]

One of the most horrifying and yet widespread of practices of female destruction is the genital mutilation which is practiced in much of East, West, and Central Africa and parts of the Middle East. Somehow the fact that this is being done to 25 to 30 million young girls *every year, right now, today* constantly seems to surprise most people. Perhaps it is so horrifying that knowledge must be suppressed. The mutilation can take the form of removal of the tip of the clitoris, complete clitoridectomy, or excision of all of the external genitalia except the labia majora and may be accompanied by infibulation—the closure of the wound by sewing with catgut or using thorns, leaving a small opening for urination and menstrual flow. Infibulation involves opening the aperture further for intercourse and childbirth and resewing at the husband's command. The practices are often carried out without anesthesia, with crude instruments, and totally without regard for sterility. Complications are rampant, as may well be imagined.[159] In Egypt "practically all" girls from eight to ten have a clitoridectomy performed. These practices are considered necessary in these cultures for a woman to be marriageable, and without marriage, a woman is worthless.[160]

A form of violence against women most in the realm of public awareness is rape. Andrea Dworkin states: "Rape is no excess, no aberration, no accident, no mistake—it embodies sexuality as the culture defines it."[161] Rape appears in many forms: sexual abuse of children, gang rape, forced intercourse with wives, sexual torture of female prisoners, intercourse with therapists, bride capture and group rape as a puberty rite, as well as the most common form.[162] Rape is "an exercise of domination and the infliction of degradation upon the victim" and serves to restrict the independence of women and remind them of their vulnerability, thereby keeping them subjugated across all patriarchal societies.[163]

Rape is a crime of violence, not sex. The recent increases of rape, assault, and murder in the United States all follow the same curve.[164] Dorothy O. Lewis and her associates found that the characteristics of rapists resemble closely those of other violent offenders.[165] A study of 133 convicted rapists in Massachusetts found that power or anger motives were dominant in all their acts of rape; sexuality was being used to express them.[166] Ann Burgess and Lynda Holmstrom, from their extensive work with rape victims and research into the problem conclude, "Although different patterns of rape are apparent, they *all* have a common motivational base: power."[167]

A final form of violence against women to be briefly mentioned is physical aggression in dating situations. Several recent studies have documented an alarming rate of violence between couples on today's college campuses; from 22.3 percent to over 60 percent of respondents reported either being victimized or perpetrating violent acts.[168] There is perhaps more reciprocity between the sexes than has been traditionally seen with wife abuse, but most of the observers are agreeing that "women are still the primary victims."[169] This particular kind of violence against women has a specific ramification in the understanding of wife abuse. It has been noted that battered women frequently (up to one-third in some samples) were attacked by their mates before marrying or living with them. Researchers have questioned if this does not mean that the women knew of probable abuse beforehand and therefore must have been accepting of it in order to go ahead with a more permanent relationship. If premarital violence is as common as these recent studies are suggesting (firsthand middle-class dating experience reveals many incidents of physical aggression from otherwise "suitable" young men), it can be understood why women would conclude that such behavior is relatively normal and of little concern. As with other forms of violence against women, society becomes inured to its occurrence. Without careful study and constant reminder, society accepts incidents as inevitable, not to be questioned, not to be decried. The myths and silences that surround such practices serve to keep women quiet about them, while the underlying fear that they engender helps to keep patriarchy intact.

A Synthesizing Conceptual Framework: Machismo

From the study of violence in general and specifically wife abuse, this author has concluded that there is a conceptual framework that can be separated out which has previously been embedded within other theoretical formulations. The concept of machismo or compulsive masculinity can be found in psychological, sociological, and anthropological literature on violence and is also mentioned in much of the wife abuse literature from all viewpoints. It can be used as a unifying concept from which to view both wifebeating and violence against women. This section will examine explanations for the occurrence of machismo, delineate characteristics associated with it, briefly describe some of the general violence literature as it relates to machismo, and explain the association of machismo with wife abuse.

Origins and Associated Characteristics

Talcott Parsons, Albert Cohen, and a few years later, Walter Miller first linked a machismo-like concept to violence. They postulated that boys seldom see their fathers and therefore have trouble making a masculine identification, but have incorporated some of the feminine characteristics of their mothers. When the boys come under social pressure to establish their own masculine identity, they reject their own feminine natures and overemphasize the traditional male values of toughness and hardness and may commit deviant acts "as a public pronouncement" that they are "real men."[170]

Psychoanalytic literature attributed

compulsive masculinity to dominating mothers, but in reality, as Beatrice Whiting states, "an individual identifies with that person who is perceived as controlling those resources that he wants."[171] Relegation of all or most early childcare to females does result in first identification with mothers, but when boys realize (after the first two to three years) that the world is obviously dominated by males, they start to try to change allegiance totally leading to inner conflict. Anthropological data from Whiting and Margaret Mead document the problems in primitive societies and polygynous cultures when fathers are completely separated from women and children, and a more violent society results from compulsive masculinity.[172] In our own country, lower-economic class white fathers have the least role in childrearing. Lower-class black males also have less of a role than middle-class fathers, but the pattern of men excluding themselves from childcare predominates over all groups.[173] All boys feel they need to prove their masculinity to some extent and reject feminine characteristics that they recognize within themselves because they see that this is not what "wins" in the patriarchal world. Even for boys from female-headed households, television, family relationships with other male adults, and a look at the "street" provide models of tough masculine behavior.[174]

Lionel Tiger postulated that a proclivity for male bonding is innate, and that machismo-type behavior originates from this instinct.[175] We can reject the idea of such an instinct by cross-cultural data indicating that such behavior is by no means universal. However, Tiger makes some interesting observations in his study of all-male groups. When they are connected with initiations and secret societies in primitive cultures, they become a factor in the breaking of ties with mothers and in maintaining dominance over and social distance from females. All-male groups in any culture tend to facilitate the expression of aggression and provide group standards for maleness such as bravery and toughness. It is easy to apply these concepts to inner-city gangs, motorcycle gangs, Ku Klux Klan, armies, and so forth.

However, male bonding cannot be regarded as a cause of machismo, only a manifestation. Anthropologists, feminists, and psychoanalysts have all noted the more or less unconscious fear and envy men have of women because of their unique and awesome ability to bear children.[176] In peaceful primitive cultures this female power is glorified and women are given rightful respect for it, but in patriarchy female power has been denied and denigrated. In patriarchy there is a basic ambivalence toward women, originating in "uterus envy" and compounded by guilt, denial, displacement, projection, and rationalization.[177] This helps to explain some of the roots of violence against women, including wife abuse.

Socialization for Machismo. The training for the male role starts early. More stringent demands are made and enforced more harshly on boys than on girls at an early age. Ronald P. Rohner found boys age two to six already more aggressive in 71 percent of the societies in a cross-cultural study, but there were great differences in the amount of that aggression depending on how the children were raised.[178] Ruth E. Hartley found kindergarten boys already restricting their interests and activities to those traditionally labeled masculine while girls took another five or more years to do so to those labeled feminine.[179] Male school and peer group activities are explicitly organized around struggle and boys are encouraged to hunt, fish, fight, and play war games by their fathers.[180] Boys at eight and eleven were found to be saying "they have to be able to fight in case a bully comes along," and they are expected "to be noisy" and "to get into trouble more than girls."[181]

Violence can be viewed "as a clandestine masculine ideal in western culture."[182] Male heroes are John Wayne types and playboy swingers, both of whom treat women with disdain. The ideal male wields authority, especially over women, has unlimited sexual prowess, is invulnerable, has competition as his guiding principle, never discloses emotion, is tough and brave, has great power, is adept at one-upsmanship, can always fight victoriously if he needs to and doesn't need anyone.[183] This is, of course, an impossible standard and creates anxiety in men because of their inability to reach it.

Characteristics of Machismo. Many characteristics have been cited as representative of machismo behavior. Whiting identifies "a preoccupation with physical strength and athletic prowess, or attempts to demonstrate daring and valor or behavior that is violent and aggressive."[184] Thrill-seeking behavior, inability to express emotions, independence, egotism, and support of the military have been noted by other authors.[185] Sexist attitudes are inherent in machismo and are demonstrated by the valuing of sexual virility, the treatment of women as commodities and conquest objects, the insistence on female subjugation, the inability to cooperate with women, and the adherence to the "unwritten law" that female sexual infidelity must be avenged.[186] The dangerousness of machismo to women is illustrated in this quote from Thelma McCormack: "Machismo is an attitude of male pride in sexual virility, a form of narcissism, that condones the sexual use and abuse of women, and, in the extreme, violence as a dimension of sexual gratification and instrumental to sexual goals."[187] Machismo, therefore, can be defined as the male attitudes and behavior arising from and supported by the patriarchal social structure which express sexism and male ownership of women, glorify violence, emphasize virility, and despise gentleness and the expression of any emotions except anger and rage.

Further Relationships of Machismo and Violence

There is considerable evidence of linkages between machismo attitudes and violent behavior. One of the additional characteristics of machismo behavior is owning and/or carrying a gun.[188] In a multistate sample of 1,504 American men and women, the most significant correlation with gun ownership was the approval of and willingness to use violence. Having been a victim of violent crime showed no correlation with gun ownership, suggesting that other variables, such as machismo, are more important than realistic fear.[189] Handguns cannot be considered as a cause of violence; however, guns in the home, ostensibly kept for defense, are at least sometimes used impulsively in the heat of an argument without death being intended by the perpetrator.

Many other indicators link violence with machismo. Two of the countries with the highest homicide rates in the world, Colombia and Mexico, also have strong machismo ethics.[190] The highest rates of homicide in the United States are found in the deep South (Mississippi, Alabama, and Louisiana) and in the West (Texas,

New Mexico, and Nevada), both areas characterized by exaggerated machismo. These six states have an average homicide rate of 13.6 per 100,000 population which is almost four times greater than the rate in all of New England, an area that less idealizes rugged masculinity.[191] Arizona, Texas, and Mississippi also have the highest number of guns per capita while New England and the eastern United States have approximately one-half the percentage of households owning guns than the South and the West.[192] Marshall Clinard and Daniel Abbott, when determining the differences between two slum areas in Kampala, Uganda, found that the area characterized by fewer negative attitudes toward fighting, more prostitution and wifebeating, was also the area of the greatly higher crime rate.[193] Richard G. Sipes found that cultures exhibiting a great deal of warlike activity were significantly more likely to engage in a great deal of combative sports activities.[194] Both John Hepburn and Howard S. Erlanger conclude from separate reviews of empirical research concerned with the subculture of violence theory that a "subculture of masculinity" better explains the evidence.[195]

Machismo and Murder. Several studies of murderers have noted machismo characteristics. Andrew K. Ruotolo described only four male murderers, but noticed that they all "confused gentleness with weakness."[196] Barry M. Maletzky examined twenty-two male subjects with long histories of violent behavior. They exhibited a variety of other characteristics, but all "appeared hypermasculine."[197] Bach-Y-Rita's group of 117 male inpatients whose chief complaint was explosive violent behavior also showed a variety of incidence of neurological symptoms, but were "generally outwardly hypermasculine and intent on physically defending their masculinity against other men."[198] In psychiatric exams of 367 men accused of murder in Scotland, Hunter Gillies found evidence of tolerance of brutality, drunkenness, wifebeating, robbery, murder, and rape. One hundred and one of these men had killed women.[199]

Machismo and Aggressive Behavior. A series of laboratory experiments also show the connection between aggressiveness and machismo characteristics. David G. Perry and Louise C. Perry found that aggressive boys are likely to perceive signs of suffering as indications of success of their aggression. They found that when a victim did not express pain, these boys became very hostile and gave increasingly intensive shocks.[200] Stuart P. Taylor and Ian Smith found that male students exhibiting traditionally dominant attitudes toward women also showed more aggressive behavior toward both males and females.[201] Using electronically measured pillow clubs, David M. Young et al. showed that young men favoring subordinate status for women were less aggressive toward female opponents when the women were passive and only defended themselves. However, when the females attacked, the traditionalists increased significantly the intensity of blows, much more so than the egalitarian males.[202] Dogmatism (measuring authoritarianism) was related to aggression and hostility for males, but only to hostility in females in yet another study.[203] Although caution must be exercised in applying laboratory data on aggression to real life, these studies add to the support of the association of various characteristics of machismo with aggression in males.

Machismo and Culture. Machismo is present to some extent in most men, but its outward display is more prevalent in lower-class males. There is also empirical evidence for the idea that machismo is especially evident in our country, in black males.[204] Black gang members were more likely to rate images of sexual virility, approval of pimping (objectification of females), and defense of a fighting or tough reputation higher than middle- or lower-class black or white teenaged boys.[205] As Michele Wallace points out, machismo attitudes in black men are not a result of racial characteristics or the family heritage of slavery; they resulted from the systematic degradation of black men (and equally so, black women) by white racist society, which was revolted against by black men in the 1960s with an image of strength and violence.[206] Along with this image came sexism which was in part an adoption of white male patriarchal values (it works for them), partially a result of encouragement for this sentiment by white racists, and somewhat a scapegoating mechanism. "Black Macho" has been fostered by the continuing powerlessness of the black male.

Curtis has developed a theory to explain the prevalence of criminal violence in poor black young men.[207] He first identifies subcultural values of the majority of people who are black and poor. They are different from the values of the dominant culture (which includes middle-class blacks), but they do not include violence. However, there is a group of poor black males who hold different and opposing values to the dominant culture that Curtis identifies as a violent contraculture. These men have found it impossible to express the characteristics of the ideal male through economic or occupational roles, and rather than accepting their fate or turning hostility inward through mental illness or drug addiction, they have accepted attitudes that foster violence. These include an "emphasis on physical prowess and toughness," on "sexual prowess and exploitation . . . on shrewdness and manipulativeness," and on "thrill seeking and change." These can be identified as machismo values. Curtis also conceptualizes that the high rate of intra-male black violence further reflects the acceptance of a violent resolution of conflict, the prevalence of jealousy, a "brittle sensitivity," and the abundance of gun carrying by these men.

Lest it be forgotten that machismo is widespread in middle-class white society, the images of women being sexually and physically abused in pornography, on record albums, in fashion magazines and in men's magazines, and on billboards are rampant.[208] Seven out of ten American men think it is a good idea for their sons to engage in fistfights.[209] Machismo is not a characteristic of only poor black men, but it is often more directly expressed in that culture because white, racist patriarchal society has rendered those men powerless except on the street and in their own homes. This can at least partially explain both the high rate of black male violence in the ghetto and also the higher rate of black female homicide victims and wife abuse victims than that of white female victims.[210]

Machismo can thus be seen to be substantially linked to violence in our culture and cross-culturally. Machismo attitudes are often strongest where other forms of violence against women are the most violent and patriarchy the strongest. The machismo ethic is very similar to the "honor code" of many Arab and other Mediterranean cultures, wherein the woman is defined as property, and the man must defend that property with violence if necessary toward other men and/or toward the woman.[211] One of the forms that this violence may take is wife abuse; the male who holds strong machismo values will usually consider it his right to beat his wife.

Machismo and Abuse of Female Partners

The nature of the patriarchal system and resulting sexist machismo attitudes toward women and especially female partners is deeply embedded in our culture and can be argued to be the root cause of wife abuse. Dobash and Dobash express the idea in the following phrase: ". . . the legacy of the patriarchy continues to generate the conditions and relationships that lead to a husband's use of force against his wife."[212] The other contributing factors which have been previously reviewed can be understood within this context. Alcohol can be seen as a disinhibiting agent which weakens the social prescription against doing physical harm to women at least in certain situations. Intoxication can then be used as a convenient excuse for battering a woman since our society teaches that such behavior is less reprehensible when under the influence. Alcohol, therefore, can give a man the courage, the excuse, and the convenient loss of social veneer necessary to behaviorally express his need for power and macho attitudes.

Social Learning, Wife Abuse, and Machismo. Machismo also fits into social learning theory and the idea that stresses and/or frustration may result in wife abuse. It is the patriarchal family arrangement that teaches the men who it is appropriate to express his frustration toward. Steinmetz and Straus point out that husbands who hit wives are "carrying out a role model learned from parents and brought into play when social stresses become intolerable."[213] Actually the model is the one learned from the father, an identification with the aggressor. In Gayford's study, 41.6 percent of the abusive husbands saw their father being violent, while only 6.9 percent experienced a violent mother.[214] Carroll also found only male sex linkages, between violent fathers and battering sons, in the intergenerational transmission of violence.[215] Dobash and Dobash further explain social learning when they state, "Thus, all men see themselves as controllers of women, and because they are socialized into the use of violence, they are (all) potential aggressors against their wives."[216]

Television is also replete with male heroes using violence to achieve goals without negative sanctions. In a survey of programming from 1967 to 1975, it was found that the "good" guys were most likely to be the killers. Women were the most often killed, and the heroes treat women with disdain.[217] Even the commercials show male authority.[218] Children's books (including classroom texts) and movies display the same theme.[219]

Machismo and Powerlessness. William Goode relates family violence to the theoretical framework of social systems and social stratification.[220] He views the family as a power system like all other social units, which "all rest to some degree on force and its threat" to operate. Goode points out that there are four ways by which people can be made to serve the ends of those in authority: (1) force and its threat (power); (2) economic variables; (3) prestige or respect; and (4) likability, attractiveness, friendship, or love. Within the marriage relationship, a combination of these factors is used to preserve male dominance. The threat of force is used more frequently than, and in conjunction with, actual violence.[221] Physical abuse enters into the picture more often, according to Goode, when the other three persuasive mechanisms fail or when the male feels his authority is threatened.[222] Thus battering behavior is more likely to appear when the man's control and therefore his macho pride is challenged by the woman's job, pregnancy, or the possibility of infidelity and if the man feels insecure about his own power from other means. As Anthony Storr states: "It is the insecure and inadequate who most easily feel threatened and who resort to violence as a primitive way of restoring dominance."[223]

The man who feels any sort of inadequacy or is powerless in the male world is most likely to use force and violence where he can, in the home and in his neighborhood. Karl Bednarik finds modern men generally in a crisis of masculinity.[224] Only a few men actually achieve dominance in work and economically, and their traditional male role in the home is being threatened. He describes the symptoms of this crisis as "impotent anger" demonstrated by outbursts of blind rage and mysterious acts of violence, and the transfer of women into a sexual commodity. The lower-class male is the least powerful man and the farthest from the ideal in society and is therefore likely to be more overt in his machismo and violent behavior. Andrew Tolson notes that working-class masculinity is characterized by an "impulsive, aggressive style" more so than middle-class masculinity. Normal masculinity in the lower class is a threatening demeanor and "drunken violence is the last line of defense."[225] The lower-class male is more likely to *insist* on his "conjugal right" to authority in the home, and violence is used when his power seems to be slipping.[226] The data on unemployment, poverty, lack of skills, and lower levels of education in many battering men is an illustration of this mechanism. It has also been suggested that the high incidence of child abuse or excessive physical punishment in the background of many wifebeaters has contributed to a basic sense of inadequacy and problems in identification with the father in these men which is later expressed as compulsive masculinity.[227] Violence against wives usually has aspects of enforcing or reasserting the control of one particular man in a relationship, and it thereby reinforces the whole of patriarchy. Most wife abusers are staunch supporters of the traditional male role of dominance and authority, and their behavior is designed to perpetuate that role both at home and in society.[228] As Terry Davidson notes, "the wifebeater intends to cause injury and pain" and assumes that there will be no retaliation from male-oriented society. She finds three common attitudes in most wife abusers: (1) the behavior is acceptable and/or justified, (2) the man is unsure of the reasons for the battering other than it is a continuation of a ritual, (3) there is a lack of guilt and shame and a mystification that the law should object.[229]

Asserting Control through Abuse. The purposeful nature of wife abuse is shown in many ways. The wife-beaters' justifications are often trivial. For example, Martin cites these cases: a woman broke the egg yolk when frying her husband's breakfast, another wife wore her hair in a ponytail, and a third served a casserole instead of fresh meat. As Martin points out, these are only excuses, not reasons for beatings.[230] Several authors have noted that wife abuse is not always preceded by verbal argument or conflict at all.[231] Walker found that "it is not uncommon for the batterer to wake the woman out of a deep sleep to begin his assault." She also states that "although these women often did or said things to make the batterer angry, it was obvious he would have beaten her anyway."[232]

Hilberman and Munson drew the following conclusion from their interviews: "Violence erupted in any situation in which the husband did not immediately get his way." They also found that the majority of the men in their sample were "making active and successful efforts to keep their wives ignorant and isolated" and therefore more submissive.[233] In Gelles's study, many of the men tried to control their wives' activities by restricting or trying to restrict their access to the car and/or money. If the wife rebelled or disobeyed, a beating resulted, being used as a "last means of controlling the behavior of his wife."[234] Dobash and Dobash found that the courtship phase of the abusive marriage was characterized by increasing isolation of the woman and increasing possessiveness of her by the man.[235] The few incidents of battering during courtship (experienced by 23 percent of the women) were sparked by issues of male possession and authority. Upon marriage, most of any remaining independent social activity by the wife swiftly ended, while the man retained his habits of going out with his friends. The first beating usually occurred within the first six months of marriage showing the husband's attempt to establish complete control early.

When a woman gets married in patriarchy, her primary responsibility becomes childrearing, domestic labor, and "personal and psychic service" to her mate. The household responsibilities are seen as a service to the person in authority, the husband, and how well they are done is a symbol of "commitment and subservience."[236] This helps to explain the often trivial nature of the incident preceding battering; it is often over the woman's performance of a small household chore. If performed poorly or reluctantly in the perception of the man, it is a symbol of some spark of rebellion against his total dominance. Such possible revolt must be quelled swiftly, with force if necessary, and such force has great symbolic meaning for the future.

Returning to Goode's basic premises, other characteristics of wife abuse can be explored. In order to use the third and fourth means of influence, prestige or love, a husband needs to be verbally persuasive. Several authors have listed poor communication skills as a factor predisposing to abuse.[237] Goode postulates that lower-class males may have fewer verbal skills as well as less prestige and decreased economic resources, and they therefore have to rely more frequently on brute power to maintain their position in the family. He contrasts this to the middle-class male whom he characterizes in the following way: "The greater the other resources an individual can command, the more force he can muster, but the less he will actually deploy or use force in an overt manner." Goode goes on to note that the middle-class male has been taught to avoid the use of force by his childhood training.[238] Whitehurst maintains that the only difference according to class is in terms of degree and frequency; the issue is still control and dominance. The middle-class husband is more likely to hit his wife only once at a time and then regain his control as he considers the consequences to his position if he were known as a batterer.[239] Yet even one blow is a powerful symbol of force and authority. As Stark and her coauthors describe, the most probable interpretation of these characteristics of wifebeating is that: "Complex social factors may determine whether and in what combination physical, ideological, political and economic force will be used to control women. . . ."[240]

Jealousy and Machismo. Jealousy, noted by almost all authors as a major cause of the wifebeater's behavior, and also as a major cause of husbands killing wives, is most logically viewed within the context of the husband's effort to maintain control over his wife and his machismo attitude. One of the dictionary definitions of jealous is "zealous in guarding."[241] Ownership is implied. Because women are considered the possession of a husband, real or imagined sexual infidelity is the gravest threat to male dominance. Sixty-six of Gayford's sample of 100 abused women cited their husband's jealousy as the main cause of abuse, while only 17 had ever actually been unfaithful in comparison to 44 of the husbands.[242] The beaten wives in Walker's study "almost universally reported irrational jealousy" shown by the males.[243] This author's research on twenty-eight homicides of women in intimate relationships revealed that male jealousy was the major cause cited in 64.3 percent of the killings; male dominance issues sparked another 17.9 percent. Whitehurst concluded from his study of 100 court cases: "At the core of nearly all the cases involving physical violence, the husband responded out of frustration at being unable to control the wife, often accusing her of being a whore or having an affair with another male, usually without justification."[244] In a review of all wife abuse literature, Sydney Brandon found that jealousy was second only to alcohol in frequency, when causes of wife battering were enumerated.[245] Renvoize illustrates well the connection between jealousy and dominance when she states: "The jealousy so often manifested by battering husbands may be one aspect of the need for one partner to have complete power over the other."[246]

Other aspects of jealousy connected with wife abuse have also been discovered. Walker finds that the "batterer's need to possess his woman totally" often causes her to leave or lose her job. The man becomes jealous of her work relationships even when she feels her home role is most important, lets him control all her earnings, and tries hard to convince him that he is still head of the family.[247] Other authors have also noted that the abusive husband is threatened when the wife wants to get a job.[248] Battering men also frequently limit the wife's visits with even female friends and relatives.[249]

The frequent wifebeating that occurs when the woman is pregnant may also express jealousy and possessiveness more than anything else; a child can divert some of a wife's attention and loyalty away from the husband.[250] Walker found that most of the women she interviewed reported more severe and more frequent violence during pregnancy and, importantly, during the child's early infancy. She also concludes that this phenomenon is directly related to the husband's possessiveness.[251] All these kinds of jealousy, cited so often as a cause of wife abuse in and of themselves, are seen from a machismo viewpoint to be part of the larger, overall cause of the patriarchal system and its substrates, the need for male dominance and sexism.

Sexual Relationships as an Outgrowth of Machismo. The machismo attitudes of wifebeaters is also shown in their sexual relationships with their wives. Martin notes that these men see conquest as an integral part of sex.[252] Several samples have shown sexual abuse as a part of the pattern of victimization.[253] Stark et al. felt that the deliberate, sexual nature of wife abuse is shown in the predominance of injuries to the face, chest, breast, and abdomen.[254] Walker found that the majority of abusing men in her sample used sex as an act of aggression: many had mutilated their wives sexually, some forced their wives into extraordinary sex practices, and most of the women felt as if they had been raped at least once during the marriage. She also notes: "The violence and brutality in the sexual relationship seem to escalate over time."[255] Other researchers have noted that when the wife refuses sex, it becomes a provocation to the husband.[256] This can be viewed as a part of the need for sexual dominance in the machismo syndrome, and when seen in the context of the frequent sexual abuse, refusal of sex seems to be a reasonable action on the part of the wives.

In summary, the concept of machismo can be seen to link a proposed root of wife abuse, the patriarchal system, with the behaviors of violent men, and wife abusers. Data from mainly descriptive studies have been used to document that wifebeaters are frequently virulently possessive and desperately trying to maintain control over their wives. For instance, Alexandra Symonds reports that the largest group of wife abusers can be categorized by a machismo attitude, little guilt, a violent character structure, and a pathological need for control.[257] These men have learned that it is appropriate to use physical aggression and to direct that force against their wives. Stress and threats to macho pride may spark such expressions of violence; alcohol may facilitate it. There is cultural support and historical precedent from patriarchal society to batter women, especially for men in the lower socioeconomic class and certain cultures where machismo is more widespread. Machismo cannot be said to be proven as a direct cause of wife abuse, but it is a useful concept for helping to understand the phenomenon.

Theoretical Frameworks Explaining Continuation

One of the most difficult dynamics of wife abuse for professionals and the general public alike to understand is why a battered wife would stay with her spouse, sometimes for many years. The problem has been addressed from several standpoints, and several well-developed theoretical frameworks have been advanced. This section will examine the formulations under three major headings: (1) societal response to victims, (2) psychological responses of abused women, and (3) Mildred Daley Pagelow's work which tested several variables previously advanced as affecting the wife's length of stay in a battering relationship.

Societal Response to Victims

Many authors have noted that a primary obstacle to an abused wife's leaving the situation is the lack of support she receives from society's institutions. As we have examined earlier, generally, the health profession has not been very helpful to the battered woman. She is likely to be perceived as mentally ill if she seeks help from traditional mental health facilities and although the emergency room and family physicians will treat her physical symptoms, they generally do not help with the actual abuse situation.

Other sources of help are equally problematical. The clergy usually emphasize the sanctity of the family.[258] In Prescott and Letko's sample, of ten women who contacted a minister or priest for advice, only one found him or her helpful.[259] The 109 wives in the Dobash and Dobash research were most likely to seek help from parents, relatives, and friends, but were usually advised on how to cope, not leave. These women were least likely to seek help from social agencies because of fear of condemnation and the cultural prohibition against seeing social workers for marital problems.[260] Walker reports that in England, physicians, service professionals, and the police have the highest incidence of abusers within professional categories.[261] This gives us an idea of what kind of attitudes abused women may encounter when they seek help from these men.

The police would ordinarily be the first agency called when assault occurs and are thought to generally protect a citizen from further harm from an attacker. Yet police do not always respond when they receive a call from an abused wife, and when they do the woman frequently finds them ineffective. Consequently, battered women seldom even call the police because they anticipate little help and fear retaliation after the police leave. Because of recent efforts of police officials such as James Bannon, this grim picture is beginning to change. The relationship of wife abuse and the police is further explored in Chapter 12. The other part of the law enforcement system, the courts, has also traditionally been of little help to abused women. The problems in the legal system and recent changes in the laws are examined in Chapter 14.

If, in spite of her terror and despair, in spite of the knowledge that the courts and police are unlikely to protect her from further retaliation, in spite of the principle that she shouldn't have to be the one to leave, she finds the courage to pack up herself and her children and leave, where is the battered woman supposed to go? She usually lacks independent financial resources and her family frequently will encourage her to return.[262] The consensus of the chief circuit judges in Florida was that abused wives stay in the relationship because usually there are no viable alternatives.[263] Housing authorities have not seen wives who have left their assaultive husbands as technically homeless, and therefore do not always provide public housing or assistance in obtaining shelter.[264] Because battering incidents usually happen at night or on the weekend, few social agencies are open. Fortunately, shelters for abused victims are beginning to stay open twenty-four hours a day in this country and in England, but as yet there are not enough. Almost 100 percent of the 150 abused women who called a crisis hot line said they would have used a shelter if one were available; unfortunately, there weren't any in that community.[265]

Even though it is difficult, battered women do try to leave their husbands. Of the 100 women in Gayford's sample, 81 had left on more than one occasion. Thirty-six of them had left more than four times. The majority had returned because their husbands had found them and promised to reform or had threatened and/or demonstrated further violence.[266] Dobash and Dobash interpret this behavior of leaving temporarily and returning as part of a process of testing the outside resources and gathering resolve to make a final break.[267] Unfortunately, the women find most of the rest of the world unsympathetic to their plight and divorce difficult and still a stigma.

Societal Myths. It is interesting to note some of the mechanisms that may operate in society to perpetuate the continued unhelpful response to wife abuse victims. As Martin Symonds notes, "There seems to be a marked reluctance and resistance to accept the innocence" of all victims of violence.[268] Most people's response, generated by the need to have rational explanations for horrible occurrences, is to imply that victims could have somehow avoided their misfortune. Without such rationalizations there are feelings of vulnerability, that if the victim is not somehow to blame, then the same kind of thing may happen to them. There is also the irrational fear of some sort of contamination, and the tendency to put the victim out of sight and out of mind. Myths have therefore arisen that blame the victim and/or explain away the facts and thus avoid the real issues—that society is in itself to blame and therefore each individual member thereof.

Some of the myths perpetuated about wifebeating are women are masochistic and ask for abuse, battered women are crazy, abused wives are free to leave at any time, and these women deserve to get beaten.[269] Victims are encouraged to internalize these myths, and, indeed, Walker found that her sample of battered women believed all the myths of wifebeating. These myths have influenced the behavior of and are perpetuated by the police, the courts, and many of the helping professionals who help to keep the abused women trapped. Walker has also identified prejudicial myths that are prevalent regarding other areas of violence against women: rape, incest, pornography, prostitution, job-related sexual harassment, and sexual relations between clients and male psychotherapists.[270] When taken in conjunction with the commonly held false beliefs about wife abuse, these myths serve to keep women from feeling the full outrage about their persecution. They all emphasize the woman's part in her own victimization and thereby mask the blame of the abusers and of society.

Learned Helplessness— the Psychological Responses of Abused Women

Walker has analyzed the psychological and behavioral reaction of battered women in terms of the "learned helplessness" theory. This phenomenon was first seen in dogs, but has been replicated in humans in experimental laboratory settings and is described as the behavior resulting when an "organism has learned that outcomes are uncontrollable by his responses and is seriously debilitated by this knowledge." When taught that a painful experience occurs randomly and whether or not anything is done to try to avoid or stop it, a person or animal becomes less motivated to try measures to end the pain; has trouble learning that responding controls outcomes generally; and exhibits anxiety, depression, and dependence.[271] Wife abuse usually also occurs randomly and whether or not the victim does anything to precipitate it or does anything to stop it. "Once the women are operating from a belief of helplessness, the perception becomes reality, and they become passive, submissive and helpless."[272] The emotional state of battered women thus may allow their further subjugation and also impedes their leaving.

There is empirical support for the idea of learned helplessness at least in terms of the reported depression of abused women. As well as Walker's own work, most of the samples of battered women describe a significant incidence of depression. Rounsaville found that 77 percent of his sample who were depressed had their first psychiatric contact after being abused, suggesting that the symptoms were related to the beating, not to general pathology. He also found that the women were "relatively unimpaired in work, child care, and relationships with family of origin," again suggesting that the depression was specific to the abuse.[273]

The Cycle of Violence. Walker has also identified a cycle theory of violence from her exploratory interviews and questionnaires from battered women.[274] The first phase, or "tension-building phase" is characterized by minor battering incidents to which the woman usually responds by being compliant, trying desperately to avoid serious incidents. Her feelings of helplessness and fear escalate as the incidents get worse over time. This phase may last for weeks or even years, until the tension has mounted to the breaking point. Phase two, "the acute battering incident," is the outbreak of serious violence that may last from two to twenty-four hours. The woman is powerless to affect the outcome of the stage and can only try to protect herself or hide. In the third stage, the aftermath, the man becomes contrite, loving, and promises to reform. This phase reinforces the woman's hope that the beatings will end. Unfortunately, the cycle almost always repeats itself.

Drake, in her small sample of abused women (twelve) has found independent corroboration for the cycle of violence.[275] However, several authors have not always found the contrite behavior Walker describes as characteristic of the third stage. Dobash and Dobash report that remorse was *not* typical according to their sample of battered women, that only 14 percent of the 109 batterers even apologized after the worst incident.[276] Apparently some men do reinforce the woman staying with promises of no more violence, but this is not always the case.

Other Psychological Responses to Abuse. Walker and other authors have noted several different psychological mechanisms that may operate in the victim of wife abuse and leave her less able to escape the situation. The realistic fear of further injury and death has already been explored in relation to homicide. Seventy-one percent of Rounsaville's sample reported that the partner had threatened to kill them if they left, and all but one said that "on at least one occasion they feared that he would kill them."[277]

Most of the authors have also remarked upon the low self-esteem of the wives caught in abuse relationships. This is understandable in terms of how married women in patriarchy are taught to define their sense of worth in terms of their domestic work and family service. As Walker found, most battered women are traditionalists and believe strongly in the prescribed feminine sex role stereotype.[278] When her husband beats her, it is a "powerful statement of her worthlessness," which, when repeated often enough, is devastating to self-esteem.[279] An authentic sense of self-esteem is necessary for self-determination and movement toward independence.

The extreme fear of these victims interacts with the low self-esteem to create a psychological state of "paralyzing terror." Hilberman and Munson described this reaction as one of unending stress, chronic apprehension of doom, overwhelming passivity, and a pervasive sense of hopelessness.[280] Alexandra Symonds has likened this state to the reaction seen in victims after natural disasters or war-caused catastrophes when they become paralyzed by terror or mental confusion and exhibit passivity and apathy. She also compares the wife of an abuser to victims of other violent crimes who have been noted to show shock and denial, appeasement behavior and/or depression, withdrawal and guilt.[281] In such an emotional state the woman is likely to turn her natural retaliatory aggression inward and blame herself. She knows that to retaliate will bring worse punishment.[282] It is not uncommon for abused women to make suicidal attempts or gestures and to feel guilty.[283]

Whatever psychological operations may be operating to keep women in the battering situation, it is important to keep in mind their psychological strengths and basic normalcy. Clinical experience with battered women has generally found them to be basically emotionally healthy women whose problems are stemming from an almost impossible situation that they have done nothing to create, not from pathology within. Linda S. Labell's large sample of 512 abused women revealed that 72 percent had sought help from outside sources and 74.2 percent had separated from their husbands at least once before going to the shelter from where she drew her sample.[284] A complex assortment of factors, both external and internal, apparently determine whether or not the abused wife is able to extricate herself from the situation.

Sorting Out the Factors: Some Empirical Evidence

Mildred Daley Pagelow has used a sample of 350 battered women to try to test some of the reasons that have been advanced for women staying in abusive relationships.[285] She tested the hypothesis that

> the fewer the resources, the more negative the institutional response, and the more intense the traditional ideology of women who have been battered, the more likely they are to remain in relationships with the batterers and the less likely they are to perform acts that significantly alter the situation in a positive direction.

She found that the strongest set of predictors were the personal resources of the woman, such as age (youth an obvious advantage) and home ownership (suggesting some financial resources). Institutional response explained very little of the length of time in the relationship but may have been confounded by what the women perceived as helpful responses from professionals; it may have been advice to stay. Traditional ideology had a somewhat greater explanatory power, but this was still low, perhaps because the variables used did not really measure traditional values. Pagelow's data also refuted the idea that childhood experience with violence is an important determinant in the wife's abuse and did *not* support the contention that severity and frequency of beatings will force a woman to leave sooner. Pagelow's study is a commendable attempt to use more sophisticated methods of data analysis to try to support carefully constructed and testable hypotheses concerning why women stay in such relationships.

Dennis Marsden has mentioned several other factors besides those already discussed that may influence the abused woman's freedom to leave her situation. These include "her emotional investment in the ideals of marriage and motherhood, contrasting with the alternate identities available to her as a lone mother or worker; her social status in the circle of her friends and how this depends upon her marriage; . . .the possibilities and stigma of gaining alternate income from social security or legal processes."[286] The wife has much to lose as well as much to fear when she leaves her marriage or cohabiting arrangement. She is frequently concerned about the effects on the children as well as on herself. The choices are difficult and serious and compounded by the psychological battering she is receiving as well as the lack of support typically given for her efforts.

Summary

Abuse of female partners has been shown to be a health problem of considerable magnitude which has a great deal of potential for nursing intervention. Even though its significance is only just beginning to be realized, the historical background to the problem is considerable. In considering the theoretical frameworks that have been advanced to explain its causes, the roles of intrapsychic factors, alcohol, stress, socialization for abuse, and cultural support have been examined. Wife abuse was also placed in the wider perspective of violence against women in general. The concept of machismo was seen to be important in explaining wifebeaters' behavior. It has been proposed that the social organization of patriarchy, from which arise the historical roots of wife abuse, cultural support for the phenomenon, and machismo, may be said to set the stage for stress to precipitate violence against wives in men who have learned abusive behavior. The formulations that propose explanations for the continuation of abusive behavior in a relationship, societal responses, and psychological factors were also explored. The theoretical frameworks which have been examined provide the basis for nursing care of battered women, but further research is needed in all the areas examined as well as research to further elucidate the relationships between the abuse of female partners and the wider problem, violence in the family.

Chapter 4

1. J. J. Gayford, "The Aetiology of Repeated Serious Physical Assaults by Husbands on Wives," *Medicine, Science, and the Law* 19 (January 1979): 19.
2. R. Emerson Dobash and Russell Dobash, *Violence Against Wives* (New York: The Free Press, 1979: p. 248.
3. Evan Stark et al., "Medicine and Patriarchal Violence," *International Journal of Health Services*): 9 (1979): 461–493, p. 465.

Abuse of Female Partners

4. Virginia Koch Drake, "Battered Women: A Health Care Problem in Disguise," *Image* 14 (June, 1982), pp. 40-47, p. 45.

5. Lenore Walker, *The Battered Woman* (New York: Harper & Row, 1979), p. 15.

6. Suzanne Steinmetz, *The Cycle of Violence: Assertive, Aggressive and Abusive Family Interaction* (New York: Praeger Publishers, 1977), pp. 499, 6, 9, 89.

7. Suzanne Steinmetz, "The Battered Husband Syndrome," *Victimology* 2 (Fall-Winter 1977-78): pp. 499, 502.

8. Elaine Hilberman and Kit Munson, "Sixty Battered Women," *Victimology* 2 (Fall-Winter, 1977-78): 460-470. p. 461.

9. Murray Straus, "Wife Beating: How Common and Why?" *Victimology* 2 (Fall-Winter, 1977-78): 443-458, p. 444.

10. Richard J. Gelles, *The Violent Home* (Beverly Hills, Calif.: Sage Publications, 1972): 21.

11. Dobash and Dobash, *Violence Against Wives*, p. 19. See also Gelles, *Violent Home*, pp. 51, 74.

12. George Levinger, "Source of Marital Dissatisfaction among Applicants for Divorce," *American Journal of Orthopsychiatry* 36 (October 1966): 803-807.

13. Dobash and Dobash, *Violence Against Wives*, p. 247.

14. Ibid., p. 120.

15. Gayford, "Aetiology of Repeated Serious Physical Assaults," p. 19.

16. Dobash and Dobash, *Violence Against Wives*, p. 120; Walker, *Battered Woman*, pp. 105, 108, 111.

17. Hilberman and Munson, "Sixty Battered Women," p. 462.

18. Dobash and Dobash, *Violence Against Wives*, p. 108.

19. Steinmetz, *Cycle of Violence*, p. 90.

20. John Flynn, "Recent Findings Related to Wife Abuse," *Social Casework* 63 (January 1977): 16.

21. William H. Webster, *FBI Uniform Crime Reports* (Washington, D.C.: U.S. Department of Justice, 1981), p. 11.

22. Martin Wolfgang, "Victim Precipitated Criminal Violence," *Journal of Criminal Law, Criminology, and Political Science* 48 (May-June, 1957): 2.

23. Dobash and Dobash, *Violence Against Wives*, p. 265.

24. Jerrold K. Footlick and Elaine Sciolino, "Wives Who Batter Back," *Newsweek* 90 (30 January 1978); 54.

25. Alan D. Eisenberg and Earl J. Seymour, "The Self-Defense Plea and Battered Women," *Trial* 14 (July 1978): 36.

26. Ibid, p. 34; Footlick and Sciolino, "Wives Who Batter Back," p. 54.

27. Walker, *Battered Woman*, p. 70.

28. Dobash and Dobash, *Violence Against Wives*, pp. 12, 120, 237, 248.

29. Webster, *FBI Uniform Crime Reports*, p. 11.

30. Margaret Gregory, "Battered Wives," in *Violence in the Family*, ed. Marie Borland (Atlantic Highlands, N.J.: Humanities Press, 1976), pp. 107-28, 107.

31. Del Martin, "Battered Women: Society's Problem," in *Victimization of Women*, ed. Jane R. Chapman and Margaret Gates (Beverly Hills, Calif,: Sage Publications, 1978), p. 115.

32. Dobash and Dobash, *Violence Against Wives*, p. 17.

33. P. D. Scott, "Battered Wives," *British Journal of Psychiatry* 125 (November 1974): 439.

34. Gelles, *Violent Home*, p. 21.

35. Walker, *Battered Woman*, p. 27.

36. Jacquelyn Campbell, "Misogyny and Homicide of Women," *Advances in Nursing Science* 3 (January 1981): 78.
37. Ibid., p. 77.
38. Walker, *Battered Woman*, p. 75.
39. Maria Roy, "A Research Project Probing a Cross-Section of Battered Wives," in Roy, *Battered Women*, p. 31.
40. Campbell, "Misogyny and Homicide of Women," p. 79.
41. Richard Makman, "Some Clinical Aspects of Inter-Spousal Violence," in *Family Violence*, ed. John M. Eekelaar and Sanford N. Katz (Toronto: Butterworth & Co., 1978), p. 56.
42. Margaret Elbow, "Theoretical Considerations of Violent Marriages," *Social Casework* 58 (November 1977): 515.
43. Langley and Levy, *Wife Beating*, p. 3.
44. Suzanne Steinmetz, "Wifebeating, Husband-beating—A Comparison of the Use of Physical Violence between Spouses to Resolve Marital Fights," in Roy, *Battered Women*, p. 63.
45. Straus, "Wife Beating," p. 445.
46. Patricia Iyer, "The Battered Wife," *Nursing '80* 10 (July 1980): 53; Federal Bureau of Investigation, *Crime in the United States* (Washington, D.C.: U.S. Department of Science, 1980).
47. Sarah Heffner, "Wife Abuse in West Germany, *Victimology* 2 (Fall-Winter, 1977-78): 472. Robert Chester and Jane Streather, "Cruelty in English Divorce: Some Empirical Findings," *Journal of Marriage and the Family* 34 (November 1972): 709.
48. Stark et al., "Medicine and Patriarchal Violence," p. 469.
49. Drake, "Battered Women," p. 46.
50. Doreen J. DeBlick "Prevalence of Domestic Violence Reported by Female Psychiatric Inpatients" (unpublished field study, Wayne State University, 1981), pp. 39, 40.
51. J. J. Gayford, "Wife Battering: A Preliminary Survey of 100 Cases," *British Medical Journal* 1 (25 January 1975): 195.
52. Drake, "Battered Women," p. 45.
53. Flynn, "Recent Findings," p. 18.
54. Walker, *Battered Woman*, p. 105.
55. Dobash and Dobash, *Violence Against Wives*, p. 31.
56. Terry Davidson, "Wifebeating: A Recurring Phenomenon throughout History," in Roy, *Battered Women*, pp. 2-21; Margaret May, "Violence in the Family: An Historical Perspective," in Martin, *Violence and the Family*, pp. 135-163; Dobash and Dobash, *Violence Against Wives*, pp. 34-75.
57. Davidson, "Wifebeating," p. 8.
58. Dobash and Dobash, *Violence Against Wives*, p. 37.
59. Davidson, "Wifebeating," pp. 10, 11.
60. Dobash and Dobash, *Violence Against Wives*, p. 46.
61. Davidson, "Wifebeating," pp. 1, 11.
62. Dobash and Dobash, *Violence Against Wives*, pp. 44, 48-49.
63. Ibid., p. 52.
64. Davidson, "Wifebeating," p. 14.
65. Dobash and Dobash, *Violence Against Wives*, pp. 54, 55.

66. May, "Violence in the Family," p. 138.
67. Ibid.
68. Davidson, "Wifebeating," pp. 14-16.
69. Christopher Herold, *The Age of Napoleon*, as quoted in Davidson, "Wifebeating" p. 15.
70. Davidson, "Wifebeating," p. 14.
71. Marielouise Janssen-Jurreit, *Sexism: The Male Monopoly on History and Thought*, trans. Verne Moberg, (New York: Farrar, Straus & Giroux, 1982), pp. 225-26.
72. Dobash and Dobash, *Violence Against Wives*, pp. 14, 74.
73. May, "Violence in the Family," p. 140.
74. Davidson, "Wifebeating," pp. 18-19.
75. Dobash and Dobash, *Violence Against Wives*, p. 74; May, "Violence in the Family," p. 139.
76. Davidson, "Wifebeating," p. 2.
77. Dobash and Dobash, *Violence Against Wives*, p. 31.
78. John Snell et al., "The Wifebeater's Wife," *Archives of General Psychiatry* 11 (1964): 110.
79. Renvoize, *Web of Violence*, p. 34.
80. Natalie Shainess, "Vulnerability to Violence: Masochism as Process," *American Journal of Psychotherapy* 33 (April 1979): 174, 188.
81. Marie Borland, Introduction, in Borland, *Violence in the Family*, p. ix; Alexandra Symonds, "Violence Against Women—The Myth of Masochism," *American Journal of Psychotherapy* 33 (April 1979): 161; Walker, *Battered Woman*, p. 15.
82. M. Faulk, "Men Who Assault Their Wives," *Medicine, Science, and the Law* 14 (July 1974): 180.
83. Walker, *Battered Woman*, p. 15.
84. Faulk, "Men Who Assault," p. 183.
85. George R. Bach and Peter Wyden, *The Intimate Enemy* (New York: William Morrow & Co., 1969) pp. 1, 111.
86. Steinmetz, *Cycle of Violence*, p. 24. Dobash and Dobash, *Violence Against Wives*, pp. 98, 124. Murray Straus, "Leveling, Civility, and Violence in the Family," *Journal of Marriage and the Family* 37 (February 1974): 18.
87. Murray Straus, "Violence in the Family," *Nursing Digest* 2 (November-December 1974): 138. Richard Gelles, "No Place to Go: The Social Dynamics of Marital Violence," in Roy, *Battered Women*, pp. 46-63, 57.
88. Dobash and Dobash, *Violence Against Wives*, p. 118; Walker, *Battered Woman*, p. 24; Bonnie Carlson, "Battered Women and Their Assailants," *Social Work* 22 (November 1977): 457; Gayford, "Wife Battering," p. 195; Hilberman and Munson, "Sixty Battered Women," p. 461; Roy, "Research Project Probing a Cross-Section of Battered Wives," p. 39; Women-In-Transition, *Annual Statistical Report* (Detroit, Michigan: Women-In-Transition, 1979), p. 5.
89. Scott, "Battered Wives," p. 438.
90. John A. Byles, "Violence, Alcohol Problems, and Other Problems in Disintegrating Families," *Journal of Studies on Alcohol* 39 (March 1978): 551.
91. Gelles, *Violent Home*, p. 114.
92. Morton Bard and Joseph Zacker, "Assaultiveness and Alcohol Use in Family Disputes," *Criminology* 12 (November 1974): 282-283, 287, 292.
93. Ibid., p. 282; Gayford, "Aetiology of Assaults," p. 24.
94. Carlson, "Battered Women and Their Assailants," p. 489.

95. Gelles, *Violent Home*, pp. 114-18.
96. Walker, *Battered Woman*, p. 24.
97. Joanne Downey and Jane Howell, *Wife Battering* (Vancouver: United Way of Greater Vancouver, 1976), p. 51.
98. Straus, "Wife Beating," pp. 450, 451, 454.
99. Roy, "Research Project Probing a Cross-Section of Battered Wives," p. 30.
100. Steinmetz, *Cycle of Violence*, p. 6.
101. Carlson, "Battered Women and Their Assailants," p. 457; Gayford, "Wife Battering," p. 195; Dobash and Dobash, *Violence Against Wives*, p. 95.
102. Joseph C. Carroll, "The Integenerational Transmission of Family Violence: The Long-Term Effects of Aggressive Behavior," *Aggressive Behavior* 3 (Fall 1977): 292, 294.
103. Steinmetz, *Cycle of Violence*, p. 6.
104. Lucien Beaulieu, "Media, Violence, and the Family," in Eekelaar and Katz, *Family Violence*, p. 60-62.
105. Gelles, "No Place to Go," p. 60
106. Shainess, "Psychological Aspects of Wifebeating," in Roy, *Battered Women*, p. 116.
107. Roy, "Research Project Probing a Cross-Section of Battered Wives," p. 30.
108. Walker, *Battered Woman*, p. 35.
109. Gayford, "Wife Battering," p. 195.
110. Carroll, "Intergenerational Transmission of Family Violence," p. 297.
111. Dobash and Dobash, *Violence Against Wives*, p. 95.
112. Mildred Daley Pagelow, *Woman-Battering* (Beverly Hills: Sage Publications, 1981), pp. 166-75.
113. Barbara Star, "Comparing Battered and Non-Battered Women," *Victimology* 3 (1978): 37, 39.
114. Steinmetz, *Cycle of Violence*, p. 1.
115. Shainess, "Psychological Aspects of Wifebeating," p. 112.
116. Carlson, "Battered Women and Their Assailants," pp. 458, 456.
117. Gayford, "Aetiology of Assaults," pp. 20, 24.
118. Scott, "Battered Wives," p. 433.
119. Hilberman and Munson, "Sixty Battered Women," p. 461.
120. Chester and Streather, "Cruelty in English Divorce," p. 710.
121. Levinger, "Sources of Dissatisfaction," p. 805.
122. Deidre Gaquin, "Spouse Abuse: Data from the National Crime Survey," *Victimology* 2 (Fall-Winter 1977-78): 638.
123. Flynn, "Recent Findings," pp. 13-20, 17, 18.
124. Langley and Levy, *Wife Beating*, p. 7.
125. Carolyn Barden and Jim Barden, "The Battered Wife Syndrome," *Viva* (June 1976): 79-81, 108-110, 80.
126. Renvoize, *Web of Violence*, p. 25; Martin, *Battered Wives* p. 86; Walker, *Battered Woman* p. 24.
127. Renvoize, *Web of Violence*, p. 25.
128. Langley and Levy, *Wife Beating*, p. 53.
129. John O'Brien, "Violence in Divorce Prone Families," *Journal of Marriage and the Family* 33 (November 1971): 695.
130. Gelles, *Violent Home*, pp. 124, 132, 125.

Abuse of Female Partners

131. Suzanne Prescott and Carolyn Letko, "Battered Women: A Social Psychological Perspective," in Roy, *Battered Women* p. 89.

132. Carlson, "Battered Women and Their Assailants," p. 456.

133. Gelles, *Violent Home*, p. 185.

134. Straus, Gelles, and Steinmetz, *Behind Closed Doors*, (New York: Doubleday, 1980), pp. 203, 204, 209.

135. Suzanne Steinmetz and Murray Straus, eds. *Violence in the Family*, (New York: Harper and Row, 1974), p. 20.

136. Rodney Stark and James McEvoy, "Middle-Class Violence," *Psychology Today* 4 (November 1970): 52–56, 110–12, 52.

137. Robert Whitehurst, "Violence Potential in Extramarital Sexual Responses," *Journal of Marriage and the Family* 11 (November 1971): 688.

138. Ursula Dibble and Murray Straus, "Some Social Structure Determinants of Inconsistency between Attitudes and Behavior: The Care of Family Violence," *Journal of Marriage and the Family* 42 (February 1980): 73, 79.

139. Murray Straus, "Sexual Inequality, Cultural Norms and Wifebeating," *Victimology* 1 (Spring 1976): 62.

140. Lance R. Shotland and Margret K. Straw, "Bystander Response When a Man Attacks a Woman," *Journal of Personality and Social Psychology* 34 (November 1976): 992, 999.

141. Bruce J. Rounsaville, "Theories in Marital Violence: Evidence from a Study of Battered Women," *Victimology* (1978) 16.

142. Davidson, "Wifebeating," p. 11.

143. Whitehurst, "Violence in Husband Wife Interaction," in Steinmetz and Straus, *Violence in the Family*, p. 78.

144. Renvoize, *Web of Violence*, p. 24.

145. Dobash and Dobash, *Violence Against Wives*, p. 24.

146. David Lester, "A Cross-Culture Study of Wife Abuse," *Aggressive Behavior* 6 (1980): 362.

147. Wilfred T. Masumura, "Wife Abuse and Other Forms of Aggression," *Victimology* 4 (1979): 52.

148. Joseph C. Carroll, "Cultural-Consistency Theory of Family Violence in Mexican-American and Jewish-Ethnic Groups," in *Social Causes of Husband-Wife Violence*, ed. Murray Straus and Gerald T. Hotaling (Minneapolis: University of Minnesota Press, 1980), p. 68.

149. Dennis Marsden, "Sociological Perspectives on Family Violence," in Martin, *Violence and the Family*, p. 116.

150. Debra Kalmuss, "The Attribution of Responsibility in a Wife-Abuse Context," *Victimology* 4 (1979): 286.

151. Adrienne Rich, *On Lies, Secrets, and Silence* (New York: W. W. Norton & Co., 1979), p. 78.

152. Margarete Sandelowski, *Woman, Health and Choice* (Englewood Cliffs, N.J.: Prentice-Hall, 1980), p. 204.

153. Claudia Dreifus, ed., *Seizing Our Bodies* (New York: Vintage Books, 1977), p. xxi.

154. Mary Daly, *Gyn/Ecology: The Metaethics of Radical Feminism* (Boston: Beacon Press, 1978), pp. 114–16, 122–33; 135–54; 224–28.

155. Dreifus, *Seizing Our Bodies*.

156. Janssen-Jurreit, *Sexism*, pp. 264–65.

157. Edwin D. Driver, "Interaction and Criminal Homicide in India," *Social Forces* 60 (December 1971): 155–56.

158. Janssen-Jurreit, *Sexism*, p. 232; M. O. A. Malik and O. Salvi, "A Profile of Homicide in the Sudan," *Forensic Science* 7 (March-April 1976): 141–50.

159. Fran P. Hosken, "Female Circumcision in Africa," *Victimology* 2 (1977–78): 487–98.

160. Janssen-Jurreit, *Sexism*, p. 248.

161. Andrea Dworkin, *Our Blood: Prophecies and Discourses on Sexual Politics* (New York: Harper & Row, 1976), p. 46.

162. Susan Brownmiller, *Against Our Will: Men, Women, and Rape* (New York: Bantam Books, 1975).

163. Donna Schram, "Rape," in Chapman and Gates, *Victimization of Women*, p. 78.

164. Charles R. Hayman and Charlene Lanza, "Sexual Assault on Women and Girls," *American Journal of Obstetrics and Gynecology* 109 (February, 1971): 483.

165. Dorothy O. Lewis et al., "Juvenile Male Sexual Assaulters," *American Journal of Psychiatry* 136 (November 1977): 1194–96.

166. A. Nicholas Groth et al., "Rape: Power, Anger, and Sexuality," *The American Journal of Psychiatry* 134 (November 1977): 1239–43, 1240.

167. Ann Burgess and Lynda Holmstram, *Rape: Crisis and Recovering* (Bowie, Md.: Robert J. Brady, Co., 1979), p. 28.

168. Rodney Cate et al., "Premarital Abuse," *Journal of Family Issues* 3 (March 1982): 82; "Socko Performance on Campus," *Time* (21 September 1981), 66–67.

169. "Socko Performance," p. 67.

170. Dan C. Gibbons, *Delinquent Behavior* (Englewood Cliffs, N.J.: Prentice-Hall, 1970), p. 154; Walter Miller, "Lower Class Culture as a Generation Milieu of Gang Delinquency," *Journal of Social Issues* 14 (1958): 5–19, 8.

171. Beatrice Whiting, "Sex Identity Conflict and Physical Violence: A Comparative Study," *American Anthropologist* 67 (December 1965): 126.

172. Margaret Mead, *Male and Female* (New York: William Morrow & Co., 1949), p. 88; Whiting, "Sex Identity Conflict," p. 126.

173. Warren Ten Houtan, "The Black Family: Myth and Reality," *Psychiatry* 33 (May 1970): 170.

174. Wade Nobels, "Toward an Empirical and Theoretical Framework for Defining Black Families," *Journal of Marriage and the Family* 40 (November 1978): 687.

175. Lionel Tiger, *Men in Groups* (New York: Random House, 1969), pp. 170, 175, 182–83.

176. Wolfgang Lederer, *The Fear of Women* (New York: Harcourt Brace Jovanovich, 1968), pp. 1–10; Mead, *Male and Female*, p. 88; Phylis Chester, *About Men* (New York: Simon & Schuster, 1978) p. 38.

177. Lederer, *Fear of Women*, p. 282; Chester, *About Men*, p. 71; Joan Myers Weimer, "The Mother, the Macho, and the State," *International Journal of Women's Studies* 1 (January-February, 1978): 73.

178. Ronald P. Rohner, "Sex Differences in Aggression," *Ethos* 4 (Spring 1972): 57–72.

179. Ruth E. Hartley, "Sex-Role Pressure and the Socialization of the Male Child," in *Men and Masculinity*, ed. Joseph H. Pleck and Jack Sawyer (Englewood Cliffs, N.J.: Prentice-Hall, 1974), p. 7.

180. Andrew Tolsen, *The Limits of Masculinity* (New York: Harper & Row, 1977), p. 25.

181. Hartley, "Sex-Role Pressure," p. 10.

182. Jackson Toby, "Violence and the Masculine Ideal," *American Academy of Political and Social Science* 364 (March 1966): 19.

183. Jack O. Balswick and Charles Peck, "The Inexpressive Male: A Tragedy of American Society," *Family Coordinator* 20 (October 1971): 364; Marc Fasteau, *The Male Machine* (New York: McGraw-Hill, 1974).

184. Whiting, "Sex Identity Conflict," p. 127.

185. Robert A. Lewis, "Socialization into National Violence: Familial Correlates of Hawkish Attitudes toward War," *Journal of Marriage and the Family* 33 (November 1971): 702; Balswick and Peck, "Inexpressive Male," p. 364; Peter Greenberg, "The Thrill Seekers," *Human Behavior* 6 (April 1977): 16–23; Robert Brent Toplin, *Unchallenged Violence* (Westport, Conn.: Greenwood Press, 1975), p. 168.

186. J. William Sherwood and John H. McGrath III, "Why People Own Guns," *Journal of Communications* 26 (Fall, 1976): 613; MacDonald, *The Murderer and His Victim*, (Springfield, Ill. Charles C Thomas, 1961); Toplin, *Unchallenged Violence*, p. 167; Miller, "Lower Class Culture," p. 8; Lewis Coser, "Some Social Functions of Violence," *Annals of the American Academy of Political and Social Science* 364 (March 1966): 11; James T. Tedeschi, "Aggression and the Use of Coercive Power," *Journal of Social Issues* 33 (Winter 1977): 114; Walter Bromberg, *The Mold of Murder* (New York: Grune and Stratton, 1961) p. 29.

187. Thelma McCormack, "Machismo in Media Research: A Critical Review of Research on Violence and Pornography," *Social Problems* 25 (June 1978): 545.

188. Toplin, *Unchallenged Violence*, p. 168; James D. Wright and Linda L. Marston, "The Ownership of the Means of Destruction: Weapons in the U.S.," *Social Problems* 23 (October 1974): 101.

189. J. Sherwood Williams and John McGrath, "A Social Profile of Urban Gun Owners," in *Violent Crime*, ed. James A. Lonciardi and Anne E. Pottieger (Beverly Hills, Calif.: Sage Publications, 1978), p. 53.

190. Weimer, "Mother, the Macho, and the State," p. 73.

191. William Webster, *FBI*, pp. 40, 42.

192. Ramsey Clark, *Crime in America* (New York: Simon & Schuster, 1970), p. 104.

193. Marshall Clinard and Daniel Abbot, *Crime in Developing Countries* (New York: J. Wiley & Sons, 1973), p. 164.

194. Richard G. Sipes, "War, Sports, and Aggression: An Empirical Test of Two Rival Theories," *American Anthropologist* 75 (February 1973): 71.

195. John Hepburn, "Subcultures, Violence, and the Subculture of Violence: An Old Rut or a New Road," *Criminology* 9 (May 1971): 93; Howard S. Erlanger, "The Empirical Status of the Subculture of Violence Thesis," *Social Problems* 22 (December 1974): 289.

196. Andrew K. Ruotolo, "Neurotic Pride and Homicide," *American Journal of Psychoanalysis* 35 (Spring 1975): 16.

197. Barry M. Maletzky, "The Episodic Dyscontrol Syndrome," *Diseases of the Nervous System* 34 (March 1973): 179-80.

198. George Bach-Y-Rita, "Episodic Dyscontrol: A Study of 130 Violent Patients," *The American Journal of Psychiatry* 127 (May 1971): 1477.

199. Hunter Gillies, "Homicide in the West of Scotland," *British Journal of Psychology* 28 (February 1976): 116.

200. David G. Perry and Louise C. Perry, "Denial of Suffering in the Victim as a Stimulant to Violence in Aggresive Boys," *Child Development* 45 (March 1974): 55, 60.

201. Stuart P. Taylor and Ian Smith, "Aggression as a Function of Sex of Victim and Males' Attitude Toward Female," *Psychological Reports* 35 (December 1974): 1096-97.

202. David M. Young et al., "Is Chivalry Dead?" *Journal of Communications* 25 (Winter 1975): 63.

203. Steven Heyman, "Dogmatism, Hostility, Aggression, and Gender Roles," *Journal of Clinical Psychology* 33 (July 1977): 695.

204. Ten Houten, "Black Family," p. 160.

205. Robert Gordon et al., "Values and Gang Delinquency: A Study of Street Corner Groups," *American Journal of Sociology* 69 (September 1963): 123.

206. Michele Wallace, *Black Macho and the Myth of the Superwoman* (New York: Dial Press, 1978), pp. 13-29, 30, 36, 116, 161.

207. Lynn A. Curtis, *Violence, Race, and Culture* (Lexington, Mass.: D.C. Heath & Co., 1975), pp. 12, 23-24, 29-30, 50-52.

208. Julia Landon, "Images of Violence Against Women," *Victimology* 2 (1977-78): 510; J. J. Gayford, "Sex Magazines," *Medicine, Science, and the Law* 18 (January 1978): 48.

209. Stark and McEvoy, "Middle Class Violence," *Psychology Today* 4 (November 1970): p. 110.

210. Maxine Lercher, "Black Women and Homicide," *Lethal Aspects of Urban Violence*, ed. Harold M. Rose (Lexington, Mass.: Lexington Books, 1979), p. 84; Straus, Gelles, and Steinmetz, *Behind Closed Doors*, p. 204.

211. Peter Loizos, in Martin, *Violence and the Family*, 184.

212. Dobash and Dobash, *Violence Against Wives*, p. 9.

213. Steinmetz and Straus, *Violence in the Family*, p. 7.

214. Gayford, "Aetiology of Assaults," p. 20.

215. Carroll, "The Intergenerational Transmission of Family Violence," p. 299.

216. Dobash and Dobash, *Violence Against Wives*, p. 22.

217. George Garbner and Larry Gross, "Living with Television: The Violence Profile," *Journal of Communications* 26 (Spring 1976): 189, 190.

218. Renate L. Welch et al., "Subtle Sex-Role Cues in Children's Commercials," *Journal of Communications* 29 (Summer 1979): 207.

219. Annette Rickel and Linda Grant, "Sex Role Stereotypes in the Mass Media and Schools: Five Consistent Themes," *International Journal of Women's Studies* 2 (4 March 1979): 164-79.

220. William Goode, "Force and Violence in the Family," *Journal of Marriage and the Family* 33 (November 1971): 624.

221. Gelles, *Violent Home*, p. 74.

222. Goode, "Force and Violence in the Family," p. 635.

223. Anthony Storr, Introduction, in Eekelaar and Katz, *Family Violence*, pp. 2-8, 7.

224. Karl Bednarik, *The Male in Crisis* (New York: Alfred A. Knopf, 1970), pp. 10, 22, 24, 29.

225. Tolson, *Limits of Masculinity*, pp. 28, 30.

226. Ibid, p. 70; Mirra Komavovsky, *Blue Collar Marriage* (New York: Vintage Books, 1964), p. 235.

227. Mary Hanemann Lystaad, "Violence at Home," *American Journal of Orthopsychiatry* 45 (April 1975): 339.

228. Walker, *Battered Woman*, p. 10.

229. Davidson, *Conjugal Crime*, p. 3.

230. Martin, *Battered Wives*, p. 122.

231. Walker, *Battered Woman*, p. 14; Dobash and Dobash, *Violence Against Wives*, p. 98.

232. Walker, *Battered Woman*, pp. 14, 61.

233. Hilberman and Munson, "Sixty Battered Women," pp. 461-62.

234. Gelles, *Violent Home*, p. 140.

235. Dobash and Dobash, *Violence Against Wives*, pp. 81, 84-85, 87, 94, 98.

236. Ibid., pp. 90, 91.

237. Martin Symonds, "The Psychodynamics of Violence-Prone Marriages," *American Journal of Psychotherapy* 38 (Fall 1978): p. 219; Gelles, *Violent Home*, p. 186.

238. Goode, "Force and Violence in the Family," p. 628.

239. Whitehurst, "Violence Potential," p. 78.

240. Stark et al., "Medicine and Patriarchal Violence," p. 481.

Abuse of Female Partners

241. *Webster's Third New International Dictionary*, s.v. "jealous."
242. Gayford, "Aetiology of Assaults," p. 22.
243. Walker, *Battered Woman*, p. 114.
244. Whitehurst, "Violence Potential," p. 77.
245. Sydney Brandon, "Physical Violence in the Family: An Overview," in Borland, *Violence in the Family*, pp. 1-24, 2. See also Davidson, "Wifebeating," p. 31.
246. Renvoize, *Web of Violence*, p. 34.
247. Walker, *Battered Woman*, pp. 33-34.
248. Prescott and Letko, "Battered Women," p. 74.
249. Rounsaville, "Theories in Marital Violence," p. 21.
250. Dobash and Dobash, *Violence Against Wives*, p. 91.
251. Walker, *Battered Woman*.
252. Martin, *Battered Wives*, p. 67.
253. Prescott and Letko, p. 81; Roy, p. 28; Diana Russell, *Rape in Marriage* (New York: MacMillan, 1982); D. Finkelhor and K. Yilo, "Forced Sex in Marriage: A Preliminary Research Report," *Crime and Delinquency* 34 (1982), 459-478.
254. Stark, Flitcraft and Frazier, "Medicine and Patriarchal Violence," p. 467.
255. Walker, *Battered Woman*, pp. 105, 108, 118, 126.
256. Renvoize, *Web of Violence*, p. 48.
257. A. Symonds, "Violence Against Women," pp. 165, 170.
258. Dobash and Dobash, *Violence Against Wives*, p. 173.
259. Prescott and Letko, "Battered Women," p. 88.
260. Dobash and Dobash, *Violence Against Wives*, pp. 168, 200
261. Walker, *Battered Woman*, p. 24.
262. Dobash and Dobash, *Violence Against Wives*, p. 145; Straus, "Sexual Inequality," p. 64.
263. Barry Kutum, "Legislative Needs and Solutions," in Roy, *Battered Women*, p. 279.
264. Sarah McCabe, "A Note on the Reports of the Select Committees on Violence in Marriage and Violence in the Family," *British Journal of Criminology* 17 (July 1977): 283.
265. Roy, "A Research Project," p. 32.
266. Gayford, "Aetiology of Assaults," p. 243.
267. Dobash and Dobash, *Violence Against Wives*, p. 159.
268. Martin Symonds, "Victims of Violence: Psychological Effects and After-Effects," *American Journal of Psychoanalysis* 35 (1975): 19, 20-22; William Ryan, *Blaming the Victim* (New York: Vintage Books, 1971).
269. Walker, *Battered Woman*, p. 31.
270. Ibid., pp. 15, 31.
271. Steven Maier and Martin Seligman, "Learned Helplessness: Theory and Evidence," *Journal of Experimental Psychology* 105 (March 1976): 4, 7.
272. Walker, *Battered Woman*, p. 47.
273. Rounsaville, "Theories in Marital Violence," pp. 18-19.
274. Walker, *Battered Woman*.
275. Drake, "Battered Women," p. 44.
276. Dobash and Dobash, *Violence Against Wives*, p. 117.

277. Rounsaville, "Theories in Marital Violence," p. 16.
278. Walker, *Battered Woman*, p. 31.
279. Dobash and Dobash, *Violence Against Wives*, p. 125.
280. Hilberman and Munson, "Sixty Battered Women," p. 464.
281. Alexandra Symonds, pp. 167-69.
282. Hilberman and Munson, "Sixty Battered Women," p. 464; Dobash and Dobash, *Violence Against Wives*, p. 109.
283. Gayford, "Wife Battering"; Prescott and Letko, "Battered Women," p. 84.
284. Linda S. Labell, "Wife Abuse: A Sociological Study of Battered Women and Their Mates," *Victimology* 4 (1979): 265.
285. Pagelow, *Woman-Battering*, pp. 16, 112, 133, 139, 140, 163, 177.
286. Marsden, "Sociological Perspectives on Family Violence," p. 117.

Child Abuse

Janice Humphreys

"Thoughtless"

enjoying the lush warmth
looking forward to more
who is this
ripping thoughtlessly
tearing at my sensitive branch?
oh my tree soon to die
hurry patch it
grab a wrap
heal the wound
so my tree
may be precious
thriving and strong

    Elizabeth Roth

Reprinted from *Every Twelve Seconds*, compiled by Susan Venters (Hillsboro, Oregon: Shelter, 1981) by permission of the author.

Child abuse and neglect is a common area of concern for the nurse who cares for families. The problem is exactly that child abuse and neglect is *so* common. The literature of several different professions (nursing, law, medicine, dentistry, social work, etc.) abounds with research reports, opinions, case studies, literature reviews, incidence reports, and theories of child abuse and neglect of varying degrees of scholarliness.[1] The task for the nurse who wishes to keep current in her knowledge and practice in the area of child abuse and neglect is monumental, if not impossible. The purpose of this chapter is to provide an overview of the knowledge and controversies to date on child abuse and neglect. The theoretical foundations of child maltreatment exist in both violence and family literature. The attempt is to update the nurse on the current theoretical understanding of child abuse and neglect, and to provide a basis for development of nursing research and application to practice (see Chapter 10.)

SCOPE

The scope of the problem of child abuse is difficult to ascertain. Few people are happy to admit that they cause physical and/or psychological injury to their children. As a result, most of the available statistics have come from child protective and other agencies. A variety of biases can be attributed to child maltreatment data coming from reporting agencies. These and other difficulties with available and extrapolated incidence statistics will be discussed. Even with the limitations of the available data, some concept of the extent of the problem of child abuse and neglect is still possible and necessary.

The *National Analysis of Official Child Abuse and Neglect Reporting* for 1977 gives the figure of 507,494 cases for the year.[2] The report, however, presents and analyzes only those cases of child maltreatment that are officially reported and are subsequently submitted to the national study.[3] Further, although every state has a law mandating reporting of child abuse and neglect, variation exists from state to state as to what constitutes a "reportable case."[4]

Richard J. Gelles extrapolates that in 1975 of the 46 million children between the ages of three and seventeen years who lived with both parents, 1.0 to 1.9 million experienced physical violence (kicked, bitten, or punched) at the hands of their parents.[5] Gelles's study has particular merit in that unlike the majority of research in the area of violence against children, it involves a "healthy" sample. That is to say, Gelles interviewed and recorded the self-reports of violence from individuals who were not currently being followed by a child protective service agency.[6] The violence committed by parents against their children is also categorized (from "slapped" to "used knife or gun") and reveals a broad range of violent acts, not all generally accepted as child abuse.[7]

Gelles's study has major limitations, however.[8] Only intact families (man and woman living together in a conjugal unit) with one or more children between the ages three to seventeen years were included in the study. If, as will be later discussed, child abuse results in part from family dysfunction, then a sample of intact families may be biased against detection. Moreover, early publications suggested that the younger child and infant are at greatest risk of child abuse and neglect.[9] To limit the sample to families with children three years of age and older does not allow for data collection from the group suggested by some to be likely to experience the problem. Nevertheless, both sample restrictions and the self-report technique are merely likely to result in a low estimate of cases.

In 1974, the Children's Division of the American Humane Society (AHA)[10] documented 35,642 cases of child abuse. The cases identified, however, were only those reported by twenty-nine states to the AHA clearinghouse.

Ray E. Helfer and C. Henry Kempe estimate that 1 percent of American children are reported to be abused or neglected each year.[11] They, however, offer no basis for their estimate and acknowledge that the actual incidence of child abuse and neglect is probably much greater.

As previously identified, children under the age of five years are often reported to be the group most likely to experience child abuse and neglect. The data from the 1977 national study indicate approximately equal occurrences of abuse and neglect across all age groups.[12] Young children, according to the report, were no more likely to be abused or neglected than an older child. Several studies have identified, however, that when abused, young children were significantly more likely to be severely injured.[13] Of particular note is the approximately equal percentage of adolescents who experienced abuse and neglect. Although female adolescents were more likely than males to be abused and neglected, the percentage of cases was significant for both sexes.[14] In a separate study by Robert W. Blum and Carol Runyan, female adolescents were significantly more likely to be maltreated and experience sexual abuse.[15] The data would tend to refute the common opinion that abuse and neglect occur only to the young child.[16]

Child abuse has until recently been identified in the literature as a problem that occurred in all socioeconomic levels and therefore was estimated to occur at similar rates at every stratum.[17] Typically, child abuse and neglect have been identified as occurring more often in poor families, but only secondary to reporting source bias and the increased opportunity for "outsider" investigation uniquely associated with poverty. That is to say that in reporting the higher incidence of child abuse and neglect in poor families, researchers frequently included a disclaimer to the effect that poor people were more often involved with public agencies, used the emergency room and public clinics for health care, and were thereby more subject to professional investigation. During assessment by the professional, the poor family was also more likely to be labeled as child abusive than the middle- or upper-class family. Middle- and upper-class families have been thought to be less frequently reported as committing child abuse and neglect as the result of their use of private physicians who in turn hesitated labeling a family peer or acquaintance. Middle- or upper-class families also had the financial resources to go outside their immediate area for health care and assistance, thereby further decreasing their likelihood of identification as child abusers.

Leroy H. Pelton presents a persuasive argument as to why child abuse and neglect is not "classless."[18] In light of Pelton and other evidence, child abuse and neglect must be considered to be a problem with increased incidence in the poor.[19] The main points put forth by Pelton are outlined in the section that follows.

Families receiving general assistance have been consistently reported as experiencing more child abuse and neglect than those not.[20] In particular, some studies reported that the very poor had an even higher incidence of child abuse and neglect than those still at the poverty level but with more income: as poverty increased so did child abuse and neglect.[21]

As child abuse and neglect reporting laws have come into existence and public awareness has grown, the incidence of reported child abuse and neglect has also increased. It would be expected that not just the public agency professional but every concerned citizen would be more likely to report child abuse and neglect and thereby increase the percentage of non-poor reported cases. The socioeconomic data over time, however, have remained relatively unchanged.[22] The poor continue to be overrepresented in child abuse and neglect statistics. In the cases of child abuse and neglect that resulted in death, a difficult fact to hide at any socioeconomic level, the poor continue to contribute an unequal number of cases.[23]

According to Pelton, the reason for the persistence of the "myth of classlessness" lies with the individuals who are supposedly working for the public good, health professionals who practice in the context of a medical model, and politicians.[24] Failure to associate child abuse and neglect with being poor, according to Pelton, increases the likelihood of monies available to "search out the real cause" and avoids the identification of the problem with something unlikely to get many votes, poverty.[25]

Concerned health professionals may have some difficulty in accepting Pelton's treatise. A great many labels already are attached to people at the bottom of the socioeconomic stratum. Acknowledging the high incidence of child abuse and neglect among the poor at first looks like just another label to keep "the poor in their place." On the other hand, if poverty is viewed as a large contributor to the stress experienced (see Theoretical Frameworks) by the child abuse and neglect family, the high incidence can be understood and no "blame" attached. In two recent studies examining child health and social status, the number and degree of severity of specific health problems (other than abuse) was also significantly associated with poverty.[26] If poverty is a major factor inhibiting the ability of individuals to achieve and maintain life, health, and well-being, failure to acknowledge its role will prevent the identification of truly helpful interventions.[27]

Women more often than men are reported to have abused or neglected their children.[28] The higher incidence of child abuse and neglect committed by women is usually explained by acknowledging that mothers spend more time with their children than do fathers. If denying that poor people are more likely to abuse or neglect their children is a disservice, then attributing the higher rate of child abuse to the propinquity of women is an equal injustice.

In almost 34 percent of the reported cases of child abuse and neglect in 1977 the mother or a mother substitute was the only adult in the home.[29] The women in these homes probably had to spend a preponderance of their *time* with their children because they had total *responsibility* for those children. In two-parent homes, women are generally still the primary caretakers of children, a task that involves more than just minutes and hours.

Women who work in the United States earn significantly less income on the average than men. The woman who works all day at a job must go home and likely work some more as a parent. For the woman to work at all she must, additionally and with sufficient advanced planning, find an adequate baby-sitter, daycare center, or other source of childcare.

For the single female parent this again adds the stress of being able to afford the price of childcare. When she finally returns home she may or may not receive assistance in childcare from a spouse. It is interesting to note that Marc F. Maden and David F. Wrench in a review of the literature, found that if the father is unemployed he is as likely as the mother to abuse their children.[30] David G. Gil reports that when the data are adjusted to allow for homes where no father or father substitute is present, mothers actually perpetrated child abuse only one-third of the time. Fathers or father substitutes committed the majority of child abuse.[31]

Adolescent mothers are also often reported to be more likely to abuse or neglect their children. More recently the relationship between adolescent mothers and child abuse and neglect has been called into question.[32] It is, however, true that many adolescent mothers are also poor; one study found that families who had experienced an adolescent birth to be existing on a mean annual income of $6,608.

The plight of the woman who abuses or neglects her child is difficult. She is likely the primary caretaker, young, and probably poor. Poverty and its stresses are multiplied in the case of women.

DEFINITION OF CHILD ABUSE AND NEGLECT

Another factor that contributes to confusion and inconsistent statistics is the difficulty in defining child abuse and neglect. The spectrum of maltreatment of children is broad and often defined by time, perpetrator, situation, professional conducting the study, and the law (see Chapter 15).

The most severe form of child abuse was most notably identified by C. Henry Kempe et al. in 1961 and labeled "the battered child syndrome."[33] The purpose of coining the phrase "battered child syndrome" was to increase the public awareness of the maltreatment of children and to spur them to action.[34] Kempe et. al were certainly effective as will be discussed in the next section.

Limitations to the phrase, "battered child" include the fact that many consider only the severely physically assaulted child to have experienced abuse.[35] Helfer and

Kempe have recently even altered their definition, asserting that "the battered child is any child who received nonaccidental physical injury (or injuries) as a result of acts (or omissions) on the part of his parents or guardians."[36]

Eli H. Newberger and Richard Bourne assert that for professionals to view child abuse as only physical battering is a disservice to the children they set out to assist. By identifying severe physical abuse from the medical perspective, many of the maltreated children do not receive the multifaceted care they need.[37] Theories of causation and interventions are also based on a limited and medical model. The reality is that the severely battered, tortured child is at the extreme end of the spectrum.[38] Unfortunately, it is often only when the discovery of such profoundly abused children is reported in the media that some people give thought to the general maltreatment of children.

Richard J. Gelles and Murray A. Straus in their investigations do not even use the phrase "child abuse." Rather, they define violence as "an act carried out with the intention or perceived intention of physically hurting another person."[39] Their reasoning in using this broad definition was to include in their study those acts such as slapping or spanking that many people might consider to be appropriate as discipline. If such acts were to be carried out against someone not in the family they would be considered assaultive.[40] Further, their concern was also primarily the act of violence and not the outcome which can vary. Such a broad definition of maltreatment is useful if the researchers, Gelles and Straus, are interested in the tendency of violence to escalate within the family. Although broad in its definition of violence, Gelles and Straus's definition completely overlooks nonviolent neglect of children. Therefore, the usefulness of such a definition on a day-to-day basis for the practitioner is limited.

To look at all acts of violence against children and consider them in some manner equally damaging is an attitude that is not generally accepted or practical. What then is meant by child abuse? The state of Michigan defines child abuse as "harm or threatened harm to a child's health or welfare by a person responsible for the child's health or welfare which occurs through nonaccidental physical or mental injury, sexual abuse, or maltreatment."[41] In Michigan, and many other states, child abuse means actual physical violence against a child or the threat of such an act. The child need not experience physical injury to be considered abused. In addition, the injury to the child need not be physical; it can be mental or emotional. Here the problem of defining just what is mental or emotional abuse becomes evident. Certainly a child who is locked up and physically isolated from all human contact for years has experienced great psychological harm. However, the child who is repeatedly told she is "bad" or "no good" is more difficult to label. Lack of praise, and constant criticism can likely result in low self-esteem in the developing child. Is the responsible adult guilty of mental abuse? It is difficult to determine.

Equally difficult to define is child neglect. To use the Child Protection Law in Michigan as an example, "child neglect" means "harm to a child's health or welfare by a person responsible for the child's health or welfare which occurs through negligent treatment, including the failure to provide adequate clothing, shelter, or medical care."[42] The child who is obviously abandoned by its parents is undoubtedly neglected. The child, however, who has not received quite enough food to satisfy its hunger may not be considered neglected. If, in addition, the reason for the lack of food is the extreme poverty of the family, who is at fault? Must the parent of a child provide adequate shelter, food, clothing at any cost? The problem is difficult.

The few examples presented should not be construed as being typical. Child abuse and neglect are on a continuum from the extreme to the mild and every degree in between. Child maltreatment exists, is well documented, and unfortunately professionals spend much of their time trying to decide what it is and is not. As Gil states, "The inability to reach closure on the issue of defining abuse (particularly moving beyond the restricted phenomenon of physical injury to include 'emotional' abuse and other operationally ambiguous concepts) reveals the lack of coherent pro-child ideology among Americans."[43] Further hesitancy about a commitment to one definition of child abuse and neglect may be due to deeper insecurities.[44] "The broader the definition of abuse, the more clear is its relation to 'normal' caregivers and their behavior with children, and the more serious the 'indictment' against society and its institutions."[45]

For the purpose of this and subsequent chapters by this author the definitions of child abuse and neglect quoted from the State of Michigan Child Protection Law will be adopted. Further, it is the author's opinion that harm to a child can begin at the moment of birth if less than an ideal environment (love, stimulation, nutrition, shelter, etc.) is not provided to the developing human being. The purpose in such a broad interpretation of child abuse and neglect is not to indict every adult who has ever had responsibility for a child. Rather, the desire is to acknowledge the right of every human being (child and adult) to life, health, and well-being and to provide a basis for professional nursing care.

HISTORICAL BACKGROUND ON THE MALTREATMENT OF CHILDREN

Children have been mistreated by adults historically, for a variety of reasons. Sacrifice of children to please the God of their parents was a common practice among certain ancient cultures.[46] Children who were born with a birth defect were killed to protect the parents as it was thought that the child surely had been affected by some demon to have acquired such an anomaly.[47] Children who experienced seizures, were mentally retarded, or mentally ill were also often thought to be possessed or in some form controlled by evil.[48] These children were most likely exposed to all kinds of torture under the guise of "ridding their bodies of demons."

More contemporary is the notion that physical abuse of children is important in the education process. The idea of "beating some sense into him" was considered necessary to insure that the child learned the lesson. Recently even the Supreme Court (*Ingram v. Wright*) ruled that schools had the right to corporally punish disobedient students.[49] The implication is that although adult criminals have some safeguards against the administration of cruel and unusual punishment, children's rights are distinctly different.

Treatment of Children in the Middle Ages

In reviewing artwork Philippe Ariès observes "medieval art until the twelfth century did not know childhood or did not attempt to portray it. It is hard to believe that this neglect was due to incompetence or incapacity; it seems more probable that there was no place for childhood in the medieval world."[50] Children were not particularly valued during this time and therefore, their images and activities were not worthy of reproduction in art. Their treatment by adults in daily life reflected the low value placed on childhood.[51]

The rearing of children during the seventeenth century is reported to have routinely included the practice of playing with the child's genitals. The stroking of the genitals and exhibiting them to various family members and neighbors was considered acceptable and necessary for the young child.[52] Circumcision of males was treated as a festival and for religious reasons a joyous occasion. Children during this time were treated, according to Ariès, as if they were incapable of being aware of or affected by sex.[53] Such treatment and low opinion of children implies that until the time of puberty, children are not worthy of the same considerations given to adults.

Childhood during the seventeenth century was virtually not acknowledged. Instead, "the idea of childhood was bound up with the idea of dependence."[54] Terms like "boy" and "lad" were used to describe even adults who were not independent, and therefore not really "men." Further, adolescence was not recognized as being any different from the rest of childhood. Until the individual was able to independently function and literally protect themself, he or she was not accorded equal treatment and certainly not protected by adults. When childhood finally began to be accepted as a time of life different from adulthood it was to no advantage to children. "The concept of the separate nature of childhood, of its difference from the world of adults, began with the elementary concept of its weakness, which brought it down to the level of the lowest social strata."[55] Elements of the continued low value placed upon childhood in the past can still be seen.

Child Labor

According to the 1879 census, approximately one in eight children between ten and fifteen years of age was employed in the United States. By 1900, one in six children was employed, 60 percent in agriculture and 40 percent in industry. Over one-half of the children employed were of immigrant families.[56] The growing number of children who were sent to work resulted from the rapid industrialization America experienced after the Civil War. More than one-half of the child labor force was between ten and thirteen years of age; many were under age ten.[57] Although the majority of children were employed in agriculture it was the general understanding of most Americans that child labor was a problem predominately of urban industry.

The work done by children was as difficult if not more difficult than that done by adults. Al Priddy describes part of his job in a mill at approximately thirteen years of age.

> The mule-room atmosphere was kept at from eighty-five to ninety degrees of heat. The hardwood floor burned my bare feet. I had to gasp quick, short gasps to get air into my lungs at all. My face seemed swathed in continual fire. The tobacco chewers expectorated on the floor, and left little pools for me to wade through. Oil and hot grease dripped down behind the mules, sometimes falling on my scalp or making yellow splotches on my overalls or feet. . . . To open a window was a great crime, as the cotton fiber was so sensitive to wind that it would spoil. (Poor cotton fiber!)[58]

The pay was also much less for the work done by children. The younger siblings of the paid, employed child might be found "helping their brothers and sisters," an explanation that provided numerous unpaid assistants.[59]

From the 1880s to the depression of the 1930s efforts to curb child labor held the attention of the American public. By 1899, twenty-eight states had passed some legislation regulating child labor; however, most legislation applied only to manufacturing and set the age limit to twelve years.[60] The majority of children, those older than twelve years working in agriculture, remained unaffected by legislation.

Efforts continued until by the twentieth century opposition to child labor became an organized crusade. In 1904 the National Child Labor Committee was formed by several prominent people in the reform movement. The committee was successful to the extent that "by 1914 35 states had a fourteen-year age limit and an eight hour day for workers under sixteen; 34 states prohibited night work under age sixteen, and 36 states had appointed factory inspectors to enforce the laws."[61] The attempt to pass a constitutional amendment was unsuccessful. However, in 1916 the Keating-Owen Act was passed and established federal law prohibiting child labor in manufacturing for children under the age of sixteen.[62]

The difficulties faced by child advocates who attempted to stop child labor are somewhat reminiscent of more recent efforts to improve the plight of children and families. According to Robert H. Bremner,

> One of the major difficulties of child labor reform in the early twentieth century was the cultural and economic gap between middle class reformers, who in their zeal to refute the stereotype of the poor widow dependent on her little boy's earnings, may have underestimated the economic necessity of child labor among large segments of the working class. . . The attack on child labor was one of the converging lines of reform which, even before the Great Depression, led to realization that solving problems of childhood required *comprehensive efforts to promote economic security for families* (my emphasis).[63]

(For a detailed outlining of childhood in America from 1600 to 1932 the reader is referred to the extensive two-volume work edited by Robert H. Bremner.)

CULTURE AND CHILD MALTREATMENT

Culturally justified mutilation is another example of the pain and injury done to children by adults. As recently as 1940, female infants of high-ranking Chinese families were routinely inflicted with binding of the feet. The goal was to keep the feet compressed, small, and "dainty." The result was deformed, barely useful feet that were painful and greatly restricted the movement of the adult woman.[64] Jill Korbin describes the case of an African woman of the Yoruba tribe who slashed the faces of her two sons and rubbed charcoal into the wounds. This mutilating act was considered child abuse in 1974 London although it is traditionally practiced in some rural areas of Nigeria.[65] Samoan childrearing practices include a number of actions that may seem questionable to Americans: "children do not sit in a house until the adults are seated; do not speak to adults unless given permission; and eat only after the adults, particularly the male adults, have had first choice of the food available."[66] Within their own cultures each of these behaviors is deemed appropriate, even necessary.

Certainly culture has a tremendous impact upon childrearing practices and the value placed upon children. However, lest the impression be given that only "uncivilized" cultures inflict pain on their offspring, keep in mind some common, generally accepted contemporary American practices. Newborn males are often routinely circumcised without anesthesia before discharge from the hospital. The value of this procedure has recently been questioned.[67] Other routine, painful procedures administered to children are ear piercing and orthodontic bands on the teeth. The point to be made here is not whether such cosmetic procedures should be discontinued, but rather that they are culturally dictated, and continue to be painfully administered to children by adults who supposedly love them—their parents. Certainly childrearing practices and the value placed on childhood are culturally defined phenomenons. Culturally appropriate definitions of child abuse and neglect are necessary within the guidelines of the best interests of the child. For a thorough discussion of these issues, the reader is referred to anthropological texts on the topic.[68]

CHILD PROTECTION IN THE UNITED STATES

The origin in the United States of societies concerned about the pathetic lot of many children begins with the historic case in April 1874 of Mary Ellen Wilson. Briefly, organized efforts for the protection of children developed as an outgrowth of humane work for animals. Mary Ellen, age eight years, was taken away from her adoptive parents who routinely beat, starved, imprisoned, and kept her in rags. Neighbors were up in arms over the child's mistreatment and feared the family would move away before action could be taken on Mary Ellen's behalf. None of the several institutions contacted by concerned neighbors would take Mary Ellen from the abusive home. As a last resort the Society for the Prevention of Cruelty to Animals (SPCA) was contacted. Henry Bergh, founder and president of the SPCA, acknowledged that "though the case was not within the scope of the special act to prevent cruelty to animals, [it was] recognized as being clearly within the general laws of humanity. . . ."[69] Mary Ellen was removed from her adoptive parents. Subsequently, in December 1874 the New York Society for the Prevention of Cruelty to Children (NYSPCC) was organized.

From the NYSPCC grew many organizations in other cities. Initially SPCC actions were policelike; the representatives wore "badges and were duly constituted officers of the law."[70] Originally, the SPCC supported institutional care for abused and neglected children. After the turn of the century, however, the goal of cruelty and humane societies was aimed more toward case finding and rehabilitation of parents and the return of the child to the home.[71] In 1882, Massachusetts enacted a "neglect law," no longer limiting the community's concern to the severely physically abused child.[72]

Studies concerned with the plight of the physically abused child reached the professional literature in 1946 when Dr. John Caffey identified curious X-rays of certain children.[73] The article was entitled "Multiple Fractures in the Long Bones of Infants Suffering from Chronic Subdural Hematoma" and gives no evidence as to possible causes of the multiple injuries.

In 1962, C. Henry Kempe, a physician, is given credit for having introduced the "Battered Child Syndrome"[74] to the American Academy of Pediatrics. Many attribute Kempe's "call to arms" with having brought about the passage of laws in all fifty states within a four-year period mandating identification and reporting of suspected victims of abuse.[75] The Child Abuse and Treatment Act of 1974 (PL–93–237) went even farther and called for a full and complete study on the incidence of child abuse and neglect. Some results of the national study and problems associated with its findings have already been reported in the section in this chapter headed "Scope."

Public Concern in the Seventies

Social scientists explain the increased concern about violence committed by parents against children in the 1970s differently. According to Straus, the public's concern about violence in general was the result of three cultural and social forces.[76] First, the public and social scientists were exposed daily to the violence of Southeast Asia, assassinations, civil disturbances, and increasing homicide rates. Second, the women's movement increased the public's awareness of violence against women and children. Third, social scientists were moving toward the conflict or social action model to examine phenomenon. The result of the combination of these forces was said to be the identification, examination, and systematic study of violence in families. The consciousness of professionals and the public alike were raised and brought to action.

THEORETICAL FRAMEWORKS

Mental Illness Model

The mental illness model or psychiatric approach was probably the first contemporary theory used to deal with parents who abused their children. In reviewing the literature, many examples of its continued use are still evident.[77]

Essentially the mental illness model theorizes that parents who abuse their children are mentally ill. The adult who inflicts bodily harm on his or her child is a psychologically "sick" person. No other factor is considered to contribute to the occurrence of child abuse and neglect, and the obvious goal of treatment is to "cure." The implication in the mental illness model is that the fault for the abuse inflicted upon the child rests in a personality flaw in the individual adult. In turn, the prospect for overcoming this weakness in the parent rests within the parent. The professional, most likely a psychiatrist or psychologist, is merely assisting the parent in his or her treatment. To some extent, organizations like Parents Anonymous still label abusive parents as "sick" and responsible for their own cure.[78]

With the publication of an increasing number of investigations in the area of child abuse and neglect, the actual incidence of psychosis among abusive parents was found to be quite small, 5 percent.[79] There is little doubt that some mentally ill adults do abuse their children. Evidence of current modes of treatment of mentally ill abusive parents are still found in the literature.[80] However, the majority of abusive parents are not psychotic. To attribute all cases of child abuse and neglect to mental illness will greatly lessen the number of interventions by and the effectiveness of the nurse.

Environmental-Stress Model

The environmental-stress model or sociological approach to the understanding of child abuse and neglect focuses on the high level of violence in the United States. Within the environmental-stress model, only two factors interact, the violent environment and stress.

According to the environmental-stress model, the environment of the abusive parent is generally violent and approves of the use of physical violence against children under certain circumstances. (See Chapter 2 for a discussion of aggression in America.) A particularly unruly child or a child who has committed an act of great danger to himself may appropriately be physically punished. Murray Straus, Richard Gelles, and Suzanne Steinmetz report that 70 percent of the Americans in their study viewed spanking and slapping a twelve-year-old as necessary, normal, and good.[81] The environment accepts that parents must at times use physical punishment for the child's own good.

Stress, as the other necessary factor for child abuse, may be chronic or acute. The parent may experience a limitless number and/or variety of stresses. The child may or may not contribute to these stresses on the parent.[82] In any case, the stress experienced by the parent reaches a point of unmanageability. The parent can no longer control himself or herself and in an environment that at times approves of violence against children under certain circumstances, the desperate parent relieves the stress by physically abusing his or her child.[83] There is some evidence to suggest that an interaction exists between stress and environmental violence. Rand D. Conger, Robert L. Burgess and Carol Barrett in their investigation found that abusive parents were far more likely than controls to experience both rapid life change and a history of punitive childrearing. The data suggest that it is primarily when parents are subject to rapid life changes that a punitive childhood history correlates with abusive or neglectful behavior in adulthood.[84]

The environmental-stress model does not approve of child abuse nor does the culture in which it occurs. Rather, the approved level of violence and aggression in the culture on a day-to-day basis is so great as to imply that violence is an acceptable means of problem solving. Child abuse or the physical harming of a child for no good reason is not socially acceptable. Instead, according to the environmental-stress model, it is postulated to be inevitable when stress becomes too great. Kevin J. Gully, Harold A. Dengerink, Mary Pepping, and Douglas Bergstrom in a study of the recollections of familial violence from 216 subjects (none known abusers), identify that even a sibling's vicarious experiencing of violence can result in an individual who considers physical violence against children as acceptable under certain circumstances.[85]

The environmental-stress model does gain support when American violence and child abuse statistics are compared with less violent societies. The incidence of child abuse in Japan, for example, is much less than in the United States.[86] If poverty is considered as a source of a great many stressors then according to the environmental-stress model, it would be expected that the poor would experience a higher incidence of child abuse. Statistics reported earlier in this chapter support the greater number of cases of reported child abuse at the poverty level.

Problems exist with the environmental-stress model's explanation of the dynamics of child abuse. Being poor exposes parents to a large number of varied stressors over long periods of time and yet the majority of poor people do not abuse their children. Many parents who were abused or neglected as children maltreat their own offspring. However, many abused parents do not use violence against their children.[87] There is no doubt that violence and aggression are daily demonstrated in the media as methods of dealing with stress and/or problem solving. Nevertheless, many American parents never use aggression or violence of any kind in dealing with their children. Jay Belsky suggests that tolerance for stress and the ability of a family to call upon resources allow nonabusive/neglectful families to function without maltreatment of children.[88] The environmental-stress model does not consider the role of family functioning or stress tolerance in its framework.

The environmental-stress model cannot explain the nonabusive or the non-neglectful parent. The factors it identifies, environment and stress, are of major concern and are seen in other models. To restrict the explanation of the cause of child abuse to two factors is simplistic and limited in its usefulness.

Social–Psychological Models

The Helfer and Kempe theoretical framework of child abuse and neglect is probably among the best known.[89] They have combined both social and psychological variables in explaining why child abuse and neglect occur.

In order for a parent to abuse a child Helfer and Kempe hypothesize that three factors must be present:

1. a special parent
2. a special child
3. stress[90]

A special parent is an adult with any number of characteristics that predispose him or her to abuse.[91] The adult may be immature, inexperienced, lack self-esteem, have unrealistic expectations of the child, and so forth. Studies of abusive parents have identified that they frequently have such characteristics. (See Patterns of Behavior.)

The special child may be perceived as special by the parent, or the child may actually be "special."[92] "Special children" may be handicapped,[93] small at birth,[94] chronically ill,[95] or may in some other way require unique parent skills. For example, some authors have noted that abused children are described as more difficult to care for[96] and more demanding or aggressive than other children.[97] It is also suggested by others that delayed mother-child contact after birth, after premature delivery, or unplanned pregnancy may cause problems in the formation of a bond between mother and child and thereby make the child "special" in either parent's mind.[98] Children perceived to be special are equally easy for the nurse to identify; she need only listen to the parent who will frequently make statements like "he's not like the rest of my kids," "she's always been different," and so forth.

The stress, identified by Helfer and Kempe, may be acute or chronic.[99] Stress is as it is perceived by the parent. The necessary amount, kind, and timing of the necessary stress varies in the individual. An intermingling can occur between the three factors. For example, an adolescent parent may abuse her premature six-month-old who will not stop crying in the middle of the night so the mother can go to sleep. It is easy in the example to identify several sources of stress (parenthood, adolescence, prematurity, lack of sleep, crying, etc.).

Helfer and Kempe do acknowledge the role of more than one variable in the occurrence of child abuse and neglect. Both the parent and the child contribute to child abuse and neglect however unwittingly. They do not, however, consider the influence of culture on child abuse and neglect. A. H. Green added a fourth factor necessary for child abuse and neglect, cultural tolerance for familial use of corporal punishment.[100]

Social Learning Model

The social learning model attempts to explain child abuse based upon the same principles previously used to describe aggression (see Chapter 2). Briefly restated, the social learning model hypothesizes that aggression is learned behavior. Learning may occur through observation or direct experience with violent or aggressive behavior. Among the best known work applying the social learning model to child abuse and neglect is that done by Straus, Gelles, and Steinmetz. Their investigations will be used to describe child abuse in terms of the social learning model. Straus, Gelles, and Steinmetz do not mention child neglect; rather, their interest is in aggression, both physical and verbal.

Straus, Gelles, and Steinmetz in 1976 conducted a study to attempt to identify the extent and dynamics of violence in the American home.[101] A nationwide sample of 1,146 adults from families with children between the ages of three and seventeen years living at home was selected. The adults were interviewed and given the "Conflict Tactics Scale."[102] Although the study has a number of weaknesses, the results are still useful in explaining child abuse in terms of social learning.

If aggressive behavior is learned, as the social learning model describes, then the use of violence against one's offspring was most likely taught through the generations. Violent parents likely experienced violence from their own parents. The data from the Straus, Gelles, and Steinmetz study supports the notion of transmission of violence through the family generations from parent to child.[103] *"Each generation learns to be violent by being a participant in a violent family.*"[104] Violence against children can be taught either through direct experience or by observation.[105] The more violent the grandparents, the more violent the parents. The more violent the parents, the more violent the siblings to each other. The investigators identify that a childhood in a violent home is particularly instructive. "Over one out of every four parents who grew up in a violent household were violent enough to risk seriously injuring a child."[106]

Violent and aggressive behavior is learned primarily, but not totally, from one's family. The social learning model also acknowledges the societal role in teaching and condoning violence.[107] The fact that violence is glorified in the media, observed on the street, and acceptable in the schools is evidence of the cultural tolerance for violence that the social learning model identifies as contributing to ongoing violence.

A major weakness of the social learning model is its inability to explain why some abused parents do not abuse their children.[108] Do some parents "unlearn" the use of violence against their children? This question remains unanswered.

The social learning model of child abuse has received a great deal of attention primarily due to the productivity of several of its proponents.[109] Much of the available data on child abuse supports the social learning model. However, more and better-designed studies are still needed.

Human Ecological Model

In 1977 James Garbarino presented a human ecological model to explain child abuse and neglect.[110] The model is based upon the general ecological model of human development,[111] is complex, and incorporates the major components deemed by many to be involved in child abuse and neglect: culture, family, parent, child, and, stress.[112] Garbarino uses the human ecological model to explain physical abuse of children "as part of a larger problem of maltreatment which includes neglect, sexual abuse, and a variety of unhealthy patterns of parent-child relations."[113] Belsky goes further to suggest that "since the parent-child system (the crucible of child maltreatment) is nested within the spousal relationship, what happens between husbands and wives—from an ecological point of view—has implications for what happens between parents and their children."[114] (See Chapter 4.)

Briefly, the human ecological model explains that "abuse is created by a confluence of forces which lead to a pathological adaptation by caregiver and (to a lesser extent) child."[115] In turn, complementary relationships on the part of other family members contribute to the existence of abuse. There are not just two malfunctioning dyads, parent and abused child within the family, but rather multiple interacting systems containing more than two persons.[116] The family then can really be viewed as a system, with patterns and abuse described as system dysfunction.[117]

Garbarino states that patterns of abuse come in two types, the kind perpetrated by pathological adults (small percentage in general but large percent of the lethal abuse),[118] and the kind of abuse that results from the compilation and intensification over time of minor parent-child problems and use of physical punishment.[119] The "healthy" parent may, according to the human ecological model, experience "situationally defined incompetence in the role of the caregiver,"[120] The parent may experience situationally defined low level of caregiver skill and/or the child's demand may not "match."[121] The abusive parent, therefore, is not, in the majority of cases, mentally ill or sick; instead, the parent who maltreats his or her child is experiencing role malfunction.[122]

To assist the adult in the transition to the role of parent, three factors have been identified: rehearsal of the role, clarity of expectations, and minimal normative change.[123] Studies that seek to identify the characteristics of abusive parents frequently identify difficulties in these three areas (see Patterns of Behavior).

Garbarino goes on to use the human ecological model to identify areas of child abuse and neglect in need of scientific research. The model to date remains untested although much evidence from previously conducted research is supportive.[124]

The human ecological model is multifactorial in its explanation of abuse and includes the major concepts generally considered to contribute. Of particular note is Garbarino's inclusion of the abused child and other family members in the explanation of child abuse. The fact that other members of the family may assist in the initiation and/or perpetuation of child maltreatment should not always be taken, though it sometimes is the case, to mean that the nonabuse members knew about the violent acts. The point Garbarino makes, and it is well taken, is that child abuse and neglect occur within a dysfunctional family. The human ecological model is the first of the models presented that considers child abuse and neglect in the larger group, the family.[125]

The major weakness of the human ecological model is that the separation of patterns of abuse into two types, the mentally ill parent and all others, seems a holdover from the psychiatric approach. If, as Garbarino states, maltreatment of children is parent role malfunction why separate out those few parents who are psychotic? Would not the individual parent's qualities and difficulties be identified at the time of assessment by the professional? Each parent is unique and would require individualized interventions whether psychotic or not. To put abusive parents on a continuum from situationally incompetent to the chronically abusive and then to separate out the mentally ill parents seems artificial and weakens the human ecological model.

Nursing Frameworks

All previously described frameworks were developed by non-nurses and although they have been successfully used by nurses as a theoretical basis for practice none was developed with the role of nursing in mind. In 1981, Georgia Kemm Millor, a nurse researcher, described a nursing framework for research in child abuse and neglect.[126] The framework is complex and incorporates the viewpoints of other disciplines (psychology, sociology). It is however, unique in its development by and for nursing. Empirical testing of Millor's framework is currently under way although as yet unreported. The framework is presented to familiarize the reader with the current state of nursing theory on child abuse and neglect.

Millor's framework borrows from the following theories: symbolic interaction, stress, and temperament theory of personality.[127] The interaction of concepts in Millor's framework is depicted in Figure 5-1.

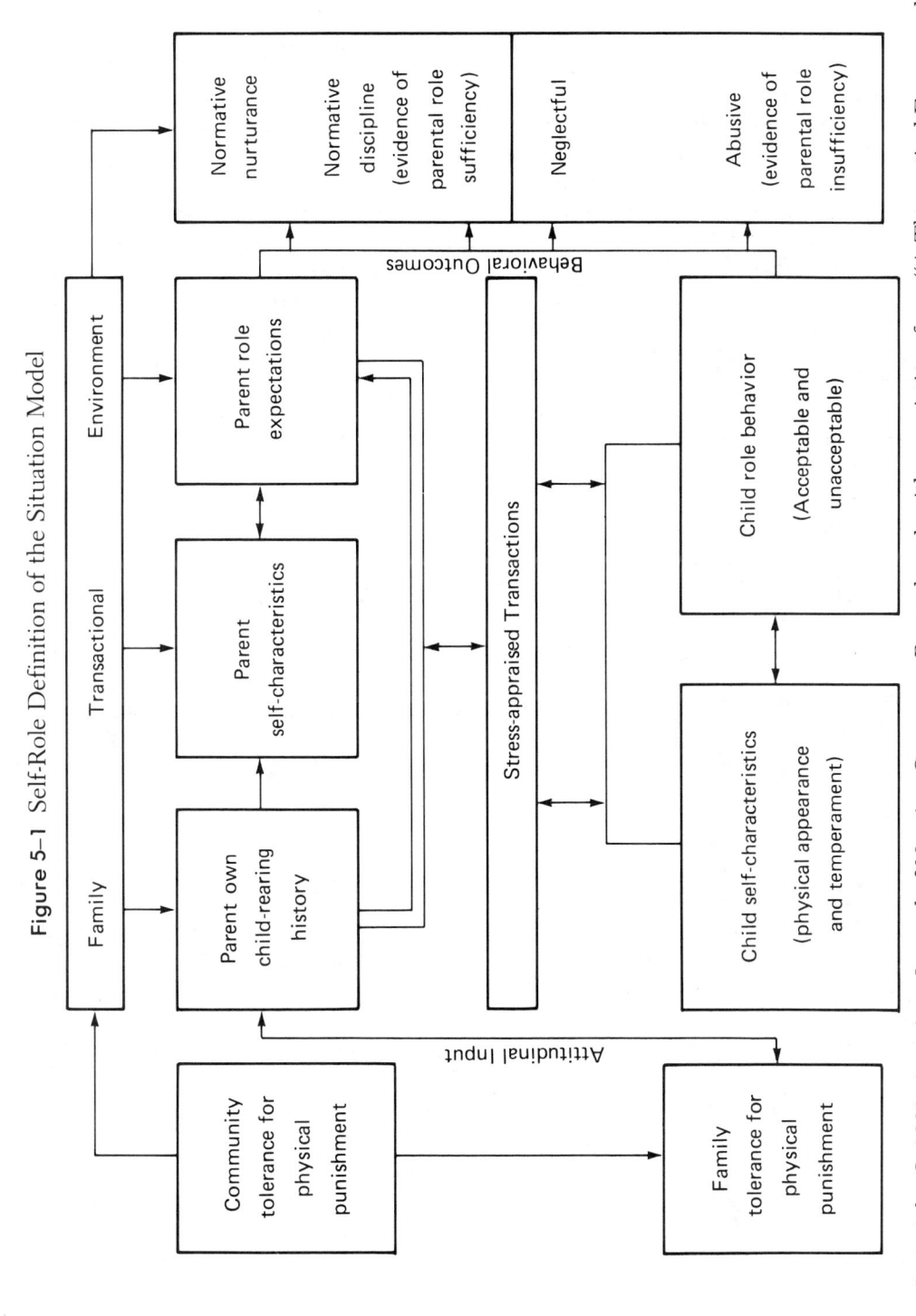

Figure 5–1 Self-Role Definition of the Situation Model

Copyright © 1981, American Journal of Nursing Company. Reproduced, with permission, from "A Theoretical Framework for Nursing Research in Child Abuse and Neglect" by Georgia Kemm Millor, *Nursing Research*, March-April, Vol. 30, no. 2. p. 80.

Millor presents child abuse and neglect as a multifactorial phenomenon within an environment (cultural tolerance for physical punishment) that results in family tolerance for physical punishment and establishes the framework for family transactions.[128] The family tolerance for physical discipline is further the result and is altered by the parent's own childrearing history and attitudes.[129] Parent experiences as a child direct the parent's own characteristics and in turn parent role expectations.[130]

Millor states that the child also plays an important part in child abuse and neglect. That is not to say that certain children "deserve to be beaten," but rather that each child brings to the parent-child interaction certain self-characteristics that interrelate with the child's role behavior (acceptable and unacceptable).[131]

According to Millor, stress is interrelated to both the parent and the child. Parents have long been identified as subject to the effects of stress;[132] Millor asserts that stress has its impact on the child as well.

The behavioral outcome of the complex interaction of culture, family, parent, child, and stress falls on a continuum, normative/nurturance, normative discipline, neglectful, abusive.[133] Millor's framework would seem to describe the interaction between non-abusive/non-neglectful, neglectful and abusive families. The "healthy" family that uses occasional physical discipline of its children need not automatically be labeled "high risk." The professional nurse may, by detailed assessment of all contributing factors of the framework, more clearly understand the strengths and resources of the families.

PATTERNS OF BEHAVIOR

Regardless of the theory or model used to explain child abuse and neglect, certain characteristics have been associated with the parent who abuses and/or neglects his or her child. Much of the research in the area of child abuse and neglect is retrospective, involves no controls, or selects "abusive families" based upon their identification by social agencies. However, parents who abuse, neglect, or occasionally use violence against their children and who are not known by public agencies generally go unexamined.

Parent Characteristics

When reviewing reports of characteristics associated with adults who abuse and/or neglect their children it is important to keep in mind that a parent is only one individual within a larger group, the family, who is experiencing difficulty.

Parent Development

Many researchers suggest that parents who abuse their children have suffered some kind of developmental trauma as children.[134] Alan L. Evans administered an instrument based upon Eriksonian developmental outcomes to twenty child abusing and twenty non-child abusing, low-income mothers.[135] The abusive mothers scored significantly lower on measures of the first six developmental stages. The study utilized a previously untested instrument and identified abusive mothers through the local protective services unit. It is not known whether having abused their children within the previous six months, having been identified by a social service agency as abusive, or having experienced some other developmental trauma resulted in the abusive mothers group's lower scores.

Marvin L. Blumberg suggests that women who maltreat their children do so because they experience "impairment of proper ego development and later super-ego evolution, leaving a basically id individual who is, therefore, prone to develop character disorders and emotional aberrations."[136] The source of the developing females' impairment is not identified. Further, the concepts of id, ego, and superego are very abstract, not verifiable in research and are more belief than conceptual formulations. Using nonpsychoanalytic terminology, however other investigators have come to similar conclusions. Many reports identify that abusive adults were themselves abused as children and therefore never received adequate parenting.[137] Much of this research looks only at parents known to be abusive. Similar results with many of the same limitations are used by other researchers to conclude that abusive adults maltreat their children because they lack knowledge of adequate childrearing practices.[138] Support for the conclusion that abusive parents are ignorant of normal child development has been provided by additional studies.[139] Systematic analysis of study results is impaired due to the many flaws apparent in the research. However, there does seem to be some evidence to suggest that abusive and neglectful parents frequently come from violent families and demonstrate inadequate parenting skills themselves.

Personality Traits

Numerous personality traits have been associated with abusive and neglectful parents. Gil, however, noted that very little consistency in the identified traits exists between reports.[140] Immaturity,[141] with poor impulse control[142] are frequently associated with adults who abuse and neglect.

An interesting study by M. A. Disbrow, H. Doerr and C. Caulfield combined both parent (abusive/neglectful and control) interviews and physiologic measures. Abusive parents were found to lack empathy and to have lower self-esteem than either neglectful parents or controls.[143] Other studies have also identified the abusive parents' low self-esteem and difficulty empathizing with others.[144] Audrey Berger states "The suggestion that abusing parents have difficulty empathizing with others is intriguing in light of Feshbach and Feshbach's (1969) findings that the inhibitory effect of pain cues on aggression may depend upon the development of empathy."[145]

Environmental Factors

Abusive and neglectful parents are frequently identified as experiencing excessive stress. Poverty, as previously discussed, is associated with numerous stresses and correlates strongly with child maltreatment. Parents who abuse and/or neglect their children are also often described as isolated,[146] with a corresponding lack of support systems.[147] The occurrence of abuse and neglect in a family requires the parent to hide the act and contributes to further isolation.

Alcohol and Child Maltreatment

The connection between substance abuse and child abuse is unclear. Certainly parents who are continually intoxicated are unable to care for their children. Margaret Cork, in interviews with 115 children of alcoholic parents reported that many of the children felt neglected by both parents, alcoholic and nonalcoholic.[148] The majority of alcoholic parents do not abuse their children. Certain characteristics, however, are very similar between alcoholic and abusive parents.[149] The relationship between child abuse and substance abuse requires further study.

Summary

In summary, child abuse and neglect is a complex area of study. Difficulties arise at the very attempt to define the terms. In its most narrow interpretation, child abuse entails severe physical harming of a child by a variety of methods. In the broadest possible definition, child abuse and neglect is committed when a child is in any way inhibited from reaching his or her maximum potential. The historical background of child maltreatment is long-standing and evolving with its definition. Theoretical frameworks that seek to explain child abuse and neglect include the mental illness model, environmental stress model, and several social-psychological models. A recently developed nursing model has been proposed as a framework for nursing theory development and research. Finally, the patterns of behavior associated with abusive parents were reviewed with a note of caution due to the methods of research in the area. Together theories of causation and empirical validation through research contribute to nursing knowledge of child abuse and neglect. The next step is the incorporation of this new knowledge into nursing practice. Theory and research are thus the basis for the direct application of care to children and families experiencing violence.

Chapter 5

1. F. G. Bolton, Roy H. Laner, Dorothy S. Gai, and Sandra P. Kane, "The 'Study' of Child Maltreatment", *Journal of Family Issues* 2, no. 4 (December 1981), 531-32. Jay Belsky, "Child Maltreatment: An Ecological Integration," *American Psychologist* 35, no. 4 (April 1980): 320-35.
2. *National Analysis of Official Child Abuse and Neglect Reporting: 1977*, DHEW Publication No. (OHDS) 79-30232 (1979), p. 28.
3. Ibid., p. 18.
4. Ibid.
5. Richard J. Gelles, "Violence Toward Children in the United States", *American Journal of Orthopsychiatry* 48, no. 4 (October 1978), 586.
6. Ibid., pp. 583-84.
7. Ibid., p. 584.

8. Leroy H. Pelton, "Interpreting Family Violence Data," *American Journal of Orthopsychiatry* 49, no. 2 (April 1979): 194, 372-74.

9. C. Henry Kempe et al., "Battered Child Syndrome," *Journal of the American Medical Association* 181, no.1 (1962), pp. 17-24.

10. American Humane Association, "Highlights of the 1974 National Data," (Denver: American Humane Association, 1974).

11. Ray E. Helfer and C. Henry Kempe, *Child Abuse and Neglect* (Cambridge, Ma.: Harper & Row Publishers, Inc., Ballinger Publishing Company, 1976), p. XVII.

12. *National Analysis: 1977*, p. 45.

13. David G. Gil, "Violence Against Children," *Journal of Marriage and the Family* 32, no. 11 (November 1971), p. 642. James R. Seaberg, "Predictors of Injury Severity," *Journal of Social Service Research* 1, no. 1 (Fall 1977), pp. 63-76.

14. *National Analysis: 1977*, p. 45.

15. Robert Blum and Carol Runyan. "Adolescent Abuse," *Journal of Adolescent Health* 1, no. 2 (December 1980), pp. 121-26.

16. *National Analysis: 1977*, p. 45.

17. Ibid., p. 33.

18. Leroy Pelton, "Child Abuse and Neglect," *American Journal of Orthopsychiatry* 48, no. 4 (October), pp. 608-617.

19. Gil, "Violence Against Children," p. 641; Elizabeth Elmer, "Follow-up Study of Traumatized Children," *Pediatrics* 59, no. 2 (February 1977), pp. 273-79; Ursula Dibble and Murray Straus, "Some Social Structure Determinants of Inconsistency between Attitudes and Behavior: The Case of Family Violence," *Journal of Marriage and the Family* 42, no. 1 (February 1980): 77-79 Abraham Morse, et al., "Environmental Correlates," p. 615; L. Young, *Wednesday's Child* (New York: McGraw-Hill, 1971).

20. Gil, "Violence Against Children," p. 647; Young, *Wednesday's Child*.

21. J. Giovannono and A. Billingsley, "Child Neglect Among the Poor," *Child Welfare* 49 (1970) pp. 196-204.

22. Pelton, "Child Abuse and Neglect," p. 610.

23. Ibid., p. 612.

24. Ibid., p. 613.

25. Ibid.

26. Elmer, "Follow-up Study of Traumatized Children," pp. 273-79. Lisa Egbuonu and Barbara Starfield, "Child Health and Social Status," *Pediatrics* 69, no. 5 (May 1982), 550-57.

27. J. Michael Cupoli and Eli H. Newberger, "Optimism or Pessimism for the Victim of Child Abuse?" *Pediatrics* 59, no. 2 (February 1977): 312.

28. *National Analysis: 1977*, p. 42; Gil, "Violence Against Children," p. 641; Marvin L. Blumberg "The Abusing Mother—Criminal, Psycopath, or Victim of Circumstances?" *American Journal of Psychotherapy* 34, no. 3 (July 1980): 352.

29. *National Analysis: 1977*, pp. 34-35.

30. Marc F. Maden and David F. Wrench, "Significant Findings in Child Abuse Research," *Victimology* 2 (Summer 1977): 197.

31. Gil, "Violence Against Children," p. 641.

32. F. G. Bolton, Roy H. Laner, and Sandra P. Kane "Child Maltreatment Risk among Adolescent Mothers,"

pp. 489–504; Gil, "Violence Against Children," p. 640; E. Milling Kinard and Lorraine V. Klerman, "Teenage Parenting and Child Abuse: Are They Related?" *American Journal of Orthopsychiatry* 50, no. 3 (July 1980): 481–88.

33. Kempe et al., "Battered Child Syndrome," pp. 17–24.

34. Ibid.

35. Helfer and Kempe, *Child Abuse and Neglect*, p. XIX.

36. C. Henry Kempe and Ray E. Helfer, ed., *Helping the Battered Child and His Family* (Philadelphia: J. B. Lippincott Co., 1972), p. XI.

37. Eli H. Newberger and Richard Bourne, "The Medicalization and Legalization of Child Abuse," *American Journal of Orthopsychiatry* 48, no. 4, (October 1978).

38. *National Analysis: 1977*, p. 54.

39. Richard J. Gelles and Murray A. Straus, "Violence in the American Family," *Journal of Social Issues* 35, no. 2, (1979): 20.

40. Ibid.

41. "Child Protection Law," Department of Social Services Publication, 3 (rev. 10-75), Lansing, Mich.

42. Ibid.

43. Gil, "Primary Prevention of Child Abuse," p. 30.

44. Ibid, pp. 30–34.

45. James Garbarino, "The Human Ecology of Child Maltreatment," *Journal of Marriage and the Family* 39 (November 1977): 722.

46. Samuel X. Radbill, "Children in a World of Violence: A History of Child Abuse," on *Battered Child*, 3rd ed., ed. C. Henry Kempe and Ray E. Helfer (Chicago: The University of Chicago Press, 1980), p. 6.

47. Ibid.

48. Ibid.

49. J. Knitzer, "Spare the Rod and Spoil the Child Revisited," *American Journal of Orthopsychiatry* 47, no. 3 (July 1977): 372–73.

50. Philippe Aries, *Centuries of Childhood: A Social History of Family Life*, trans. Robert Baldick (New York: Random House, Vintage Books, 1962), p. 33.

51. Ibid., pp. 33–36.

52. Ibid., p. 103.

53. Ibid., p. 106.

54. Ibid., p. 26.

55. Ibid., p. 262.

56. Bremner, *Children and Youth in America*, (Cambridge, Ma.: Harvard University Press, 1971), p. 601.

57. Ibid.

58. Ibid., p. 616.

59. Ibid., p. 615.

60. Ibid., p. 601.

61. Ibid., p. 603.

62. Ibid., p. 703.

63. Ibid., p. 604.

64. Jill E. Korbin, "Very Few Cases: Child Abuse and Neglect in the People's Republic of China," in *Child Abuse and Neglect*, ed. Jill E. Korbin (Berkeley: University of California Press, 1981), p. 173.

65. Jill Korbin, "Anthropological Contributions to the Study of Child Abuse," *International Child Welfare Review* 35 (December 1977): 23.

66. John Bond, "The Samoans," in *Child Abuse, Neglect, and the Family Within a Cultural Context*, Protective Services Resource Institute, Rutgers Medical School, 2, No. 7 (1977), 6.

67. Lula O. Lubchenco, "Routine Neonatal Circumcision: A Surgical Anachronism," *Clinical Obstetrics and Gynecology* 23, no. 4, (December 1980): 1135–40.

68. Korbin, *Child Abuse and Neglect*; Jill E. Korbin, "A Cross-Cultural Perspective on the Role of the Community in Child Abuse and Neglect," *Child Abuse and Neglect: The International Journal* 3 (1979): 9–18; Jill E. Korbin "Anthropological Contributions to the Study of Child Abuse," *Child Abuse and Neglect: The International Journal* 1 (1976): 7–24.

69. Bremner, *Children and Youth in America* 2: 186.

70. Ibid., p. 116.

71. Ibid., p. 118.

72. Ibid., p. 207.

73. John Caffey, "Multiple Fractures in the Long Bones of Infants Suffering from Chronic Subdural Hematoma," *American Journal of Roentgenology* 56 (1946): 163–73.

74. Kempe et al., "Battered Child Syndrome," pp. 17–24.

75. Newberger and Bourne, "Medicalization and Legalization of Child Abuse," p. 597.

76. Murray A. Straus, Forward, in Richard J. Gelles, *The Violent Home: A Study of Physical Aggression Between Husbands and Wives* (Beverly Hills, Calif.: Sage, 1974), pp. 13–17.

77. Blumberg, "Abusing Mother," pp. 351–62. J. J. Spinetta and D. Rigler, "The Child Abusing Parent: A Psychological Review," *Psychological Bulletin* 77 (1972): 296–304; Brant Steele, "Psychodynamic Factors in Child Abuse," in Kempe, *Battered Child*, pp. 49–85.

78. Newberger and Bourne, "Medicalization and Legalization of Child Abuse," p. 603.

79. Blair Justice and Rita Justice, *The Abusing Family* (New York: Human Sciences Press, 1976), p. 48.

80. Barry M. Panter, "Lithium in the Treatment of a Child Abuser," *American Journal of Psychiatry* 134, no. 12 (December 1977): 1436–37.

81. Murray Straus, Richard J. Gelles, and Suzanne Steinmetz, *Behind Closed Doors; Violence in the American Family* (New York: Doubleday, Anchor Press, 1980), p. 55.

82. William N. Friedrich and Jerry A. Boriskin, "The Role of the Child in Abuse: A Review of the Literature," *American Journal of Orthopsychiatry* 46, no. 4 (October 1976): 580–90; Audrey Berger, "The Child Abusing Family: II", *The American Journal of Family Therapy* 8 (Winter 1980): 52–68.

83. Morse et al., "Environmental Correlates of Pediatric Social Illness," pp. 612–14.

84. Rand D. Conger, Robert L. Burgess, and Carol Barrett, "Child Abuse Related to Life Change and Perceptions of Illness: Some Preliminary Findings," *The Family Coordinator* 28, no. 1 (January 1979): 73–78.

85. Kevin J. Gully, Harold A. Dengerink, Mary Pepping, and Douglas Bergsrom, "Research Note: Sibling Contribution to Violent Behavior," *Journal of Marriage and the Family* 43, no. 2 (1981): 333–37.

86. Wagatsuma Hiroshi, "Child Abandonment and Infanticide: A Japanese Case," in Korbin, *Child Abuse and Neglect*, p. 120.

87. Straus, Gelles, and Steinmetz, *Behind Closed Doors*, p. 122.

88. Belsky, "Child Maltreatment," p. 326.
89. Helfer, "Etiology of Child Abuse," pp. 777-79.
90. Ibid., p. 777.
91. Ibid., p. 777-78.
92. Ibid., p. 778-79.
93. Friedrich and Boriskin, "Role of the Child in Abuse," pp. 583-86.
94. Edward Goldson, Michael J. Fitch, Theodore A. Wendell, and Gary Knapp, "Child Abuse: Its Relationship to Birthweight, Apgar Score, and Developmental Testing," *American Journal of Diseases of Children* 132 (August 1978): 790-93.
95. Berger, "Child Abusing Family: II," pp. 55-56; Friedrich and Boriskin, "Role of the Child in Abuse," pp. 84-85.
96. Friedrich and Boriskin, "Role of the Child in Abuse," pp. 580-90; Mary Main, "Abusive and Rejecting Infants," in *Psychological Approaches to Child Abuse*, ed. Neil Frude, (Totowa, N.J.: Rowman & Littlefield, 1981), pp. 19-38.
97. Carol George and Mary Main, "Social Interactions of Young Abused Children: Approach, Avoidance, and Aggression," *Child Development* 50 (1979): 306-18.
98. Marshall H. Klaus and John Kennell, *Maternal-Infant Bonding* (Saint Louis, Mo.: C.V. Mosby Company, 1976), pp. 3, 8.
99. Berger, "Child Abusing Family: II," pp. 60-61; Helfer, "Etiology of Child Abuse," p. 777.
100. A. H. Green, "Self-Destructive Behavior in Physically Abused Schizophrenic Children," *Archives of General Psychiatry* 19 (August 1968): 171-79.
101. Straus, Gelles, and Steinmetz, *Behind Closed Doors*, pp. 24-26.
102. Murray A. Straus, "Measuring Intrafamily Conflict and Violence: The Conflict Tactics (CT) Scales," *Journal of Marriage and the Family* 41, no.1 (February 1979): 75-88.
103. Richard J. Gelles and Murray A. Straus, "Violence in the American Family," *Journal of Social Issues* 35, no. 2 (1979): 29.
104. Straus, Gelles, and Steinmetz, *Behind Closed Doors*, p. 121.
105. Suzanne K. Steinmetz, "The Use of Force for Resolving Family Conflict: The Training Ground for Abuse," *Family Coordinator* 26 (January 1977): 20; Patricia Ulbrich and Joan Huber, "Observing Parental Violence: Distribution and Effects," *Journal of Marriage and the Family* 43, no. 3 (August 1981): 623-31.
106. Straus, Gelles, and Steinmetz, *Behind Closed Doors*, p. 122.
107. Ibid., p. 237.
108. Rosemary S. Hunter and Nancy Kilstrom, "Breaking the Cycle in Abusive Families," *American Journal of Psychiatry* 136, no. 10 (October 1970): 1320-22.
109. Gelles, "Violence Toward Children in the United States," pp. 580-92; Gelles, "Violence in the Family,"; Gelles and Straus, "Violence in the American Family," pp. 15-39; Straus, "Measuring Intrafamily Conflict," pp. 75-88; Dibble and Straus, "Some Social Structure Determinants," pp. 71-80; Suzanne K. Steinmetz, "Occupation and Physical Punishment: A Response to Straus," *Journal of Marriage and the Family* 33 (November 1971): 664-65; Suzanne K. Steinmetz and Murray A. Straus, ed. *Violence in Family* (New York: Harper & Row, 1974).
110. Garbarino, "Human Ecology of Child Maltreatment," pp. 721-36.
111. U. Bronfenbrenner, *The Ecology of Human Development*, (Cambridge, Ma.: Harvard University Press, 1979).

112. Belsky, "Child Maltreatment," pp. 320, 326.

113. Garbarino, "Human Ecology of Child Maltreatment," p. 721.

114. Belsky, "Child Maltreatment," p. 326.

115. Garbarino, "Human Ecology of Child Maltreatment," p. 723.

116. Ibid.

117. Ibid.

118. Phillip J. Resnick, "Child Murder by Parents: A Psychiatric Review of Filicide," *American Journal of Psychiatry* 126 (September 1969): 330.

119. Garbarino, "Human Ecology of Child Maltreatment," p. 723.

120. D. McClelland, "Testing for Competence Rather than Intelligence," *American Psychologist* 28 (January 1973): 1-14.

121. A. Green, "Self-Destruction in Physically Abused Schizophrenic Children," *Archives of General Psychiatry* 19 (April 1968): 171-97; Belsky, "Child Maltreatment," p. 324.

122. Garbarino, "Human Ecology of Child Maltreatment," p. 723.

123. G. Elder, "Family History and the Life Course," *Journal of Family History* 2, no. 4 (Winter 1977): 279-304.

124. Gil, "Violence Against Children," pp. 637-48; Belsky, "Child Maltreatment," pp. 320-35; Mary Hanemann Lystad, "Violence at Home: A Review of the Literature," *American Journal of Orthopsychiatry* 45, no.3 (April 1975): 328-45.

125. Garbarino, "Human Ecology of Child Maltreatment," p. 724.

126. Georgia Kemm Millor, "Theoretical Framework for Nursing Research in Child Abuse and Neglect," *Nursing Research* 30, no. 2 (March-April 1981), 78-83.

127. Ibid., p. 80.

128. Ibid.

129. Ibid., p. 81.

130. Ibid.

131. Ibid., p. 82.

132. Ibid., p. 81.

133. Ibid., p. 82.

134. P. Butterfield, W. vanDoornick, P. Dawson, and H. Alexander, "Early Identification of Dysparenting," cited in Belsky, "Child Maltreatment," p. 322.

135. Alan L. Evans, "An Eriksonian Measure of Personality Development in Child-Abusing Mothers," *Psychological Reports* 44 (1979): 963-66.

136. Blumberg, "Abusing Mother," p. 353.

137. Margaret Varma, "Battered Women: Battered Children," in Roy, *Battered Women*, p. 268; Phyllis A. Jameson and Cynthia Shellenback, "Sociological and Psychological Factors in the Background of Men and Women Perpetrators of Child Abuse," *Child Abuse and Neglect: The International Journal* 1 (1979): 80; Kempe et al., "Battered Child Syndrome," p. 106; Gil, "Violence Against Children," p. 641; Helfer, "Etiology of Child Abuse," p. 777.

138. Thomas J. Hunt, Ray Hepner, and Karen W. Seaton, "Childhood Lead Poisoning and Inadequate Child Care," *American Journal of Diseases of Children* 136, no. 6 (June 1982): 538-42; Belsky, "Child Maltreatment," pp. 323-24; Berger, "Child Abusing Family: I," p. 60; Berger, "Child Abusing Family: II," p. 58; Young, *Wednesday's Child*.

139. Marvin Blumberg, "Psychopathology of the Abusing Parent," *American Journal of Psychotherapy* 28

(1974): 21-29; Elizabeth Elmer, *Fragile Families, Troubled Children* (Pittsburgh: University of Pittsburgh Press, 1977); Selwyn Smith and Ruth Hanson, "Interpersonal Relationships and Child-Rearing Practices in 214 Parents of Battered Children," *British Journal of Psychiatry* 127 (December 1975): 523.

140. David G. Gil, *Violence Against Children: Physical Abuse in the United States* (Cambridge: Harvard University Press, 1970).

141. Blumberg, "Psychopathology of the Abusing Parent," pp. 21-29; Barton D. Schmitt, "Battered Child Syndrome," in *Current Pediatric Diagnosis and Treatment*, 5th ed., edited by C. Henry Kempe, Henry Silver and Donough O'Brien (Los Altos, Calif.: Lange Medical Publications, 1978), p. 852.

142. Gil, "Violence Against Children," p. 645; Blumberg, "Psychopathology of the Abusing Parent," pp. 21-29.

143. M. A. Disgrow, H. Doerr, and C. Caulfield, "Measuring the Components of Parents' Potential for Child Abuse and Neglect," *Child Abuse and Neglect: The International Journal* 1 (1977): 279-96.

144. B. Melnick and J. R. Hurley, "Distinctive Personality Attributes of Child Abusing Mothers," *Journal of Consulting and Clinical Psychology* 33, no. 6 (1969): 746-49; A. M. Frodi and M. E. Lamb, "Psychophysiological Responses to Infant Signals in Abusive Mothers and Mothers of Premature Infants," cited in Berger, "Child Abusing Family: I," p. 59.

145. Berger, "Child Abusing Family: I," p. 59; N. Feshbach and S. Feshbach, "The Relationship between Empathy and Aggression in Two Age Groups," *Developmental Psychology* 1 (1969): 102-107.

146. Norman A. Polansky, Mary Ann Chalmers, Elizabeth Buttenwieser, and David P. Williams, "Isolation of the Neglectful Family," *American Journal of Orthopsychiatry* 49, no. 1 (January 1979): 151; Belsky, "Child Maltreatment," pp. 327-28.

147. Gil, "Violence Against Children," p. 645; Polansky, "Isolation of the Neglectful Family," p. 150; Elizabeth Elmer, *Fragile Families, Troubled Children* (Pittsburgh: The University of Pittsburgh Press, 1977); Belsky, "Child Maltreatment," p. 328.

148. Margaret Cork, *The Forgotten Child* (Toronto: Paperjacks in association with Addition Research Foundation, 1969).

149. Margaret Hindman, "Child Abuse and Neglect: The Alcohol Connection," *Alcohol Health and Research World* (Spring 1977): 2-7.

Domestic Abuse of the Elderly

Mary C. Sengstock
and
Sara Barrett

When I was a laddie
I lived with my granny
And many a hiding ma granny di'ed me.
Now I am a man
And I live with my granny
And do to my granny
What she did to me.

(Traditional rhyme, anonymous)

Strong preference is expressed on the part of many elders, and of their families as well, to maintain the care of aged persons in their own homes or in the homes of relatives for as long as possible.[1] This preference is based, in large part, upon the assumption that the family is seen as "a center of solidarity and love,"[2] and is believed to be a preferable alternative to the formalized care obtained in nursing homes or homes for the aged. However, this assumption concerning the type of care that exists in the family setting has been called into question in recent years as research has indicated that some elderly persons are subjected to neglect or outright abuse by the members of the family who are responsible for their care.[3]

This awareness of the wrongful treatment of the aged by their families is only part of a larger recognition of what Suzanne K. Steinmetz and Murray A. Straus call "the myth of family consensus and harmony."[4] Families are presumed to be loving and harmonious. Family members are supposed to be kind, loving, and helpful to one another. That this is not necessarily the case is illustrated by a number of studies indicating that a substantial amount of aggression and violence is present in the American family, and that some of it is directed toward its elderly members.

This chapter reviews some of the findings to date concerning elder abuse and is based upon existing theories and previous research in the field, with special reference to a study in which both authors participated, one as principal investigator (Sengstock), and the other as chief research assistant (Barrett).[5] This study was conducted by the Institute of Gerontology (IG), Wayne State University in Detroit, Michigan, under a grant from the Andrus Foundation. It will henceforth be known as the IG study. In the IG study, questionnaires and interviews were completed with medical, social, and mental health agencies in the Detroit metropolitan area. As the result of these contacts, reports of seventy-seven cases of abused elders were reported to the project, and detailed information about each case was obtained. In addition, twenty of the victims and six members of their families were interviewed. In this chapter, five major topics will be considered:

1. Characteristics and frequency of domestic abuse of the aged,

2. Characteristics of abused and abuser,

3. Proposed causes of elder abuse,

4. Means used by agencies in identifying and serving abused aged,

5. And suggested nursing care for elder abuse victims.

CHARACTERISTICS AND FREQUENCY OF DOMESTIC ABUSE OF THE AGED

Types of Elder Abuse

Previous research has indicated that elder abuse is actually a variety of behaviors, all of which threaten the health, comfort, and possibly even the lives of elderly people. However, the nature of the threat and its effect on aged persons' health and comfort may take very different forms. Studies of child and spouse abuse have tended to focus on physical abuse alone.[6] Elder abuse research, however, has focused on a much broader range of behaviors, including the following six major categories of abuse and neglect.[7]

1. *Direct Physical Abuse* includes actions which are direct attacks, are apparently deliberate, and can cause actual physical injury. Included in this category are direct physical assaults (slaps, punches, beatings, pushes, etc.), as well as threats in which a weapon, such as a knife or gun, is directly involved.

2. *Physical Neglect* includes the failure to provide an aged and dependent individual with the necessities of life: food, shelter, clothing, medical care. In fact, such neglect may be as injurious and life-threatening as a direct attack.[8] However, the major difference between direct abuse and neglect lies in the fact that neglect does not appear to involve a deliberate attempt to injure.

3. *Financial Abuse* includes the theft or misuse of an aged individual's money or property. Examples would include taking money from a bank account without the elder's consent; sale of a home without knowledge or permission; cashing a Social Security check and not returning the money to the recipient; and so on.

4. *Psychological or Emotional Abuse* involves assault or the infliction of pain through verbal or emotional means rather than physical means. Examples are verbal assault (screaming, yelling, berating) and threats which induce fear, but do not involve use of a weapon.

5. *Emotional Neglect* includes isolation or ignoring the elder.

6. *Violation of Rights* includes acts such as forcing a person to move into a nursing home against his or her will, prohibiting him or her from marrying, or preventing free use of the elder's own money.[9]

Frequency of Elder Abuse

Before discussing the frequency of elder abuse, it is necessary to note that the major studies on the topic present serious limitations in establishing reliable statistics. Sample sizes are generally too small to establish any significant generalizations concerning the characteristics and extent of this problem—Elizabeth Lau and Jordan Kosberg, N=39;[10] Marilyn R. Block and Jan D. Sinnott, N=26.[11] All the studies are analyses of whatever cases the researchers have been able to uncover, and none can be considered to be representative of the aged population.[12] Further, one major study[13] does not examine case-related data, but rather relies upon service providers' general impressions of the nature of the problem.

As a result of these limitations, accurate reports of the frequency of elder abuse are not available. The frequency can only be estimated from existing data. In Marvin Wolfgang's famous analysis of homicides in Philadelphia, he notes that 4 percent of the cases of homicides involving relatives were parents killed by their children.[14] He also found that 20 percent of homicide victims were over fifty years of age, while only 9 percent of offenders were in this age group, suggesting that in this most extreme form of attack, elders are victimized by persons younger than themselves.[15] In most cases, the attacker was much younger, for Wolfgang also found that where there was a difference of twenty-five years or more in the ages of the offender and the victim, three-fourths of the time the victim was the elder.[16]

Homicide, of course, represents only the most extreme aspect of the problem. Less extreme types of abuse are certainly much more common. Although available data are highly tentative, estimates of the amount of elder abuse may be obtained from some recent studies. Steinmetz suggests that approximately 11 percent of the population may be vulnerable to elder abuse,[17] and Block and Sinnott estimate that abuse is an actual problem for at least 4 percent of the elderly population.[18] Lau and Kosberg found 39 cases of abuse among 484 elderly persons in their sample, a rate of 80.58 per 1,000.[19] Because their sample was designed to uncover abuse known to professionals, this rate is probably far too high. Another estimate based on the frequency of child-to-parent violence can be found in the work of Murray H. Straus, Richard G. Gelles, and Suzanne K. Steinmetz.[20] In their national survey of violence in American families, they found that 18 percent of parents reported having been struck by a child. Although their respondents were primarily under sixty-five, it is likely that violent patterns developed early in life may continue when the parent is aged.

Using the Department of Justice's National Crime Survey (NCS) we note that one in five aged victims of violent crimes were victimized by someone they knew.[21] Since the rate for personal crimes against the elderly (assaults or robbery, for example) is 12.44 per 1,000, the rate of personal victimization of the elderly by people they know, would be 2.49 per 1,000.[22] This should be considered to be a minimum, since the NCS questionnaires are less likely to elicit reports of domestic abuse, and it is known that victims of domestic abuse often try to hide the abuse.[23] A somewhat higher rate was reported by Block and Sinnot who had several samples, including a sample of 443 elderly; in this sample they discovered three cases, a rate of 6.772 per 1,000.[24] Hence their data would suggest that domestic abuse of the aged is about one-half as frequent as the overall rate of personal crime against the aged. These studies suggest that the threat of abuse in the home is nearly as serious a threat as is that of the personal crime which elders fear so much. Some suggest it may be more serious since these are crimes which the victim cannot escape.[25]

Frequency of Various Abuse Types

The frequency of each type of elder abuse which has been identified tends to vary in different studies. Some studies have found psychological abuse to be most prevalent,[26]

Domestic Abuse of the Elderly

while others have noted that physical abuse was the most common form of abuse.[27] It has been noted that these findings might reflect the observation that agencies tend to identify forms of abuse which most closely correspond to the forms of treatment which they offer.[28] Thus Block and Sinnott's finding might reflect the fact that most professionals reporting cases of abuse to them were social workers, professionals concerned primarily with the psychological status of clients.[29] At the same time, Lau and Kosberg's samples of abused elders was derived from case records of persons who were seen at a chronic disease center for a medical malady.[30] Consequently, this might account for the strong tendency toward physical abuse in the cases which were identified by their research.

The frequency with which each type of abuse and/or neglect appeared in the IG study is shown in Table 6–1.[31] Similar to Block and Sinnott's findings, psychological or emotional abuse was the most frequent type of abuse of the elderly, with 81.8 percent of cases suffering some type of emotional abuse or neglect.[32] This pattern should be understood in context, however. As Lau and Kosberg reported, most victims suffered from more than one form of abuse, a pattern which appeared in the IG study as well.[33] In fact, while emotional or psychological abuse occurred independently in a few cases, it almost always accompanied other forms of abuse. Hence it is not surprising that it has been found to be the most common type of elder abuse. Since emotional or psychological abuse or neglect often accompanies other types of abuse, there is a great need for service providers to look further in cases in which these abuse types are found; for it is quite possible that another type of abuse may also be present.

Direct emotional abuse was found to be more common than emotional neglect/deprivation of rights (58.4 percent versus 23.4 percent of the cases). An early concern of the project had been the fear that a large number of "imaginary" abuse cases would be generated—elderly individuals who were unnecessarily demanding upon their families and defined themselves as abused when their demands were not met. The small percentage of cases in this category suggests that this was an unfounded concern; most of the cases referred to the study appear to be genuine cases of abuse or severe neglect.

Table 6–1 *Type of Abuse Suffered by Aged Abuse Victims*

Type of Abuse (N = 77)	Number and Percent of Cases (%)	
Direct Physical Abuse	15 (19.5)	Total
Physical Neglect	18 (23.5)	Physical: 33 (42.9%)
Financial Abuse	42 (54.5)	
Psychological/Emotional Abuse	45 (58.4)	Total
Emotional Neglect/ Deprivation of Rights	18 (23.4)	Emotional: 63 (81.8%)

The second most frequent type of abuse was found to be financial abuse, suffered by about one-half of the cases in the IG study. The high prevalence of cases of financial abuse in this sample may arise, in part, from the fact that a legal aid agency reported the largest number of cases to the project. This is the type of agency that would most likely be consulted by aged persons with various financial concerns, such as the claim that someone has stolen money or misused property.

Physical abuse and/or neglect proved to be the least frequent type of abuse suffered by the victims in the IG study. However, this type of victimization, with abuse and neglect combined, was still suffered by nearly half of the victims in the IG sample (42.9 percent). Of this group, slightly less than one-half (19.5 percent of the sample as a whole) suffered direct physical abuse. The rest (23.5 percent of the sample) suffered physical neglect.

Most of the cases referred to the IG study were cases of current abuse. Nearly two-thirds of the victims were found to have suffered the most recent incident during 1981, the year of the study. One-fourth had suffered the most recent incident during the immediately preceding year, 1980. And less than 10 percent had suffered the most recent incident prior to 1980. It was also clear that abuse or neglect rarely occurred as an isolated incident. Two-thirds of the workers said that prior incidents had occurred. Most workers could not specify an exact number of prior incidents, but stated that "several" incidents had preceded the most recent one.

The enduring character of the abuse becomes more clear when one looks at the length of time over which the abuse has occurred. One-fourth of the victims had suffered abuse for one year or less. Twelve percent were said to have suffered abuse for one to two years, while nearly 17 percent were reported to have endured abuse for more than two years. Again, the workers in about one-third of the cases were unable to specify any definite time period for the abuse, but could only comment that, to their knowledge, the abuse had continued for a substantial period of time. If it may be assumed that "a long time" probably indicates at least one year, then it would appear that about 60 percent of these victims have endured abusive family situations for a period of one year or longer.

Unlike other categories of domestic abuse, elder abuse tends to include more than direct physical violence. Six types of abusive behavior are commonly included: direct physical abuse, physical neglect, financial abuse, emotional abuse, emotional neglect, and deprivation of rights.

No firm generalizations can be made about the frequency of elder abuse or of each specific subtype. A variety of studies cited suggest that the rate of domestic abuse of the aged may range from about 2.5 to about 6 or 7 per 1,000 aged persons. Because of the difficulty in uncovering this behavior, such figures may be underestimations. Some studies have shown psychological abuse to be more frequent while others find a prevalence of physical abuse. Several studies have noted that elder abuse often involves multiple types in a single case. Elder abuse cases which have been studied also tend to involve a substantial number of separate incidents of abuse which have taken place over a considerable period of time, often lasting for months or even years.

One cannot conclude, on the basis of existing data, that elder abuse is a widespread problem. The majority of the aged probably have satisfactory relationships with their children and other relatives. For those few aged who are abused, however, the abuse tends to be persistent, serious, and urgently requires attention.

CHARACTERISTICS OF ABUSED AND ABUSERS

Who is a likely victim of elder abuse? And who is most likely to be an abuser? In this section we will discuss the demographic characteristics which have been found to be associated with abuse and neglect of the aged by their families. We will consider first the characteristics of the victim, moving then to characteristics of the abuser.

Demographic Characteristics of Victims

The demographic characteristics of the victims are summarized in Table 6-2. As the table indicates, 90 percent of the victims were between fifty-nine and ninety years of age, evenly divided between the three decades, with about thirty percent of the sample in each. Only three victims (3.9 percent) were ninety or over.[34] This wide age distribution differs from earlier research, which has found the preponderance of victims to be very old.[35]

Previous studies have also suggested that the majority of elder abuse victims are women.[36] This predominance of female victims was true of the IG study as well, with three-fourths of the cases reported involving female victims, as opposed to only one-fourth male victims. In terms of race, other researchers have found most victims to be white.[37] In the IG study, however, the victims were almost evenly divided between blacks (about 40 percent) and whites (about 56 percent). Agency workers were not always able to identify the religion of the victims. For those cases in which the religion was known, there was a clear predominance of Protestants (about 35 percent of the sample), with about 17 percent Catholics, and only one Jewish victim (1.3 percent).

It is clear that the victims in the IG sample tend to be lower-income persons, with nearly 60 percent of them reporting an income of less than $5,000 a year. This contrasts with Block and Sinnott, who found that victims were evenly divided between lower and middle class.[38] Another 25 percent of the IG study reported an income of from $5,000 to $9,999 per year. Hence over 50 percent of the victims had to live on less than $10,000 per year. It is easy to see why they would feel quite dependent upon their families and unable to escape the abusive situation. It should be noted, however, that the wealthy are not immune to the problems of domestic abuse, although they may be better able to hide these problems from authorities.[39] Five of the victims had incomes of over $10,000 per year, and of these, two had incomes in excess of $20,000 per year.

Over 80 percent of the victims resided in the city of Detroit, as opposed to the suburbs. In part this probably reflects the fact that older persons are more likely to reside in the central city than are younger persons.[40] It may also reflect the location and case concentrations of the agencies participating, although several agencies in suburban areas were contacted for possible participation in the project. The majority of the victims either lived alone (31.2

Table 6-2 Demographic Characteristics of Aged Abuse Victims (N = 77)

	Number of Cases	Percent
Age of Victim:		
58-59	2	2.6%
60-69	24	31.2
70-79	25	32.5
80-89	23	29.9
90+	3	3.9
Sex of Victim:		
Male	20	26.0
Female	57	74.0
Race of Victim:		
White	43	55.8
Black	31	40.3
Unknown	3	3.9
Religion of Victim:		
Roman Catholic	13	16.9
Protestant	27	35.1
Jewish	1	1.3
Unknown	36	46.8
Victim's Annual Income:		
$<5,000	44	57.1
$ 5- 9,999	19	24.7
$10-14,999	2	2.6
$15-19,999	1	1.3
$20-24,999	2	2.6
Unknown	9	11.7

percent) or with one other person (42.9 percent). Fourteen victims (18.2 percent) lived with two other people; six lived with three or more other people, including one aged victim in a household which included six other persons. It should be noted that living alone does not preclude the existence of abuse on the part of family members, who may abuse the aged person during visits, or subject them to neglect or isolation.

One interesting pattern that appeared with these aged victims was their number of contacts outside their own households. Most have family contacts, but these consist mainly of a visit or phone call every week or less. They are less likely to have friends, but those who do tend to have closer contact with them than most victims have with their families. One might suggest that the picture which emerges is similar to that which Blair Justice and Rita Justice found with families in which child abuse was a problem.[41] They described the abusing family as one in which the members had very limited contact outside the family. This made it impossible for the members to get outside support in times of trouble, leaving no one to intervene if abuse occurs.

One of the conclusions which has been drawn in other studies of elder abuse is that persons with some type of physical or mental disability are more likely to be abused than those who are physically strong.[42] The IG study did not find this to be true in the majority of cases.[43] Agency workers reported physical and/or emotional impairment in only seventeen cases (22.1 percent). The most frequently reported type of impairment was some degree of emotional impairment. Other disabilities were the inability to prepare food and the inability to perform personal hygiene. Smaller numbers of victims were reported to be unable to prepare their own medicine, were totally bedridden, or had other types of impairments. It has also been noted that medication may itself be a means of abuse, as some elders are given excessive doses of drugs by their doctors or their families in order to make them more manageable.[44]

Portrait of the Abuser

Previous studies of elder abuse have suggested that the abuser is most likely to be a family member of the victim, usually one of the victim's own children.[45] It has also been found that the abuser is most often forty years of age or older.[46] Block and Sinnott also found that most abusers were female, a situation very likely brought about by the fact that women are most frequently the caretakers in constant contact with the incapacitated elderly.[47]

According to Block and Sinnott, most abusers acted because of psychological (58 percent) rather than economic (31 percent) or unknown reasons.[48] They also found most abusers to be white (88 percent), middle class (65 percent), and middle-aged (53 percent).[49] This pattern contrasts with child and spouse abuse, as both have been characterized as phenomena which are more common among the lower classes.[50]

In the IG study, it was found that the abuser is more likely to be a member of the victim's household than to live elsewhere; this was the case in 60 percent of the cases.[51] The suggestion that aged persons are more likely to be abused by their own children was also borne out in the study: one-half of the abusers were the children of the victim. However, this study did not confirm the picture of the daughter as the most common abuser (Table 6-3). Children who abused their parents were almost equally divided between sons (26 percent) and daughters (23.4 percent). It should be noted that spouse abuse is not unknown among the aged. Twelve percent of the abusers were the spouse of the victim. Grandchildren were the abusers in 3.9 percent of the cases. Sisters were more likely to be abusers than brothers (5.2 percent versus 1.3 percent). Other relatives (nieces, nephews, cousins) accounted for 7.8 percent of the cases. In 13 percent of the cases the abuser was not a relative. These included friends (5.2 percent), roomers (6.5 percent), and landlords (1.3 percent).

The picture of the abuser as somewhat advanced in age was also supported in the IG data. Two-thirds of the abusers were forty years of age or over, with 24 percent

Table 6-3 Characteristics of the Abuser

	Number of Cases	Percent
Residence of Abuser:		
Lives in victim's household	46	59.7%
Not in victim's household	26	33.8
Unknown	5	6.5
Abuser's Relationship to Victim:		
Son	20	26.0
Daughter	18	23.4
Spouse	9	11.7
Grandchild	3	3.9
Sister	4	5.2
Brother	1	1.3
Other relative	6	7.8
Friend	4	5.2
Roomer	5	6.5
Landlord	1	1.3
Unknown	4	5.2
Age of Abuser (N = 50 cases in which age is known):		
< 20	1	2.0
20-29	9	18.0
30-39	4	8.0
40-49	12	24.0
50-59	10	20.0
60-69	11	22.0
70+	3	6.0

in their forties and 20 percent in their fifties. Twenty-two percent of the abusers were in their sixties and 6 percent were seventy years of age or older—well into the category of being classified as elderly themselves. Conversely, only 8 percent of the abusers were in their thirties; 18 percent in their twenties; and 2 percent less than twenty years of age.

One issue which should be considered is the relationship between types of abuse and the abuser. Certain types of abuse were more likely to be inflicted by specific types of abusers (Table 6-4). Thus most physical abuse was inflicted by sons, who were the suspected abusers in over one-half of these cases. This finding is contrary to the Block and Sinnott study, which found that most elder abuse was perpetrated by women; their study also found a prevalence of psychological abuse, the form of abuse in which daughters appear more likely to be involved.[52] The remaining physical abuse was rather evenly divided among daughters, spouses, other relatives, and unrelated persons, each of which has one or two perpetrators. No siblings were involved in physical abuse.

Domestic Abuse of the Elderly

Table 6-4 Abuse Type by Suspected Abuser

Suspected Abuser	Physical Abuse	Physical Neglect	Emotional Neglect/ Deprivation of Rights	Emotional Abuse	Financial Abuse
Spouse	(1) 6.7%	(1) 8.3%	(1) 11.1%	(4) 9.1%	(3) 7.3%
Daughter	(2) 13.3	(2) 16.7	(4) 44.4	(10) 22.7	(11) 26.8
Son	(7) 53.3	(3) 25.0	-0-	(13) 29.5	(11) 26.8
Sibling	-0-	(3) 25.0	(3) 33.3	(4) 9.1	(2) 4.9
Other Relative	(2) 13.3	(1) 8.3	(1) 11.1	(6) 13.6	(7) 17.0
Unrelated	(2) 13.3	(2) 16.7	-0-	(7) 15.0	(7) 17.0
Totals	(14)	(12)	(9)	(44)	(41)

Physical neglect was more likely to be perpetrated either by sons or siblings, but differences are very small.

The abusers most likely to be involved in emotional neglect/deprivation of rights were daughters (44.4 percent) and siblings (33.3 percent). It is interesting to note that no sons or unrelated persons were believed to be guilty of emotional neglect. It might be suggested that the persons accused of emotional neglect—daughters and siblings—are persons from whom the elderly would be most likely to believe they can expect emotional support. This would be particularly true of daughters. Emotional support, on the other hand, is not usually thought to be the responsibility of men, so parents would not be likely to express disappointment if their sons failed to provide such support. Neither would they be likely to expect such help from unrelated persons. Hence we suggest that the prevalence in this category of daughters and siblings may be due primarily to the expectations of the elderly rather than to a different type of behavior on the part of the alleged abusers.

Direct emotional abuse, on the other hand, was more characteristic of sons, who made up the major portion (29.5 percent) of the alleged abusers in this category. This type of abuse includes more direct action—verbal assaults, creating fear—which many people might consider to be more appropriate masculine behavior. This might account for the greater representation of sons in emotional abuse than in the more passive emotional neglect. Daughters, however, were almost as likely to engage in direct emotional abuse as their brothers (22.7 percent versus 29.5 percent). Unrelated persons (15 percent) and other relatives (13.6 percent) also appeared in considerable numbers. Sons and daughters were also the most likely to engage in financial abuse, with each representing about one-fourth of the cases. Other relatives and unrelated persons were the next most frequent offenders (17.1 percent each).

The data suggest that sons and daughters are the major perpetrators of most types of abuse, as they are of elder abuse as a whole. It was noted, however, that sons were more likely to engage in active, direct abuse. They were responsible for two-thirds of the physical abuse and nearly 30 percent of the emotional abuse. Daughters were also responsible for direct emotional abuse and were accused of a great deal of the indirect emotional neglect (44.4 percent). Other relatives and unrelated persons tended to appear as suspected abusers primarily in instances of direct abuse. They were less likely to be accused of neglect, probably because the aged victims do not depend upon them for help and would not recognize its absence as neglect.

PROPOSED CAUSES OF ELDER ABUSE

There is no lack of theory to explain the existence of family violence and abuse. Theories abound that purport to explain why parents abuse their children and husbands beat their wives. As interest in elder abuse has increased, so also have the number of theories that claim to explain why adults abuse their aging parents. Unfortunately, most of these explanations remain at the level of untested hypotheses. Many have some research to support their claims. Others are simply assertions of variables that appear to be important.

In this section we will examine some of the proposed explanations for elder abuse, together with references to whatever research data are available to support each. However, it must be emphasized that none of these theories can be considered to be well-established as accurate explanations of the problem. Certainly, no single theory yet developed is adequate to explain the existence and nature of elder abuse.

Nonetheless, such theories can provide professionals with valuable indicators of the probability of abuse. Most theories of domestic abuse have been developed as a result of associating specific instances of known abuse with other factors in the social-psychological environment of the victim and his or her family. Consequently, such theories suggest the types of factors which may be related to abuse, and which should be viewed as "danger signals" by nurses and other persons who work with elderly patients. They can, therefore, suggest the need for further inquiry on the part of concerned professionals. Two categories of theories will be examined: general theories of family violence, and explanations of abuse relating directly to the aging process.

General Theories of Family Violence

One point that has been stressed with regard to characteristics of the elderly is the continuity of personality and behavior throughout life.[53] Gerontologists who espouse this view emphasize the fact that most individuals exhibit a constant pattern of personality characteristics and behavior patterns from youth through middle age and into old age. Radical changes, either in personality or behavior, once one reaches old age, are rare. This theory suggests that the family problems of the aged, including potentially abusive behavior, may be very similar to those of younger persons. Consequently, it may be very useful to examine theories of family violence which have been found useful in analyzing child and spouse abuse, in order to determine the degree to which they may be applicable to abuse of the aged as well.

Three types of general theories of domestic abuse will be considered. These are:

1. Abuser-focused theories,
2. Situational stress theories,
3. Theories focusing on the nature of family relationships.

Abuser-focused Theories

Domestic abuse in general has often been explained as being related to the psychopathological state of the abuser.[54] In essence, these theories suggest that the abusive individual is essentially mentally ill and the abusive behavior is the result of this mental illness. A closely related theory associates domestic abuse with the misuse of alcohol or other substances.[55] This approach is often taken by persons with a serious concern about substance abuse. They suggest that persons who are alcoholics or drug addicts are highly likely to engage in abusive behavior. In contrast, some theorists suggest that the alcohol is not the basic cause of the abusive behavior; rather the substance abuse is used by the abuser as a "cover-up" for abusive tendencies that are already present.[56]

In either instance, the cause of the abuse is sought in the psychological state of the abuser. He or she is thought to be mentally ill or under the influence of alcohol or drugs, and therefore incapable of controlling behavior. This approach seems highly tempting since it provides an obvious factor which is responsible for the abuse, and also an equally obvious solution: cure the psychopathological problem and the abuse will cease.

Unfortunately, studies of domestic abuse rarely have access to independent evidence of mental illness and substance abuse. Hence it is difficult to ascertain with accuracy the percent of cases in which either or both of these factors exist. In the IG study, for example, case workers were asked to indicate whether they had noted the presence of these factors in each instance of abuse reported.[57] Workers noted the presence of mental illness and/or substance abuse in a relatively small percentage of the cases. In only 5 cases (6 percent) was the abuser described as an alcoholic; in one case the abuser was known to be a drug addict; in another three cases (4 percent) the abuser had been diagnosed as mentally ill. This leaves a total of only nine, or 12 percent of the cases, in which the abuser could be clearly said to possess a psychic state which made behavior control difficult or impossible. Hence there is specific mention of the psychopathological state of the abuser in relatively few cases of elder abuse.

It should be noted, however, that the failure of such causal factors to appear in studies of abuse may well be due to the inability of the researchers to uncover the evidence. Either the data collection instruments may fail to elicit this information from the professional workers, or in some cases, undiagnosed mental illness, alcoholism, or drug abuse may be present and the agency workers themselves may not yet be aware of it.

Those cases of elder abuse in which mental illness or substance abuse is present appear particularly serious or difficult to control. In one instance, an alcoholic daughter subjected her recently widowed mother, a heart patient, to constant verbal abuse. She also depended upon her mother to care for her three active children since her alcoholism had forced her to relinquish custody. Another woman was subjected to constant threats and emotional abuse by her elderly alcoholic husband. Still another woman had an alcoholic grandson who constantly stole money she had given him to pay her bills.

Even more serious abuse occurs in cases in which mental or emotional illness is present. One aged woman had been severely beaten by her schizophrenic son who lived with her. She was also deprived of the companionship of her daughter, who avoided visiting her mother out of fear of her brother, who had beaten his sister in the past. In another case, the aged victim had evicted her emotionally ill son from her home. Yet the son continued to return home, often breaking into the home while the mother was at work. The victim had sought legal assistance from a legal aid agency and the county prosecutor in order to protect herself from her son's abusive behavior.

In terms of providing service to victims, it does not appear to be advisable to rely heavily on the notion that the abuse is caused by such factors as mental illness or substance abuse. If an agency should find such problems to be present in an instance of elder abuse then, of course, it is imperative that these problems be treated as a part of the entire family problem. However, an assumption that such factors must be involved whenever elder abuse occurs would prevent workers from looking for other factors that are likely to be present as causal variables in the majority of cases.

Such factors can, however, be of value to service providers in that they may serve as "danger signals." Elder abuse may occur in many cases where mental illness, or drug or alcohol abuse are not present, and these factors may not always lead to abuse of aged members of the family. But the risk of abuse in such cases is sufficiently great that agency workers should make additional inquiries in order to determine the possible presence of abusive behavior. This would be necessary even if the alcoholic, drug addict, or mentally ill individual was an aged person. For these patterns can be associated with abuse in a variety of ways. The psychologically disturbed individual may abuse others, and he or she may be abused by others as a reaction to the disturbing behavior patterns. And, as indicated elsewhere, some elder abuse is actually elder-elder abuse. Hence aged alcoholics or drug abusers may be abusing their own aged relatives.

Situational Stress Theories

One of the factors frequently cited as a cause of family abuse is the prevalence of stress in the family. Proponents of this view point out that situational factors such as poverty, isolation, or occupational stress may cause people to abuse members of their families. It has consistently been found that child and spouse abuse occur more frequently, though not exclusively, in lower-class groups, which are presumed to experience greater stress due to economic deprivation.[58]

Perhaps the primary proponent of the situational stress model is David G. Gil, who believes that there would be no child abuse if it were not for such factors as poverty or job stress.[59] Expanding on this approach to child abuse, Blair Justice and Rita Justice noted that families that have considerable numbers of other problems are more likely to abuse their children.[60] In their sample of abusing parents, they found an unusually high frequency of persons who had undergone a "prolonged series of changes"—economic crises, illnesses, death, accidents. They emphasize that it is the prolonged series of stressful situations, rather than a single stressful event, that promotes violence. It has also been noted that abusive families are unlikely to have social resources to call upon when stressful situations occur. A high association with social isolation was found both among abusive parents[61] and among abused elders.[62]

It has been found that professionals who work with abused elders are divided in their views as to the importance of life crises or situational stress factors in reference to abuse of the aged.[63] Other authorities have suggested that the problems associated with care of an aged person may create stress promoting abuse.[64] Such age-specific factors will be discussed in a later section. In this section, we will discuss some more general, non-age-related stress factors that may tend to promote elder abuse.

As has been indicated, one theory suggests that a family is more likely to engage in abusive behavior toward their children if they have had a number of problems to deal with in a short period of time.[65] It is possible that a similar situation may exist in families characterized by elder abuse. That is, abuse of the elderly may exist in families plagued with a large number of problems, serious and otherwise.

Consequently, some authorities employ stress scales to differentiate abusive from nonabusive families.[66] In the IG study,[67] victims interviewed were asked to respond to a modified version of the Holmes and Rahe stress scale,[68] indicating whether they or members of their families had experienced any of a list of forty-six possible problems in the past year. The problems included such items as death of a spouse or other family member, the existence of debts both large and small, change in or loss of job, changes in living arrangements, and so on.

One striking characteristic of these victims was the large number of problems they or their families had experienced. Twenty percent of the interviewees stated that members of their families had experienced twenty or more of these problems in the past year. Another 30 percent reported having had from eleven to nineteen problems; 35 percent had from five to nine problems; and only 15 percent had had less than five.

These victims' families are clearly "multiproblem" families. It is probable that the abuse of the aged person could not be corrected until the accompanying problems and tensions in the family had been alleviated as well. As has been found with other types of domestic violence, treatment of the entire family and its problems is necessary.

The situational stress theory of domestic abuse has been subjected to severe criticism. It has often been noted that situational stress is inadequate in explaining child abuse, since it fails to show why some families react to stress and frustration by abusing their children, while others, subjected to the same stress, do not.[69] Similarly, a stress model does not totally explain why some adults, when faced with severe family stress, would react by abusing an aged member while others do not.[70] However, the stress model does call attention to the fact that factors outside of the abuser must be considered in explaining the abusive behavior. Thus Justice and Justice conclude that the abuser is an individual with serious personal problems.[71] In working with abusive parents, they contend that the problems of the abuser must be dealt with sympathetically before the relationship with the child can be rebuilt on a nonviolent basis. They further contend that the family must be dealt with as a unit, lest the abuser go back to his or her abusive behavior once family problems and the interactions of other family members reassert themselves.[72] As therapists, they attempt to provide support to the abusing parent.[73]

Theories Focusing on The Nature of Family Relationships

Another approach to the analysis of family violence which has received considerable support is a model that views domestic abuse in the context of general family relationships. This approach suggests that the existence of a well-established pattern of violent behavior on the part of an individual need not necessarily suggest the existence of either situational or psychopathological state.[74] Rather, such behavior, like nonviolent behavior, can be learned in early life. The IG study found evidence to suggest that the elderly victims in our study, as well as the members of their families, may indeed be persons for whom abusive behavior has been learned as an appropriate approach to the solution of life's problems.[75]

Normative Violence

It has been suggested by some authors that domestic abuse is part of a general pattern of "normative violence," in which violent behavior is accepted, even approved, as a normal part of family life. This was an area which was investigated in the IG study. Are these victims persons who are more likely to use and approve of violent behavior, especially in family relationships?

Victims were asked if they were ever punched or hit, or if they had ever been threatened with a knife or gun. Responses could include the abuse reported, other family incidents, or incidents outside the family. Nearly one-half of these elderly people reported that they had been punched or hit. Ten percent had been threatened by another person wielding a knife. What was most shocking was the fact that 35 percent of these aged persons had, at one time or another, been threatened with a gun. In contrast, a study of domestic violence using a national random sample found that 10 percent of persons had been hit or kicked some time during their marriages, and 4 percent had been threatened with a knife or gun.[76] Although the studies are not totally comparable, the national data do suggest that our victims had considerably more violence in their backgrounds. Some even created a sense of discomfort in our interviewers by indicating they were armed at the time of the interview. If these people were part of a "subculture of violence," it would not be surprising if they had come to accept violent action as "normative" or appropriate.[77]

Many of the victims expressed their belief that physical punishment of children was appropriate and necessary. This belief may cause children to grow up with the idea that physical responses are appropriate in instances in which a larger, stronger person has his or her will thwarted by a smaller, weaker person. It would not be surprising if abuse victims learned the lesson that such behavior was appropriate when and if they should move into such a position in reference to their parents. In effect, the aged parents, through their actions when their children were small, may have taught them that abusive behavior was appropriate.

It was also noted that the abusive behavior is closely related to the social role which is generally associated with certain types of abusers. As was noted, sons were more likely to engage in direct abuse, while daughters were more likely to be responsible for emotional abuse or neglectful behavior. Such differences suggest that abuse may be learned as a part of normal sex role patterns, in which men are expected to react in a direct, physical manner, and women to react with emotional outbursts and withholding of affection and support. Hence the data provide some support for the learning theory of domestic abuse.

Long-standing Patterns of Family Violence

When attitudes and behaviors that support the use of violence and force are firmly established in a family, it is likely that such force will be turned against those family members least able to defend themselves. These victims are, therefore, more likely to include children or the aged. In the IG study, the most tragic cases were those showing evidence of a long-term abusive pattern in the family. In these cases, abusive behavior may continue for the entire duration of a marriage, or the victims of abuse may alternate between one generation and another. As Straus, Gelles, and Steinmetz point out, abusive behavior patterns are highly likely to be passed on from parents to children.[78] Several cases will illustrate this type of pattern.

A stroke victim with partial paralysis was hospitalized following an "accident" in which she had allegedly fallen down the stairs. Actually, her husband, who had abused her for most of her married life, had pushed her down the stairs. As a child she had also been abused by her mother. In planning for her release from the hospital, the hospital staff arranged for this victim to live with her daughter instead of returning to her abusive husband. However, it was found that the daughter's husband was also abusive. Hence this family is now in its third generation of abuse, and is rearing a fourth generation of young people who view abuse as a well-established and seemingly appropriate dimension of family life.

In another case, a woman had had her children removed from her custody because she had abused them. Subsequent to the removal of her children, she assumed a role in the care of her invalid father. This case came to light when the daughter poured boiling water over her father, scalding him badly.

Cases such as these suggest that the common pattern of removing a victim from an abusive situation often does little to resolve the situation. While it may protect the specific individual victimized at a given time, it does nothing to assist the abuser in controlling his or her behavior. As a result the abuse may simply be transferred to another likely victim: from child to aged parent, from aged parent to spouse, or perhaps to an unsuspecting friend or neighbor.

Although abuse by children was more common, the IG study found several instances of abuse in marital or pseudomarital relationships. This type of abuse was especially common in cases in which one member of a couple was either considerably older or more infirm then the other. The example of an aged woman whose husband pushed her down the stairs has already been noted. In several cases, however, the usual domestic violence sex roles were reversed, with the woman being the abuser and the man the victim. In two separate cases, children removed an infirm father from the home because they saw evidence that their mother was abusing their father, either physically or emotionally, or both. In both instances the mother claimed that her children were abusing her because they had deprived her of her husband's presence in the home. Yet in one instance a medical examination showed clear evidence of malnutrition in the father, whose condition improved greatly after being removed from his wife's care. A case worker reported that one of these women had stated that her husband had made her suffer for most of her life, and it was now his turn to suffer. In still a third case, the wife and children together took the husband's money and abandoned him.

Victim Precipitation Among the Elderly

A common explanation usually given for domestic abuse is that of victim precipitation: the victim "asked for it." That is, through his or her own misbehavior or goading, the victim forced the offender to take revenge. This view is found often with regard to spouse abuse.[79] The IG study found evidence of this situation among the aged victims we studied. Only eight of the cases gave clear evidence of mutual abuse; in another twenty-five it was unclear as to whether mutual abuse had occurred. However, these cases together constitute 33 percent in which there is a possibility of mutual abuse, and these merit some attention.

Some service providers believed abuse was precipitated by the victim, at least in part, when an aged parent attempted to retain more control over his or her children than most young adults were likely to allow. In one case the mother and her abusive son had a mutually dependent relationship, which was threatened by the son's impending marriage. The abuse of the mother occurred when the mother attempted to block the marriage. In another mother-son case, the mother was an extremely religious woman who wished to convert her son. She constantly berated her son for his sins and he responded by abusing her psychologically. In such cases, agency workers suggested that the abuse would probably not have occurred, or would not have been so severe, if the elders had not engaged in the provocative behavior. It is also clear that the abuse is not likely to cease unless the elderly person can be induced to give up, at least to a degree, the behavior that provokes the abuse.

Family Financial Issues

A considerable amount of the abuse that the IG study uncovered appeared to be provoked by financial difficulties on the part of one or more members of the family. The time of death and the distribution of the decedent's property seemed to be a particularly vulnerable time for an elderly person to be victimized in this way. Abusers included siblings, spouses, grandchildren, and unrelated persons, as well as children.

The most frequent abusers in this type of setting were still the children, however. In one instance a son was known to have taken $80,000 from his father's bank account while his widowed father was in a nursing home. The son also attempted to block his father's remarriage in order to protect any remaining property. Another man who spoke only Spanish, was tricked into signing over his home to his son, who then mortgaged the home and forced his

Domestic Abuse of the Elderly

father to make the payments. In a third case, the abuser was a twenty-year-old woman who made frequent visits to her great-grandmother; during the visits she stole the lady's bank books and emptied her great-grandmother's accounts.

In a few of these cases it appears that there may indeed be true financial need on the part of one or more members of the family which occasions the temptation to take money from the aged person, who is probably seen as having little use for it. In many instances, however, such as the case of the son who had already taken $80,000 and still wanted to insure that he would receive the rest, it is difficult to avoid the conclusion that greed motivates the actions. Observation of this factor could be an important part of the clinical assessment process. Clinical personnel would be wise to investigate the possibility of abuse in cases in which family members appear inordinately concerned about the financial assets of an elder or their possible depletion through medical expenses.

Explanations of Abuse Relating to the Aging Process

Normal family relations can by their very nature be tense and stressful.[80] However, some analysts of elder abuse suggest that the very nature of the aging process creates additional stress and tension in a family. Thus Block and Sinnott list five major factors related to the aging process which they believe may be possible causes of elder abuse.[81] In this section these five factors listed by Block and Sinnott, as well as some manifestations of these and other factors as indicated in the IG data, will be described.

Demographic and Economic Changes

There are no clear data to indicate whether the current cases of elder abuse represent either an increase or a decrease as compared with such problems in the past. Firm statistics are lacking concerning the frequency of elder abuse at the present time; statistics on the prevalence of elder abuse in past decades are impossible to reconstruct. Thus one cannot make any claims that elder abuse is more frequent today than in past generations.

It is suggested, however, that the present demographic and economic patterns are such that they help to promote the likelihood of elder abuse by making it increasingly difficult for adult children to provide necessary care for aged parents.[82] In the past, families were considerably larger, and the life expectancy of the elderly was substantially shorter. Consequently, there were several children in a family who could share the responsibilities of caring for an aged parent. Furthermore, the period of time during which an aged parent would suffer a debilitating illness and require constant care was likely to be only a few years, perhaps a decade at most.

Changes in the medical care available to the aged have greatly increased their life span, with the result that many elderly may live two or more decades during which they require constantly more and more assistance from their children. And the trend toward smaller families means that this increased responsibility falls upon the shoulders of fewer and fewer children. Such factors may make it difficult for even the best-intentioned children to care adequately for their aged parents.[83] Furthermore, the increased life span has been accomplished largely thanks to modern medicine with all of its attendant costs. In families already pressed by the high cost of living, the cost of medical care for an aged parent can "often go beyond the resources of both the elderly parent and the adult children."[84] It is the existence of factors such as these which probably accounts, in large part, for the prevalence of abuse among the aged infirm.[85] Consequently, some authorities believe that elder abuse results from the absence of services to assist families in the care of their aged members.[86]

Changes in the Elderly Person's Life

Compounding the difficulties of care of an aged parent is the fact that the process of aging is often a debilitating one.[87] Many people look forward to retirement as a time of increased freedom and opportunity. However, many factors may intervene to thwart these plans. Old age can be a time of decreasing physical and mental capacity, of increased dependence upon others, of loss of independence, and of loss of social relationships and status.[88] Thus aged persons often find that the activities they were formerly able to perform for themselves—personal care, care of the home, meal preparation—are now beyond their capacity. Social roles they formerly filled—such as caring for children or grandchildren, or holding valued positions in business or community—are no longer theirs. They may have lost valued relatives or friends through illness or death. Thus they suffer great loss of self-esteem as they see themselves becoming progressively less capable. Concurrently, they become more and more dependent upon their children not only for personal care and assistance with normal household tasks, but also for most of their social needs. Such extreme dependency in several areas of life is often impossible for many families to handle, particularly since the increased life span may prolong this dependency period for decades.

Changes in the Life of the Adult Offspring

The increased care required by an aging parent also comes at a highly inopportune time in the lives of many adult offspring. Most caretaking offspring are in middle age, a time which is itself rife with conflict.[89] Men may be facing retirement and looking forward to a more leisurely lifestyle. Children may have left the home, or at least, have reached an age when they no longer need constant care. Middle-aged adults often reach the point at which they find they no longer need to obtain sitters for their children, only to discover that their mobility is now limited by the necessity of finding someone to care for an aged parent in their absence.

As Steinmetz notes, elder abuse resembles child abuse in several ways, including the fact of total dependency, as well as the existence of often severe financial, emotional, and physical stress for the caretaker.[90] With normal childcare, however, parents can usually look forward to a not-too-distant day when the child will be independent. With care of an aged parent, however, caretakers must face ever-increasing dependence for periods of indeterminable duration. There is no relief in sight.

Another problem stems from the fact

that the caretaking task has usually fallen to the women, most of whom stayed at home. In recent years, however, the increased number of women who work outside of the home, particularly after their children are in school, reduces the possibility that there will be middle-aged caretakers available in the family.[91] This caretaking period is also likely to fall at a time when the middle-aged female caretakers are reaching menopause. Hence women are often expected to assume the care of an aged parent or in-law when they themselves are not feeling at their best.

For many middle-aged women, the pressures of parent care may place them in a "no-win" situation, as they are caught between the needs of their aged parents and in-laws and those of their husbands and children. Their husbands may demand more adult time alone; their children are reaching the difficult teen years. On the other hand, their time and energies are increasingly sapped by the growing needs of their aged parents. They may often be emotionally, and even physically unable to cope with both.

It is tempting to criticize middle-aged offspring for being thoughtless and unloving when they resist caring for an aged parent, or even worse, when the person under their care suffers neglect or abuse. These problems in the caretakers' lives are very real, however, and the problem of elder abuse is not likely to be solved as long as there are inadequate supports for families dealing with such stresses.

Problems of Intergenerational Living

Several authorities have pointed out that intergenerational living can itself create stress which may bring about the propensity for abuse.[92] Even families maintaining positive relationships may be placed under severe stress by the problems of constant daily contact. Adding an additional person to a household may create problems of crowding. Adult offspring and grandchildren may be forced to give up their privacy and alter their life-styles in order to accommodate an aged person's needs. Often the caretaking child feels that he or she was forced into having the aged parent in the home. Power conflicts are also likely to occur, as the members of each generation, with their differing views, express conflicting opinions over household maintenance, childcare, and family activities.

Again it is tempting to suggest that a middle-aged offspring or grandchild who would resent making such adjustments in deference to a beloved parent or grandparent is thoughtless and unfeeling. It must be recognized, however, that no one can maintain a totally selfless demeanor for an extended period of time. The needs of all persons in a multigenerational household must be accommodated in order for such a pattern to be successful on a long-term basis. And all too often, the supports necessary for such accommodations are unavailable to the families that require them. Such supports might include, for example, daycare centers for the aged, provisions for short-term care to afford a family an occasional vacation, as well as financial supports for families that assume the responsibility of in-home care of the aged.

The Effect of Aging on Long-Standing Family Relationships

All the factors mentioned above can create serious difficulties even for the most loving of children who are anxious to provide the best of care for their aged relatives. It must be recognized, however, that many families do not resemble the image of the loving, harmonious family.[93] We have already pointed out that some elder abuse is actually an extension into old age of abusive and violent patterns that have existed in the family for years or even generations. It is also true that families that have managed to contain their conflict within bounds in earlier periods may be unable to continue to do so when faced with the problems of old age.

Children who have never had a good relationship with their parents may be able to avoid open conflict by maintaining a degree of social distance between the generations. The constant contact required by a caretaking relationship may destroy this fragile peace; conflict and possible abuse may be the result. It has also been noted that some offspring never mature to the point of accepting their parents on an adult level. They are unable to accept the new role relationship in which their parents are no longer all-powerful and are increasingly dependent upon their children.[94] The aged parent may also be unable to accept the altered role relationship and thus, the adult status of their children, and may make constant unreasonable demands and interfere with their adult children's lives and decisions.

Such parent-adult child relationships appear to be the most likely to be involved in elder abuse. As we noted earlier, however, some cases of elder abuse involve spouse abuse. Cases have already been discussed that represent a continuation of a long abusive pattern. In some instances, however, the abuse may be precipitated by problems of aging. For example, a fragile marital relationship may be unable to survive the increased contact which accompanies retirement. Couples may also find that role reversal accompanies old age. Thus a husband who is accustomed to having his wife handle all household tasks may be unable to deal with her becoming an invalid. One case of severe neglect our study uncovered involved a frail but proud old man whose invalid wife was badly in need of health care assistance; her husband, however, resisted all efforts to help, insisting they could care for themselves.

Such cases may often occur with cases of neglect of the aged, since the caretakers may themselves be aged and frail. It is not unknown for eighty- or ninety-year-old parents to be dependent for total care upon their sixty- or seventy-year-old offspring, who may be incapable of carrying out the tasks required for the care of the parent. To accuse a seventy-year-old caretaker of neglect for failing to provide the health assistance required by a bedridden parent or spouse may be highly unreasonable. Hence nursing interventions for an aged person must be planned with an eye towards assuring there is a reasonable expectation that the family is capable of carrying out the plans without undue stress being produced.

Loneliness of the Single Aged as a Cause of Abuse

When family abuse is discussed, the usual patterns involved include the traditional family relationships: spouses, children, or less frequently, grandchildren, siblings, nieces, and nephews. However, only 14 percent of aged women and 5 percent of aged men live with their children or other relatives.[95] Consequently, the majority of elderly people often find themselves alone, either without family nearby on whom they can rely, or with family who cannot or will not assist them. Hence they may be willing to trust a friendly outsider who offers assistance, perhaps more willing than might be altogether prudent. One hears a great deal about the fear of crime which pervades the aged population.[96] One would think, therefore, that the elderly would be extremely cautious in admitting unknown persons to their homes. Upon occasion, however, aged persons may be less cautious, often with sad results.

In the IG study, one case involved a stroke victim, who was unable to remain alone after her return from the hospital. She and her family arranged for a homemaking service agency to provide care in her home; but as the cost became prohibitive, they accepted the offer of a distant relative to come into the home and provide this service at a lesser cost. Unknown to the family, however, the willing housekeeper was a drug addict. She was extremely abusive to the aged lady, screaming at her and refusing to assist her in going to the bathroom or the bedroom, and even attacking her physically. Another aged woman took in a boarder who was presumed to be a good risk; however, she kept late hours and was very loud, making it difficult for the elderly landlady to sleep. Upon being asked to move, she refused and the lady had to get legal assistance to get her out of the house.

Another situation which portends a strong tendency for abuse is the life-style of the aged single male. Whether widowed, divorced, or never married, these men often find that their ability to attract women has drastically decreased; yet they still have the same sexual needs and desire for female companionship. As a result they often place themselves in situations in which they can easily be taken advantage of by younger women, who promise companionship and sexual favors and then abuse them, usually by stealing money.

Such instances make it clear that extreme caution should be exercised by aged persons before taking anyone into their home or their confidence. With family and close friends, they are likely to have at least some idea of the person's behavior patterns and the likelihood of risk. With strangers, they often will not know anything about the risk until after it is too late.

Theories of Elder Abuse as Clinical Indicators

There is no clear theory or set of theories which have been indisputably established as explanations for the existence of elder abuse. The theoretical positions that have been proposed remain largely in the nature of hypotheses. However, as was noted earlier, these theories may serve as valuable indicators of the likelihood of abuse. Aged persons who exhibit, or whose families exhibit, any of the characteristics listed here are persons whose associates or living arrangements place them in considerable danger of being abused physically or emotionally, severely neglected, or placed in a position of extreme financial disadvantage. They may be in great need of help and may not know of any alternative to their present situation. Because of the greater health needs of the aged, they may come into contact with nurses more than with most other professionals. The factors suggested by theories of domestic abuse provide symptoms which can help to identify those aged who may be in need of such help.

Because the same family patterns affect young and old alike, some explanations of domestic violence in general are equally applicable to elder abuse. Hence some aged appear to be abused because they have the misfortune to be associated with family members who have severe psychological or emotional problems lending support to abuser-focused theories. The situational stress theory appears quite promising, because a substantial number of aged abuse victims are found to come from families that have an unusually large number of serious family problems. Support can also be found for the view that elder abuse occurs in families where there is a long-term, well-established behavior pattern in which violence and abuse play an accepted role.

Authorities have also noted, however, that certain social correlates of the aging process play a special role in the development of the types of family tension which may lead to elder abuse. The increased life expectancy of the aged, with its increased years of dependency and burgeoning health care costs, places an ever-increasing burden on fewer and fewer children for a longer period of time. Such tensions often place severe stress on families already strained by crises of middle age or already tenuous family ties. Steps in preventing elder abuse must recognize the legitimacy of such family needs. Proposed solutions need to include means of relieving the tensions of the care-giving family if elder abuse is to be halted or avoided.

MEANS USED BY AGENCIES IN IDENTIFYING AND SERVING ABUSED AGED

One major problem which is encountered in providing services to victims of elder abuse is the identification of victims. Services cannot be provided until agencies become aware of the persons in need of help. And abused elders like other victims of family abuse are very difficult to identify.

Most studies have suggested that abuse of the elderly is probably greatly underreported.[97] The reasons for this include both a reluctance on the part of victims to report their abuse, and hesitance on the part of official agencies to invade the privacy of the home. It has been noted that victims of domestic violence are more reluctant to report their victimization than other victims. One commonly recognized reason is that people are embarrassed to admit that their own families depart from the presumed norm of family harmony and love.[98] An admission of family violence suggests a failure in oneself for not having achieved the ideal of family harmony. Thus a battered elder may feel that he or she has failed by having raised an abusing child. It has also been noted that a desire to maintain the family's reputation and avoid embarrassment may serve as considerations that lead the abused person to the decision of not reporting the abuse to a professional.[99]

Another reason for reluctance to report on the part of victims of domestic abuse is their fear of reprisals from the abuser. Such reprisals may involve the threat of further violence, the fear of losing support, or both. Domestic abuse victims are often dependent upon their abusers. As Gelles has pointed out, victims of domestic violence have "no place to go" where they can be free of the threat of further abuse.[100] Such fears are commonly mentioned by abused wives as the reason they do not report the abuse.[101]

Richard L. Douglass, Thomas Hickey, and Catherine Noel recognize the fear of reprisal as a reason for nonreporting.[102] Dependence of the victim upon the abuser is also mentioned by Block and Sinnott.[103] In addition, Douglass, Hickey, and Noel point out that many elderly decline to report the abuse because they fear the loss of the relationship with the abuser, who may be a beloved child and perhaps one's closest remaining relative.[104]

Many elderly victims are also reluctant to turn to professional agencies because they lack knowledge or have fear of the agencies themselves. Disorientation, senility, or a simple lack of knowledge concerning available services may render a victim incapable of reporting the fact that he or she has been abused.[105] Those victims who are aware of available resources may still resist reporting the abuse because they feel incapable of coping with the responsibilities which may ensue if they do report.[106] Possible court appearances or conversations with the police can be fear-provoking experiences in themselves.

For all of these reasons, some abuse victims are so reluctant to deal with the abuse that they will refuse professional help even if it is offered.[107] Hence, dealing with elder abuse is a task requiring great care and tact. Block and Sinnott suggest that civil rather than criminal means are more appropriate for dealing with elder abuse.[108] One reason is the lesser stigma that attaches to such a judgment, allowing both offender and victim to deal with the problem more easily.

This reluctance of victims to report abuse is especially serious in view of the fact that most agencies depend at least partially upon victim reports to identify victims. In a survey of 108 agencies, 16 of 25 agencies seeing elder abuse noted that a client report was at least one of the means by which the abusive situation was identified.[109] Seven agencies reported that they learned of the abuse through a report from another agency. Physical symptoms such as cuts and bruises were a source of identifying abused elders for 5 of the agencies, while 3 mentioned that they became aware of elderly victims from police reports. Ten agencies noted that "other" means of identifying abused elders were also used. These other means included symptoms of neglect such as malnourishment in an elder not living alone, and reports from family members, neighbors, and friends. In addition, dentists were particularly mentioned by some agencies as a source of referral. Most agencies (17) reported that two symptoms of abuse were present in cases in which they had identified abused elders.

It has also been found that some agencies, and some workers in every agency, are more likely to identify abuse cases than are other agencies or workers. In the IG study, the largest number of cases by far was reported by a legal aid agency, which reported thirty cases, or nearly 40 percent of the total.[110] There are two reasons for this prevalence: First, a legal aid agency would be very likely to be consulted by persons wth serious physical and/or financial abuse in an effort to deal with the problem. Second, it was quite clear that two workers in this agency were very concerned about the abuse, to the extent of rereading old case records in order to make accurate reports on the cases. This agency vividly illustrates the fact that agency service to elderly abuse victims is quite dependent on two factors: the nature of the agency and the interest of the individual worker.

Agency Type and the Observation of Abuse

As noted earlier, some authors suggest that agencies are more likely to observe abuse

Table 6-5 *Abuse Type by Reporting Agency*

Reporting Agency	Physical Abuse	Physical Neglect	Emotional Neglect/ Deprivation of Rights	Emotional Abuse	Financial Abuse
Health	(4)26.7%	(1) 5.6%	(5)27.8%	(8)18.2%	(2) 4.9%
Family, Mental Health	(2)13.3	(2)11.1	(2)11.1	(3) 6.8	(3) 7.3
Senior Service	(1) 6.7	(9)50.0	(7)38.9	(7)15.9	(5)12.2
Churches, Schools	(2)13.3	(1) 5.6	(1) 5.6	(2) 4.5	(2) 4.9
Law Enforcement	(1) 6.7	(1) 5.6	(1) 5.6	(2) 4.5	(1) 2.4
Legal Aid	(5)33.3	(4)22.2	(2)11.1	(22)50.0	(28)68.3
Totals	(15)	(18)	(18)	(44)	(41)

Abuse Type*

in the area they are accustomed to treating.[111] Data from the IG study provide some additional support for this view.[112] As Table 6-5 shows, one out of four instances (26.7 percent) of physical abuse was reported by the health agencies.* Only the legal aid agency, which reported the largest number of abuse cases by far, reported a larger percentage of physical abuse cases (33.3 percent). One would expect health-related agencies to be more likely to note physical abuse since they would be called upon to treat the resulting injuries and are accustomed to observing such symptoms.

Physical neglect, on the other hand, was more likely to be observed by senior service agencies, which reported one-half of these cases. Again, this is not surprising since these agencies are often called upon to assist aged persons who have need of food, shelter, or housekeeping assistance, all of which may be related to neglect. Such agencies are also more likely to observe emotional neglect (38.9 percent of the observed cases). The health agencies reported the next largest frequency of this type of case (27.8 percent).

Both direct emotional abuse and financial abuse were most frequently identified by the legal aid agency which identified one-half of the former and two-thirds of the latter cases. Legal aid attorneys would be in a particularly good position to learn of such abuse, since victims would be very likely to bring these problems to an attorney. Persons who believe they have been cheated out of money or property are likely to seek a lawyer to regain what they believe to be rightfully theirs. Seeking aid from an attorney would also seem appropriate when one is the victim of verbal assault and fears for his or her safety. In fact, the legal aid agencies appear to be highly promising as a mechanism for identifying elder abuse cases of all types, particularly those that involve direct action (for ex-

---

* In Table 6-5 each type of abuse present in multiple abuse cases was considered independently; hence, more than seventy-seven instances are considered.

ample, abuse as opposed to neglect). The legal aid attorney has the opportunity to interview a client and elicit information concerning all aspects of life, thus making it possible to uncover symptoms of abuse in all areas. Fortunately, the Federal Administration of Aging has recently made the identification of elder abuse a priority for agencies providing legal aid to the elderly.[113]

It was reported earlier that agencies tended to identify abuse victims largely through the victim's own reports. This information is confirmed by the cases the agencies reported to us. In over one-half of the cases the initial report of the abuse to the agency was made by the victim. Other sources of reports were hospitals or clinics; other social service agencies, both public and private; or public health agencies. The police were a source of referral in only two cases. Six cases came to agency attention through a referral by a member of the family and two through referral by a friend. Five cases were regular cases of the agency, and abuse was uncovered as a part of normal handling of the case.

Clearly, one factor that made identification of victims more difficult was the fact that each agency is geared up to "notice" only symptoms that characterize the problems treated by that agency. Thus hospitals are likely to observe physical abuse, but will miss psychological or financial abuse. Social agencies are more likely to observe psychological abuse, and will learn of physical abuse only by reports of the victim or if the symptoms are particularly obvious. The one agency that reported the widest variety of cases was the legal aid agency, to which persons with all types of problems were referred for possible consideration of a legal remedy. It appears likely that more abuse would be uncovered if agencies that serve the aged would become more aware of the symptoms of abuse other than those that their agency is used to observing.

Services Provided to Victims

Even if an abused victim decides to report the experience to some authority, it is not at all clear that he or she will receive any assistance in dealing with the matter. Thus Block and Sinnott found that although 95 percent of their sample reported their victimization, no victim received assistance.[114] This is similar to the pattern that appears with most domestic abuse. A tendency to "accept-and-hide" domestic violence has been encouraged by society as a whole, from friends and relatives of the violent family to official agencies. Wife abuse victims are often encouraged by their families to accept the situation.[115] Medical practitioners, who are most likely to see evidence of serious violence, often try to avoid dealing with domestic abuse, both of children[116] and adults.[117] Police and the courts, normally the avenue of redress for the victim of criminal assault and/or civil injury, have largely ignored domestic assaults.[118] This is due partly to the belief that such things are best left a private matter, and partly to the recognition that domestic disturbance calls can be very dangerous for the police.[119]

Noncriminal approaches to such domestic problems are usually recommended.[120] However, it has also been noted that traditional counseling agencies have not dealt very effectively with family violence. Marriage counselors and social workers often encourage the maintenance of family ties, even violent ones.[121] Conflicting advice is also given. Thus some counselors encourage the open expression of aggressive feelings in order to vent them in appropriate channels[122] while others believe that expressed hostility can generate even more aggressive feelings.[123]

In the cases reported to the IG study, referral or legal action were the most common types of agency responses.[124] In eighteen cases (23 percent) the client was referred to another agency, which the referring agency presumably believed was better qualified to serve the victim. In seventeen cases (22 percent) legal action was taken. These involved primarily the legal aid cases and involved action such as filing suit to remove a roomer from a home or to regain lost property.

Counseling was also commonly used. In thirteen cases (17 percent) the victim was counseled. Nearly as many attempts were made to counsel the abusing family (twelve cases or 16 percent). Other direct action was taken in 17 percent of cases. This included assisting victims in obtaining food, housekeeping services, a change in residence, financial assistance from Social Security or the Veteran's Administration, and so on.

In nearly two-thirds of the cases (62 percent) the agency workers felt that their efforts had led to a change in the situation. Another 29 percent said that they had not produced a change in the situation. The rest did not respond or did not know whether a change had occurred.

The Interest of the Individual Professional

One clear problem is the uneven quality of service provided to abuse victims by different agencies. Some medical institutions were quite likely to observe abuse while others avoided the problem; religious institutions were mentioned by some victims as being unsympathetic, yet some churches and ministers referred cases to us and were quite concerned about them. It became clear that the major factor generating effective service for abused elders was a high degree of personal concern and interest on the part of the specific professional assigned to the case. It was not enough for the agency as a whole to have a general policy of helping abused victims, because individual professionals could avoid the problem if they wished. Conversely, some providers in agencies with a clear policy of disinterest in the problem appeared to be among the most helpful, spending much time and effort to unravel the bureaucratic red tape impeding effective service to the abuse victims.

Hence certain professionals in an agency are more likely to develop an interest in the area of domestic abuse and to search for this problem among their clients. One might say these professionals have had their "consciousness raised" regarding the problem of domestic abuse. Consequently, they inquire about the family situation and are more likely to learn of abuse if it exists. Furthermore, agency providers in personal conversations told us that family abuse was a problem which was not likely to be uncovered very easily. Rather, a substantial number of visits and a considerable rapport had to be developed with a client before most clients were willing to discuss family abuse.

The professions represented by the reporters of abuse varied widely. The two most frequent reporters were legal aid attorneys, which is not surprising since this agency reported the most cases by far. Leaving these aside, however, other professionals reporting substantial numbers of cases were social workers (18 percent) and staff workers of senior centers (16 percent). Other professionals reporting were nurses (7 percent), psychologists or counselors (4 percent), and religious workers (5 percent).

Finally, it should be mentioned that some professionals, and some agencies as well, had difficulty dealing with family abuse because of a preference for viewing the topic as a "private matter," an approach which is often taken with regard to child or spouse abuse. One agency professional reported a case in which a woman was referred to a hospital for injuries suffered in an instance of physical abuse. The provider stated: "I really have no right to interfere in this case. If she wants to go back to live with her son (i.e., the abuser), then that is her right. He's her son and she wants to live with him, and that's the way she has worked out her life. I shouldn't interfere." However, the provider was not willing to consider the possibility that she might have had an obligation to suggest possible alternatives which the aged woman might not have known existed. In situations such as the above, the abuse victim sees no alternative to accepting the abuse. What is even more tragic is the fact that this professional also described another case of abuse which resulted in death.

The Need for Further Research and Planning

As a consequence, domestic abuse has been greatly neglected by service providers. This is true of child and spouse abuse as well as elder abuse. As Block and Sinnott point out, strategies of intervention must be developed primarily to end the abuse, but secondarily to help in establishing the physical and mental well-being of the entire family.[125] As noted earlier, usually the abuser is also a person with severe problems which must be solved before the abuse can be stopped. And for most abused elders, severance of the abusive relationship is not viewed as a desirable alternative.[126] Clearly, further research is necessary in order to determine the needs of aged abuse victims and the most appropriate ways of providing for them.

It has been suggested that the problems of providing care for aging family members are likely to become more severe in future years. As Block and Sinnott point out:

> Decreasing fertility and mortality rates mean that there will be more older persons and fewer children available as possible caretakers. The adult child may be faced with as many as two sets of grandparents to care for as well as aging parents.[127]

The emotional, physical, and financial resources of such caretaking offspring become depleted very quickly, leading to resentment against the aged relatives perceived to have caused the difficulty. In such settings, there is an increased possibility of abuse being directed against the aged requiring the care. Increased support for elders and their caretaking families are necessary if such abuse is to be avoided.[128]

SUGGESTED NURSING CARE FOR ELDER ABUSE VICTIMS

As has been seen in this chapter, abuse of the elderly is a topic that has only recently received attention from researchers and service providers. Due to the relative "newness" of the area, research on elder abuse is limited in several respects: most samples are small and are purposive rather than random; studies are exploratory in nature concentrating on the development of hypotheses rather than on the testing of theories in existence. These limitations make it difficult to generate a universal tool for the identification of elder abuse. Consequently, the suggestions that are made in this section must be viewed as tentative. It is fairly certain that the description of possible symptomatology is representative of elder abuse cases studies to date. The presented at-risk indicators may have to be revised, however, when more knowledge has been accumulated in this area.

Assessment

The task of obtaining an accurate assessment of abuse in an elderly client requires that the nurse overcome a number of formidable obstacles. These include the reluctance of the victim to admit abuse; the necessity of developing a strong, trusting relationship before abuse can be identified; the absence of a clearly defined symptomatology for elder abuse; and the difficulty of distinguishing symptoms of elder abuse from the normal symptoms of aging. In this section each of these difficulties, together with possible remedies, will be discussed.

Reluctance of Victims to Report

The reluctance of abuse victims to report abuse and the reasons for this reluctance, have been noted previously. Victims often fear retaliation from the abuser, loss of support, or loss of their relationship with loved ones. They may also feel guilt or shame if they have raised children who are abusive, or have maintained close social and/or familial ties with abusive relatives. They are unwilling to admit the presence of an abusive situation to someone perceived to be an authority due to fear of the possible consequences of such a report. Some elderly victims of rather severe abuse cannot admit even to themselves that a beloved relative would abuse them. Such victims are therefore incapable of reporting the abuse, since they are not really aware that abuse is occurring.

Developing Trust

Such reluctance to admit abuse may be overcome if the nurse is careful to develop a trusting relationship with the client. Admissions of abuse are not likely to be forthcoming unless the client has come to feel that the nurse is someone who accepts him or her and does not present a threat to his or her well-being. Victims must believe that the nurse does not stand in judgment of them for being in or remaining in an abusive situation. They must also believe that the nurse has a genuine desire to help them and will not reveal their difficulty to authorities against their will. Consequently, any aged patient with a possible vulnerability toward abuse must be approached by the nurse in a holistic and nonthreatening manner.

Particularly with short-term clients, it may be difficult to develop the degree of trust necessary in the nurse-client relationship in order to obtain an accurate patient assessment. Professionals interviewed by Sengstock and Barrett often stated that an abusive situation was not uncovered until the professional and client had established

Domestic Abuse of the Elderly

a long-term, trusting relationship.[129] Many of the service providers expressed concern that abuse might be overlooked in the case of the client whose presenting problem required only short-term intervention or presented at-risk indicators with which the practitioner was unfamiliar.

Ambiguous Indications

Because of the difficulty of obtaining an admission of abuse, it is often the nurse's responsibility to identify a victim of elder abuse on the basis of an observation of presenting at-risk findings. Unfortunately, however, there is no list of indicators that clearly identifies elder abuse in the absence of other verifying evidence. As can be seen from Table 6-6, a number of indicators found in the client's history may be suggestive of abuse, but when taken as independent entities may not support the suspicion that the client is being victimized by family and/or friends. For example, a chronic physical disability may not be indicative of abuse. Similarly, conditions such as poverty may not indicate that an elderly person is at risk or has been abused. Even fractures or extensive bruising may not be clear indicators of abuse. In such cases, the client should be further observed for other possible indicators of abuse.

Since there are no clear physical indicators of elder abuse, the nurse may often find that a victim of abuse must be identified on the basis of a configuration of at-risk findings. Hence extensive bruising or a chronic illness alone may not indicate abuse, but these findings, coupled with the nurse's observation of other indicators, such as overt antagonism between the client and family or friends, may lead to a suspicion of abuse. Consequently, it is imperative that the nurse obtain a thorough case history of clients in which abuse is a possible cause of the findings. A thorough assessment would include an overview of the physical, social, and psychological characteristics of the elder and his or her significant others, especially those on whom the supposed victim is dependent. Relevant factors in the case history are outlined in Table 6-7. Since it is recognized that this depth of information is often impossible to obtain, it is imperative that the nurse be prepared to obtain much of the assessment data from objective observations of the client and the client's family, social network, and environment.

Differentiating Abuse from the Normal Aging Process

The problem of using physical findings when assessing an elderly person for the presence of abuse deserves special attention. While physical indicators appear to be among the most valid symptoms of abuse or neglect in the child or middle-aged person, it has been noted that apparent symptoms of abuse in an elderly person may in fact be due to the aging process.[130] Richard Ham's discussion of the problems of identifying physical abuse of the elderly observes that the normal physiological processes which govern normal aging lead to physiological changes such as increased capillary fragility, osteoporosis, poor balance, poor vision, mental confusion, and musculoskeletal stiffness, among others. In elaborating upon these physiological changes, Ham states that the elderly may be more likely to lose their balance and fall. Since they are more likely to suffer from skeletal fractures and bleed,

Table 6-6 *Physical Examination of Elderly Persons—Indicators of Potential or Actual Elder Abuse**

Area of Assessment	At-Risk Responses
I. General Appearance	Fearful, anxious
	Marked passivity
	Malnourished looking
	Poor hygiene
	Inappropriate dress, re: weather conditions
	Physical handicap
	Antagonism and/or detachment between elder and caretaker
II. Vital Statistics	
A. Height	
B. Weight	Underweight
C. Head Circumference	
III. Skin	Excessive or unexplainable bruises, welts, scars, possibly in various stages of healing
	Decubitus ulcers
	Burns
	Infected or untreated wound
IV. Head	
V. Eyes	No prosthetic device to accommodate poor eyesight
VI. Ears	No prosthetic device to accommodate poor hearing
VII. Nose	
VIII. Mouth	Bruising, lacerations
	Gross dental caries
	No prosthetic device to accommodate loss of teeth
IX. Neck	
X. Chest	
XI. Abdomen	Abdominal distention
XII. Genital/Urinary	Vaginal lacerations
	Vaginal infection
	Urinary tract infection
XIII. Rectal	
XIV. Musculoskeletal	Skull/facial fractures
	Fractured femur
	Fractures of other parts of the body
XV. Neurological	Limited motion of extremities
	Difficulty with speech
	Difficulty with swallowing

*Symptoms listed may be symptoms of normal aging. Therefore, physical symptoms must be assessed in conjunction with the patient's personal history.

Domestic Abuse of the Elderly

Table 6-7 *History of Elder—Possible Indicators of Potential or Actual Elder Abuse*

Area of Assessment	At-Risk Responses
I. Primary Concern/Reason for Visit	Historical data that conflicts with physical findings
	Acute or chronic psychological and/or physical disability
	Inability to participate independently in activities of daily living
	Inappropriate delay in bringing elder to health care facility
	Reluctance on the part of caretaker to give information on elder's condition
	Inappropriate caretaker reaction to nurse's concern (overreacts, underreacts)
II. Family Health	
A. Elder	Grew up in a violent home (abused as child, spouse; abused children)
	Substance abuse
	Excessive dependence of elder on child(ren)
B. Child(ren) of Elder	Were abused by parents as children
	Antagonistic relationship with elder
	Excessive dependence on elder
	Substance abuse
	History of violent relationship with other siblings and/or spouse
C. Siblings	Antagonistic relationship between siblings
	Excessive dependence of one or more siblings on another or each other
D. Other Family Members and Family Relations	Other history of abuse and/or neglect or violent death
E. Household	Violence and aggression used to resolve conflicts and solve problems
	Past history of abuse and/or neglect among family members
	Poverty
	Few or no friends or neighbors or other support systems available
	Excessive number of stressful situations encountered during a short period of time (unemployment, death of a relative or significant other, etc.)

(continued)

Table 6-7 (Cont.)

Area of Assessment	At-Risk Responses
III. Health History of Elder	
A. Child	History of chronic physical and/or psychological disability
B. Midlife	History of chronic physical and/or psychological disability
C. Nutrition	History of feeding problems (G.I. disease, food preference idiosyncracies)
	Inappropriate food, drink, or drugs
	Dietary intake that does not fit with findings
	Inadequate food or fluid intake
D. Personal/Social	Caretaker has unrealistic expectations of elder
	Social isolation (little or no contact with friends, neighbors, or relatives; lack of outside activity)
	Substance abuse
	History of spouse abuse (as victim and/or abuser)
	History of antagonistic relationships among family members (between family members in general, including elder)
	Large age difference between elder and spouse
	Large number of family problems
	Excessive dependence on spouse, children, or significant others
E. Discipline	
1. Physical	Belief that the use of physical punishment is appropriate
	Threats with an instrument as a means to punish
	Use of an instrument to administer physical punishment
	Excessive, inappropriate, inconsistent physical punishment
	History of caretaker and/or others "losing control" and/or "hitting too hard"
2. Emotional/Violation of Rights	Fear provoking threats
	Infantilization
	Berating

Domestic Abuse of the Elderly

Table 6-7 *(Cont.)*

Area of Assessment	At-Risk Responses
	Screaming
	Forced move out of home
	Forced institutionalization
	Prohibiting marriage
	Prevention of free use of money
	Isolation
F. Sleep	
G. Elimination	
H. Illness	Chronic illness or handicap
	Disability requiring special treatment from caretaker and others
I. Operations/Hospitalizations	Operations or illness that required extended and/or repeated hospitalizations
	Caretaker's refusal to have elder hospitalized
	Caretaker overanxious to have elder hospitalized
J. Diagnostic Tests	Caretaker's refusal for further diagnostic tests
	Caretaker's overreaction or underreaction to diagnostic findings
K. Accidents	Repeated
	History of preceding events which do not support actual injuries
L. Safety	Appropriate safety precautions not taken, especially in elders known to be confused, disoriented, and/or with physical disabilities restricting mobility
M. Health Care Utilization	Infrequent
	Caretaker overanxious to have elder hospitalized
	Health care "shopping"
N. Review of Body Systems	

a relatively minor fall may result in numerous fractures and extensive bruising, subdural hematomas, and hemorrhage which may be fatal. In addition, Ham notes that elderly clients who are suffering from senile dementia may develop delusions concerning the treatment they receive from others. Thus physiological aging may generate complaints of mistreatment.

According to Ham, all of these findings

may mimic abuse; thus he warns against "falsely diagnosing" abuse as the cause of suspicious physical and psychological symptomatology. While his observations may be accurate, they also mask a dangerous set of assumptions that must be avoided if aged abuse victims are to be served. Research to date on elder abuse has shown that victims are often not recognized since professionals tend to observe instances of abuse only when they are actively looking for the problem.[131] Consequently, it is imperative that professionals not dismiss prematurely the possibility of abuse when suspicious findings are present.

Results of physical examination should be assessed in conjunction with historical data which the nurse has collected on the client, as noted in Table 6-7. Careful questioning on the part of the nurse may determine such things as whether a client who complains of mistreatment is exhibiting symptoms of confusion, dementia, or is in fact expressing a valid complaint of abuse, or if it is actually the result of a physical assault. Thus the importance of obtaining a thorough, objective history on elderly clients cannot be overemphasized.

Intervention

As has been noted, an elderly client may be reluctant to admit the existence of abuse even though a number of historical and physical findings point to its presence. It would be wise, therefore, for the nurse to proceed as if the client is at risk until abuse has been ruled out as at least a partial cause of the elderly individual's problem. Three factors appear to be important in the development of an adequate program of intervention. These are the establishment of a strong trusting relationship with the client; maintenance of a single individual as primary care provider; and the development of a comprehensive plan which can be followed by and coordinated with all caregivers.

Trust as a Major Component of Care

Establishing a trusting relationship appears to be the most critical component, not only in assessment, but also in the provision of adequate care to aged abuse victims. Clients, especially those who have experienced the trauma of domestic violence, are not likely to accept assistance from nurses or any other outsiders unless they believe the care provider is deserving of their trust. Such trust can be fostered if the nurse exhibits a sympathetic concern for the client and thus indicates that the client's feelings are important, that the nurse understands the victim's problems, is interested in his or her well-being, and is willing to put forth effort in the client's behalf. Such concern is especially evident in the nurse's nonjudgmental demeanor. Abuse victims are not likely to accept care if they feel that the nurse is critical either of them or of their loved ones, even if they are abusive.

Unfortunately, the establishment of a trusting relationship is particularly difficult in elder abuse cases. This difficulty arises from two factors. One is the particular barrier to the development of a trusting relationship on the part of abuse victims. The other is the lengthy time span required for the development of trust.

It has been observed that abuse victims find it particularly difficult to establish trusting relationships.[132] Many elder abuse victims have had little opportunity to maintain trusting relationships with others, since those who are closest to them are the same persons who abuse them. They are often unable to confide in family members other than the abuser, since such relatives may have difficulty relating both to the abuser and the victim. As a result, abused elders often lack the ability to trust and confide in anyone. The concerned nurse must overcome this barrier before a trusting relationship can be established with the victim-client.

Data on elder abuse gathered to date also suggest that developing a trusting relationship is a time-consuming process.[133] It is often necessary to establish a long-term relationship with a professional before a feeling of trust is exhibited by the victim. Only then is the victim able to admit that abuse is present, either as the underlying problem or as an additional problem which has been overlooked. Thus intervention in cases requiring only short-term medical attention presents nurses with a particular challenge, as they strive to attain the critical attitude of trust.

Importance of a Primary Care Provider

The utilization of a primary care nurse in order to promote continuity of care as well as to aid in the development of trust is vital. This person must be sympathetic to the problem of abuse and be someone with whom the client is able to communicate. The role of the primary care nurse can be particularly important in dealing with abuse cases since both victim and family are usually reluctant to accept outside help. Professionals who have had little contact with such persons may find them uncooperative and unwilling to accept help. The nurse who has established a trusting relationship with the client can act as a liaison between the victim and professionals from other areas.

An example of such intervention is the common instance in which the nurse refers a client to social services. In such a situation, the nurse should provide the social worker with a detailed history of the client, explain why abuse is suspected, and also discuss all factors contributing to the abusive situation. The nurse should also prepare the client concerning this intervention and preferably be present during the social worker's initial visit. While these measures might sound time-consuming and unnecessary under normal circumstances, in the case of the abused elder they are very important. It is more likely that the abused elder will accept outside assistance if it is encouraged and supported by a professional whom the victim already trusts.

Development of a Comprehensive Plan

The importance of a comprehensive plan cannot be overemphasized. Such interventions must be the result of an ongoing process, which is originally based upon an accurate assessment of the client's condition, developed as much as possible in collaboration with the victim and family, and undergoes constant reassessment and alteration as new observations about the client's needs become evident. Such a plan should prove to be an effective method in the establishment of a trusting relationship as well as in the provision of high quality care to the elder abuse patient.

This is particularly important in those cases in which only short-term care is to be provided, or in cases in which the client is to be assisted by a number of care providers. Other nurses, and other professionals involved in the care of the elder, should be fully familiarized with the plan of care for the client and should be observant concerning other at-risk findings which the client and situation exhibit. These observations should be continually added to the initial assessment of the client in order to obtain an accurate record concerning the client's overall situation.

Evaluation of Nursing Intervention

Evaluating the effectiveness of nursing intervention in elder abuse cases is also a challenging problem. Particularly in cases in which nursing intervention is short term in nature, nurses may not be able to ascertain whether or not they had a long-term effect on the well-being of an abused elderly patient. However, there are some clues which the nurse may use to help determine whether the assistance has been of value. These include client's acknowledgment of the abuse; willingness of the victim, the abuser, and the family to accept outside help; and/or removal of the victim from the abusive situation.

Victim's Acknowledgment of Abuse

As has been noted, a great many victims of elder abuse are reluctant to admit, even to themselves, that an abusive situation exists. However, assistance to an abuse victim cannot begin until there is an acknowledgment of the abuse. Hence an admission on the part of the victim that abuse exists should be considered to be an important sign that the client has made progress in dealing with the abuse. Dealing with an abusive situation often requires years of diligent work on the part of dedicated professionals. If the nurse's work leads the client to begin this process, this should be viewed as a major accomplishment.

Willingness to Accept Intervention

Another sign that the nursing intervention has been successful is an observed willingness on the part of victim, abuser, and/or other family members to accept outside intervention and needed support services. It has been hypothesized that much of the elder abuse that exists today is caused by the stress of caring for an elderly, dependent relative.[134] In such cases, daycare, meal services, and other assistance with activities of daily living can be of great benefit in alleviating the stress in the family and the resulting abuse as well. Hence the willingness of the abuser to see a counselor, the willingness of the family to reorganize family activities, or the willingness of the elderly victim to accept daycare or housekeeping services are all indications that the abuse may be on the road to resolution.

Removal of the Victim from the Abusive Situation

It has been noted, however, that some elder abuse is the result of a long-standing pattern of abuse in the lives of the victims and their families. In such situations, it is unlikely that even long-term nursing intervention will have a substantial impact on the abusive pattern. In long-term abusive patterns, the only likely solution is the separation of the abuser and the abused. In these cases, the establishment of the victim in a living situation separate from that of the abuser should be seen as a positive step. Examples would be nursing home placement or moving the victim to a senior citizens' residence. Placement with another relative may not be a positive sign in a habitually abusive family because such families tend to foster abuse in all members, and the victim may simply move from one problem situation to another.

Summary

Abuse of the elderly has been neglected by professionals and public alike. Child abuse and abuse of female partners, although also inadequately recognized, have received much more attention. Yet, the phenomenon of violence in the family is common to all three types of member maltreatment. Although the few studies that have examined the problem of elderly abuse have provided some basis for clinical practice, much theory development and research remains to be done.

It is impossible to determine accurately the exact historical and physical findings that professionals can use to diagnose the existence of elderly abuse. As has been shown, the problems of obtaining an accurate and objective history, coupled with the similarity between physiological aging and abuse symptoms, make identification of elder abuse victims a challenging responsibility for the nurse. The task of identifying and aiding such victims is also complicated by the reluctance of abuse victims to seek help. While it is unfortunate, it is also understandable that many victims of elder abuse are reluctant to trust professionals who may be able to assist them.

It is suggested, therefore, that the key element in the provision of high-quality care to elder abuse victims is the establishment of a trusting and insightful relationship between the victim and the primary care provider. Other care providers should work through this trusted professional. All components of the care must be recorded so that all professionals can follow the progress of the client in order to provide the client with continuity in care. Hopefully, as the client becomes aware of the concern of the nurses who are caring for him or her, the element of trust will grow.

In turn, these measures will enable the client to be more open with the nurse and will lead to greater insight into the elderly individual's physical, psychological, and social situations, resulting in more appropriate measures in the client's care. It should be recognized that diagnosis and treatment of this problem requires patience, and in many cases long-term intervention, before the victim will acknowledge his or her predicament and discuss it with a professional willing to help.

This makes it very difficult for the nurse to evaluate the effectiveness of the intervention. In many instances, nurses may have to be content with the recognition that they have helped the patient to begin the process of dealing with the problem, and the realization that final resolution of the problem may not occur until many years and several other professionals have intervened. Nurses willing to take up this challenge may gain satisfaction from the knowledge that they are forerunners in the development of methods of assistance to elderly abuse victims who have heretofore been neglected by other professionals in the health care arena.

Chapter 6

1. Elizabeth Lau and Jordon Kosberg, "Abuse of the Elderly by Informal Care Providers," *Aging* (Sept./Oct., 1979) pp. 10–15.

2. Suzanne K. Steinmetz and Murray A. Straus, "General Introduction: Social Myth and Social System in the Study of Intra Family Violence," in *Violence in the Family*, ed. Suzanne K. Steinmetz and Murray A. Straus (New York: Harper & Row, 1974), p. 6.

3. Marilyn R. Block and Jan D. Sinnott, *The Battered Elder Syndrome: An Exploratory Study* (College Park, Md.: Center on Aging, 1979).

4. Steinmetz and Straus, "General Introduction," p. 7.

5. Mary C. Sengstock and Jersey Liang, *Identifying and Characterizing Elder Abuse* (Detroit, Mich.: Wayne State University Institute of Gerontology, 1981); Mary C. Sengstock and Sara Barrett, "Techniques of Identifying Abused Elders," (Paper presented at the Twelfth International Congress of Gerontology, Hamburg, Germany; 1 July 1981); Mary C. Sengstock and Sara Barrett, "Legal Services for Aged Victims of Domestic Abuse: The Experience of One Legal Aid Agency," (Paper presented at the American Society of Criminology, Toronto, Ontario; November 1982).

6. Blair Justice and Rita Justice, *The Abusing Family* (New York: Human Sciences Press, 1976).

7. Richard L. Douglass, Thomas Hickey, and Catherine Noel, *A Study of Maltreatment of the Elderly and Other Vulnerable Adults* (Ann Arbor, Mich.: University of Michigan Institute of Gerontology, 1980); Mildred Krasnow and Edith Fleshner, "Parental Abuse," (Paper presented at the Twenty-third Annual Geronotological Society Meeting, Washington, D.C.; November 1979); Block and Sinnott, *Battered Elder Syndrome*.

8. Block and Sinnott, *Battered Elder Syndrome*; Lau and Kosberg, "Abuse of the Elderly."

9. Krasnow and Fleshner, "Parental Abuse."

10. Lau and Kosberg, "Abuse of the Elderly,"

11. Block and Sinnott, *Battered Elder Syndrome*.

12. Sengstock and Liang, *Identifying and Characterizing Elder Abuse*.

13. Douglass, Hickey, and Noel, *Study of Maltreatment*.

14. Marvin Wolfgang, *Patterns in Criminal Homicide* (New York: Wiley, 1958), p. 212.

15. Ibid., p. 65.

16. Ibid., p. 211.

17. Suzanne Steinmetz, "Elder Abuse," *Aging* (January/February 1981): 6–10.

18. Block and Sinnott, *Battered Elder Syndrome*.

19. Lau and Kosberg, "Abuse of the Elderly."

20. Murray A. Straus, Richard J. Gelles, and Suzanne K. Steinmetz, *Behind Closed Doors* (New York: Anchor Books, 1980), pp. 119–120.

21. U.S. Department of Justice, *Criminal Victimization in the United States, 1974* (Washington, D.C.: National Criminal Justice Information and Statistics Service, 1977), p. 36.

22. Jersey Liang and Mary C. Sengstock, *Criminal Victimization of the Elderly and Their Interaction with the Criminal Justice System* (Detroit: Institute of Gerontology, Wayne State University, 1980), p. 23.

23. Richard J. Gelles, *The Violent Home* (Beverly Hills, Calif.: Sage, 1974), p. 5.
24. Block and Sinnott, *Battered Elder Syndrome*.
25. Richard J. Gelles, "Child Abuse as Psychopathology: A Sociological Critique and Reformulation," *American Journal of Orthopsychiatry* 43 (July 1973): 611-21.
26. Block and Sinnott, *Battered Elder Syndrome*; Douglass, Hickey, and Noel, *Study of Maltreatment*.
27. Lau and Kosberg, "Abuse of the Elderly."
28. Douglass, Hickey, and Noel, *Study of Maltreatment*; Sengstock and Barrett, "Techniques of Identifying Abused Elders."
29. Block and Sinnott, *Battered Elder Syndrome*.
30. Lau and Kosberg, "Abuse of the Elderly."
31. Sengstock and Liang, *Identifying and Characterizing Elder Abuse*.
32. Block and Sinnott, *Battered Elder Syndrome*.
33. Lau and Kosberg, "Abuse of the Elderly."
34. Sengstock and Liang, *Identifying and Characterizing Elder Abuse*.
35. Block and Sinnott, *Battered Elder Syndrome*.
36. Ibid, pp. 75-76.
37. Ibid.
38. Block and Sinnott, *Battered Elder Syndrome*.
39. Steinmetz and Straus, "General Introduction."
40. Midwest Research Institute, *Crimes Against the Aging: Patterns and Prevention* (Kansas City, Mo.: Midwest Research Institute, 1977).
41. Justice and Justice, *Abusing Family*, pp. 112, 149-52.
42. Lau and Klosberg, "Abuse of the Elderly;" Block and Sinnott, *Battered Elder Syndrome*.
43. Sengstock and Liang, *Identifying and Characterizing Elder Abuse*.
44. Block and Sinnott, *Battered Elder Syndrome*, p. 51.
45. Ibid., p. 77; Lau and Klosberg, "Abuse of the Elderly."
46. Block and Sinnott, *Battered Elder Syndrome*, p. 81.
47. Ibid.
48. Ibid.
49. Ibid.
50. M. Blumberg, "When Parents Hit Out," *Twentieth Century* 173 (Winter 1964): 39-44; David Gil, "Violence Against Children," *Journal of Marriage and the Family* 33 (November), p. 645; Steinmetz and Straus, "General Introduction," pp. 7-8; G. Levinger, "Sources of Marital Dissatisfaction among Applicants for Divorce," *American Journal of Orthopsychiatry*," 26 (October 1976): 803-807.
51. Sengstock and Liang, *Identifying and Characterizing Elder Abuse*.
52. Block and Sinnott, *Battered Elder Syndrome*.
53. B. L. Neugarten, R. J. Havighurst, and S. S. Tobin, "Personality and Patterns of Aging," in *Middle Age and Aging*, ed. B. L. Neugarten (Chicago: University of Chicago Press, 1968); K. W. Back, "Personal Characteristics and Social Behavior: Theory and Method," in *Handbook of Aging and the Social Sciences*, ed. R. H. Binstock and E. Shanas (New York: Van Nostrand Reinhold, 1976).
54. Gelles, "Child Abuse."

55. Gelles, *Violent Home*, pp. 111-12.
56. Ibid, pp. 112-18.
57. Sengstock and Liang, *Identifying and Characterizing Elder Abuse.*
58. Blumberg, "When Parents Hit Out," p. 40; Gil, "Violence Against Children," p. 645; Steinmetz and Straus, "General Introduction," pp. 7-8; Levinger, "Sources of Marital Dissatisfaction."
59. Gil, "Violence Against Children."
60. Justice and Justice, *Abusing Family*, p. 30.
61. Ibid.
62. G. B. Case and G. Lesnoff-Caravaglia, "The Battered Child Grown Old" (Paper presented at the American Gerontological Society, Dallas, Texas, 1978).
63. Douglass, Hickey, and Noel, *Study of Maltreatment*, pp. 69-71.
64. Block and Sinnott, *Battered Elder Syndrome*, p. 53.
65. Justice and Justice, *Abusing Family*, pp. 25-30.
66. Ibid.
67. Sengstock and Liang, *Identifying and Characterizing Elder Abuse.*
68. Thomas Holmes and Richard Rahe, "The Social Readjustment Rating Scale," *Journal of Psychosomatic Research* 11 (1967): 213-18.
69. Justice and Justice, *Abusing Family*, p. 44; J. Spinetta and D. Rigler, "The Child Abusing Parent: A Psychological Review," *Psychological Bulletin* 77 (April 1972): 293-304.
70. J. Steuer and E. Austin, "Family Abuse of the Elderly," *Journal of the American Geriatrics Society* (August 1980) pp. 372-76.
71. Justice and Justice, *Abusing Family*, p. 110.
72. Ibid.
73. Justice and Justice, *Abusing Family*, pp. 190-91.
74. Gelles, "Child Abuse as Psychopathology."
75. Sengstock and Liang, *Identifying and Characterizing Elder Abuse.*
76. Straus, Gelles, and Steinmetz, *Behind Closed Doors*, p. 33.
77. Marvin Wolfgang and Franco Ferracuti, *The Subculture of Violence* (London: Tavistock, 1967), pp. 271-84.
78. Straus, Gelles, and Steinmetz, *Behind Closed Doors*, chap. 5.
79. Gelles, *Violent Home*, pp. 59, 85-86.
80. Steinmetz and Straus, "General Introduction," pp. 6-7.
81. Block and Sinnott, *Battered Elder Syndrome*, pp. 53-55.
82. Ibid.
83. Suzanne K. Steinmetz, "Battered Parents," *Society* (July/August, 1978), pp. 54-55.
84. Block and Sinnott, *Battered Elder Syndrome*, p. 53.
85. Ibid.; Lau and Klosberg, "Abuse of the Elderly."
86. G. R. Burston, "Do Your Elderly Parents Live in Fear of Being Battered?" *Modern Geriatrics* (November 1978): 16.
87. Block and Sinnott, *Battered Elder Syndrome*, p. 53.
88. C. Strow and R. MacKreth, "Family Group Meetings—Strengthening Partnership," *Journal of Gerontological Nursing* 3, no. 1 (1977): 31-35.
89. Sengstock and Liang, *Identifying and Characterizing Elder Abuse*, pp. 43-44.

90. Steinmetz, "Battered Parents."
91. Block and Sinnott, *Battered Elder Syndrome*, p. 53.
92. Ibid., p. 55; Jean Renvoize, *Web of Violence: A Study of Family Violence* (London: Routledge and Kegan Paul, 1978); Burston, "Do Your Elderly Parents Live in Fear."
93. Steinmetz and Straus, "General Introduction."
94. Block and Sinnott, *Battered Elder Syndrome*, p. 54.
95. Jon Hendricks and C. Davis Hendricks, *Aging in Mass Society*, 4th ed. (Cambridge, Mass.: Winthrop Publishers, 1981), p. 74.
96. Richard Sundeen and James Mathieu, "The Fear of Crime and Its Consequences among the Elderly in Three Urban Communities," *Gerontologist* 16, no. 3 (1976): 211-19.
97. Douglass, Hickey, and Noel, *Study of Maltreatment*; Lau and Kosberg, "Abuse of the Elderly."
98. Steinmetz and Straus, "General Introduction," pp. 6-7; Gelles, *Violent Home*, p. 40.
99. Lau and Kosberg, "Abuse of the Elderly."
100. Gelles, *Violent Home*, p. 93.
101. Michigan Women's Commission, *Domestic Assault* (Lansing, Mich.: State of Michigan, 1977), pp. 6-8.
102. Douglass, Hickey, and Noel, *Study of Maltreatment*.
103. Block and Sinnott, *Battered Elder Syndrome*.
104. Douglass, Hickey, and Noel, *Study of Maltreatment*.
105. Lau and Kosberg, "Abuse of the Elderly."
106. Ibid.
107. Ibid.
108. Block and Sinnott, *Battered Elder Syndrome*, p. 92.
109. Sengstock and Barrett, "Techniques of Identifying Abused Elders."
110. Sengstock and Liang, *Identifying and Characterizing Elder Abuse*; Sengstock and Barrett, "Legal Services."
111. Douglass, Hickey, and Noel, *Study of Maltreatment*.
112. Sengstock and Liang, *Identifying and Characterizing Elder Abuse*.
113. "Elder Abuse: Reported Cases Increase," *Vintage* (10 September 1981), 3.
114. Block and Sinnott, *Battered Elder Syndrome*.
115. Michigan Women's Commission, *Domestic Assault*, p. 14.
116. G. H. Kempe et al., "The Battered Child Syndrome," *JAMA* 181 (July 7, 1966), pp. 17-41.
117. Law Enforcement Assistance Administration "News Release," (Washington, D.C.: U.S. Department of Justice, 4 September 1977).
118. Martha H. Field and Henry F. Field, "Marital Violence and the Criminal Process: Neither Justice Nor Peace," *Social Service Review* 47, no. 2 (1973): 221-40; Richard J. Gelles, "No Place to Go: The Social Dynamics of Marital Violence," in Roy, *Battered Women*, p. 61; Elizabeth Truninger, "Marital Violence: The Legal Solutions," *Hastings Law Journal* 23 (November 1971): 259-76.
119. Robert Calvert, "Criminal and Civil Liability in Husband-Wife Assaults," in Steinmetz and Straus, *Violence in the Family*; Straus, Gelles and Steinmetz, *Behind Closed Doors*, pp. 232-33.
120. Block and Sinnott, *Battered Elder Syndrome*, p. 92.
121. Michigan Women's Commission, *Domestic Assault*, pp. 83-84.
122. Steinmetz and Straus, *Violence in the Family*.
123. Leonard Berkowitz, "The Case for Bottling up Rage," *Psychology Today* (July 1973): 24-31; Albert

Bandura and Richard Walters, "Catharsis—A Questionable Mode of Coping With Violence," in Steinmetz and Straus, *Violence in the Family*.

124. Sengstock and Liang, *Identifying and Characterizing Elder Abuse*.

125. Block and Sinnott, *Battered Elder Syndrome*, p. 88.

126. Douglass, Hickey, and Noel, *Study of Maltreatment*, p. 109.

127. Block and Sinnott, *Battered Elder Syndrome*, p. 93.

128. Ibid.

129. Sengstock and Barrett, "Legal Services."

130. Richard Ham, M.D., "Pitfalls in the Diagnosis of Abuse of the Elderly," in, *Abuse and Neglect of the Elderly in Illinois: Incidence and Characteristics, Legislation and Policy Recommendations*, ed. Britta B. Harris (Springfield, Ill.: State of Illinois, 1981); Sengstock and Barrett, "Techniques of Identifying Abused Elders."

131. Sengstock and Barrett, "Techniques of Identifying Abused Elders."

132. Justice and Justice, *Abusing Family*.

133. Sengstock and Barrett, "Techniques of Identifying Abused Elders."

134. Block and Sinnott, *Battered Elder Syndrome*.

Intra-familial Sexual Abuse

Ann Wolbert Burgess
(With Assistance by June Johnson and Jane Jacobs)

NIGHT VISITOR

He drools as he advances
Undressing me with his eyes.
Closer my kinsmen comes taking
his chances; but mother won't be surprised.

A pillow hushes childish screams,
souvenirs are tears and momentary pain.
How well I remember being alone. . . exposed.
Nobody saw my tears—nobody wanted to.

He's left me half dead inside and
I don't want to remember why.
Do not weep for me but for those
still living in-between.

For them, he still comes.

    K. Amanda Vaden
    Reprinted with permission from *Up the Wall*
    (Alexandria, Va.) forthcoming

Intra-familial sexual abuse is anything but exotic or rare. Both empirical research and victim surveys identify it as an everyday experience for thousands of families in every economic and cultural subgroup in the United States. Parent-child incest and spouse rape are power-based violent acts that challenge nurses in terms of assessment, diagnosis, and nursing interventions. It is generally well accepted that reported intra-familial acts are significantly less than the number of acts actually being committed. Thus, these are social problems that generally go unreported, undetected, and undisclosed to professional groups.

Recognition, belief, and support for the victims of family sexual abuse depend on an awareness of new, still-controversial data and a willingness to question a number of comforting forms of denial. Sometimes the denial is professionally based. As physician Suzanne Sgroi has said, "Recognition of sexual molestation of a child is entirely dependent on the individual's inherent willingness to entertain the possibility that the condition may exist."[1] Sgroi also emphasizes that the willingness to consider such a diagnosis often varies in inverse proportion to the professional's level of training and that the more advanced the training of some, the less willing they are to suspect molestation. Sometimes the denial is gender-based. Professor Benjamin DeMott, upon being assigned the task of reviewing sociologist Diana Russell's book, *Rape in Marriage*, begins his review with: "Well, well: Another expose of macho horror. Hasn't there been an oversupply of this lately? Perhaps we deserve a break today." Fortunately, in this case, DeMott is strongly persuaded to the victim's plight through Russell's carefully researched and skillfully written book and he reverses his initial "macho" defense.[2]

In spite of the tendency toward denial, nurses need to be aware of the pervasiveness of family sexual abuse. This chapter will first describe the various forms this kind of violence may take. The theoretical frameworks of causation are then critically analyzed, including examination of traditional approaches which have been historically based on myths about women, and contemporary views of sexual abuse emphasizing power and violence dynamics. The pattern of victim response, an area in which nursing research has made a significant impact, is then discussed. Finally, a description of a therapy group for adult victims of childhood incest is included to illustrate the responses and underscore the need for intervention.

This chapter also seeks to emphasize the opportunity nurses have for effective intervention on behalf of the family and child mental health. Research strongly argues for prevention of chronic sexually abusive situations through early case finding and intervention. In 1973, psychiatrist Joseph Peters described child sexual abuse as a "psychological time bomb" which he predicted to be totally destructive to later adult adjustment even when the child showed no immediate signs of emotional trauma.[3] While it is clear that sexual abuse of children is not the sole cause of identity crises or emotional disorders, recent empirical clinical studies inspire some radical claims. Crisis-responding therapeutic resolution of incest trauma can provide dramatic remissions of major mental illness and behavior disorders in selective cases.[4] Thus, the hypothesis of a single trauma etiology in these patients raises promise for primary prevention of mental illness from childhood sexual abuse if cases are detected and resolved early. As noted in other forms of child maltreatment, there is the generational bonus of prevention if the victim can be identified and reparented. Clinical reports are emphasizing that today's victim may be tomorrow's offender and that boy victims tend to repeat their experiences on younger boys or girls.[5]

Judith Herman and Lisa Hirschman researched forty women who had incestuous relationships with their fathers during childhood and twenty women whose fathers had been seductive, but not overtly incestuous. Their findings suggest high-risk families for incest include families in which mothers are rendered unusually powerless whether through battering, physical disability, mental illness, or the burden of repeated childbearing. Incest should be suspected, Herman and Hirschman report, as a precipitant of impulsive, self-destructive behavior such as suicide attempts, drug abuse, attempts at running away, and the so-called sexually acting out behavior of adolescent girls.[6] In a preliminary report on a study of forced sex in marriage, David Finkelhor and Kristi Yllo report that the husband's goal in many instances appears to be to humiliate and retaliate against his wife, and the abuse very often occurs near the end of the marriage and may often include anal intercourse.[7]

As R. Summit argues, uncounted numbers of children in future generations can be spared the geometric chain reaction of abuse for each link that can be broken through effective intervention and care.[8] Similarly, in spouse rape, intervention may be a means of identification of other abusive situations which in turn can free family members from secrecy toward resolution of the conflict.

FORMS OF INTRA-FAMILIAL SEXUAL ABUSE

Incest

Incest has been a social issue and problem throughout civilization. It seems that in the United States that each generation sees increasing difficulty with it. Currently there are strong social forces giving incest heightened perspective: the reemergence of the women's movement; the new children/adolescent movement and national attention to child abuse in general.

Sgroi has analyzed how clinicians have historically handled incest by denial, emphasizing that those professionals who were in the position of interveners handled incest by supporting the adult, consequently playing into the adult's misuse of power, dominance, and authority and put effort into minimizing the credibility of the child. She challenges clinicians to develop their skills and fulfill their clinical responsibility to children and intervene in a positive supportive way for the child instead of avoiding or denying the problem.[9]

Incest, like rape, is a legal term. Incest is proscribed in every state. Therefore, one way to discuss the problem is to understand that the offender, who shares a kin relationship to the victim, has a problem; for example, engaging in illegal behavior.

There is ambivalence in our societal attitude over the controversy about whether or not to involve some incest offenders in the criminal justice system. Louise Armstrong documents the incredible reluctance of court systems to give voice to the abused child.[10] Lucy Berliner and Doris Stevens note there are acts clearly agreed to be criminal and deserving of prosecution if committed by a stranger or acquaintance yet considered differently if committed by a family member.[11] That is, people have little conflict about criminal prosecution of a stranger for rape of a child; yet let that child be raped by her father and the criminal action issue becomes immensely blurred. Historically, there has been reluctance to intrude in the affairs of the family. As social scientists—especially feminists—have well observed, women and children have been considered property and that usually has meant the male adult family members could and perhaps still can do whatever they want to members of their own family.

Although statutes vary from state to state, incest usually refers to sexual intercourse between two persons so closely related that they are forbidden by law to marry. In that narrow sense, sexual intercourse between first cousins at age twenty could be legally termed incest while oral copulation of a four-year-old by his father would not be incest and could receive a different label of abuse.

Clinical definitions are more helpful to consider. Herman and Hirschman differentiated incest, any physical contact between parent and child that had to be kept secret, from seductive behaviors (for example, peeping, exhibitionism, leaving pornographic materials visible for the child, sharing detailed descriptions of the child's real or imagined sexual activities) that were clearly sexually motivated but did not include secrecy and physical contact.[12]

Incidence

The incidence of incest is significantly underestimated by all reports whether looking at psychiatric textbooks that report one case per million or official figures from court records on which textbooks base their figures.[13] Contemporary figures are best estimated from research surveys. Retrospective surveys of college-age females identify a 20 to 30 percent rate of child sexual victimization.[14] A consistent finding among the surveys that matches with clinical data, is that 70 to 80 percent of sexual offenders were known to the child with about one-half of the molesters being relatives, 22 percent residing in the child's home, and 6 percent fathers or stepfathers.[15]

High-risk families show even higher rates. Surveys of foster children, runaways, drug addicts, and prostitutes find incestuous backgrounds in the 60 to 70 percent range. Mothers in treatment centers for child abuse are reporting 80 to 90 percent prevalence in incestuous abuse in their childhoods, suggesting the correlation between child sexual abuse and abusive parenting by the victims in later life.

Summit, using Finkelhor's data, gives a conservative estimate that about 5 million women in the United States were sexually victimized by a male relative. This figure assumes approximately 10 percent of female children in incestuous relationships and assumes an adult female population of 50 million.[16]

The focus of this chapter is intergenerational incest between adult and child. Such incestuous offenses are not confined to sexual activity between a biological father and daughter, but encompass any sexual relationship in which the male adult occupies an authority role in relation to the child such as adoptive, step, foster or common-law parent. The concern is with age-power relationships, the child's sense that he or she has been sexually violated, and the betrayal of a trusted, caretaking role, rather than with the technicalities of penetration or genital touching. The position being taken is unequivocally that sexualization of a childcaring relationship is a violation of ethics. As Finkelhor argues, a child is incapable of informed consent with a controlling adult because the child has no power to say no and has no information on which to base a decision.[17] Or as Summit describes, the child is just as powerless within the intimidating or ingratiating relationship as the adult rape victim would be at the point of a knife.[18] Therefore, incest is considered here as a form of rape.

Other Forms of Sexual Abuse of Children

All victimized children stand in a relationship of power to the adult. The incidence data on child sexual assault estimates one in four females will be molested or raped by the time she reaches age twenty. The literature is fairly consistent that a female child is at risk for being sexually victimized by a family member. Numbers for male victimization by family members are even more hidden because boys are more reluctant to admit to victimization. However, clinical data are increasingly suggesting that boys may be at equal risk for sexual victimization since they are the preferred target of habitual pedophiles and child pornography collectors.[19]

The sexual abuse of boys is most frequently by men who have easy access to them and includes teachers, coaches, sports leaders, and so forth. Current research is showing that boys are often victimized through sex ring crimes.[20] The first level of ring, child sex initiation ring, is the simultaneous involvement with a number of children, ages six to fourteen, in sexual activities with an adult who capitalizes on his legitimate role in the lives of these children to recruit them into his illegal behavior. The characteristics of the ring are that the offender occupies a position of authority and familiarity to the children, and the children know each other and are aware of each other's involvement in sexual acts with the adult offender. The first level of the ring could be an intrafamilial situation for some boys. The children become programmed by the adult to provide sexual services in exchange for a variety of psychological, social, monetary, and other rewards.

The second and third levels of the ring—youth prostitution and organized pornography and the sexual services structure—may or may not involve family members. The three types of rings, depending on various factors, may constitute different stages in the evolution of child sexual abuse, from loosely formed incestuous relationships to organized or syndicated child prostitution.

Rape of Spouse

The frequency of forced sex in marriage is beginning to be addressed. Peggy Spektor in surveying 304 battered women in ten shelters in Minnesota found that 36 percent had been raped by their husband or cohabitating partner and Mildred D. Pagelow reported a figure of 37 percent on a sample of 119 women in California.[21] Diana H. Russell's study of wife rape in San Francisco, based on 930 interviews of a random sample, reports 14 percent forced sex.[22]

It is important to note that many of these studies are careful to avoid stigmatizing words such as rape in asking interview questions. Russell asked the women to describe any kind of unwanted sexual experience with a husband or former husband and then only included in her tally those encounters that met California's legal definition of rape.[22] Finkelhor and Yllo asked the question: Has your spouse or person you were living with as a couple ever used physical force or threat to try to have sex with you? Ten percent of their sample said this had happened.[23]

One of the problems in spouse rape is that public attitude has not advanced nationally to recognizing this problem. As of January 1982, only ten states recognized the rape of a wife as a prosecutable offense. Most states have a spousal exemption in their rape laws, and many states extend this exemption not just to husbands but to cohabitating lovers.[24] Such laws are effective in denying the possibility of charging a husband, regardless of the amount of violence. The laws are also based on the implicit assumption that a woman upon marrying gives permament and irrevocable consent to any and all sexual approaches a husband wishes to make.[25]

There has been vehement opposition in some locales that changing the laws to include spouse rape will result in a rash of fabricated complaints. However, evidence from countries and states where marital rape is a crime indicates few such complaints are in fact brought to court.[26]

THEORETICAL FRAMEWORKS OF CAUSATION

This section has two goals: first, to review the traditional views which have been responsible for perpetuating the stigmatizing and sex bias aspects of rape and incest, and second, to present a contemporary conceptualization of the victim experience and power and aggression themes.

Rape

Rape—forcible sexual assault—is a sexual offense, is illegal behavior, and is proscribed in the criminal code of every state. It is a felony, a capital offense punishable by varying degrees of penalties. There are three traditional views in the rape literature that have been used to do what William Ryan calls blaming the victim.[27] These views include sexual provocation, false accusation, and female masochism. These perspectives have also served to blame the victims of all forms of intrafamilial sexual abuse.

Sexual Provocation

The subject of rape is one that abounds with many misconceptions, the most insidious of which is the erroneous but popular belief that rape is motivated primarily by sexual desire and/or frustration. This assumption results in the shifting of blame for the assault from the offender to the victim: if the assailant is sexually aroused and is directing these impulses toward the victim, then it must be that she has stimulated or aroused this desire in him.

This myth has maintained its hold on the thinking and practice of clinicians who see the rape or incest victim as a seductive, young, attractive female who could have avoided being raped. As Malhah T. Notman and Carol C. Nadelson state:

> Until recently many psychiatrists have felt that rape was not a psychiatric issue, and that psychiatrists had little to offer the rape victim. They often shared the view that the victim "asked for it" and she was seen as acting out her unconscious fantasies and therefore not a "true victim." Thus, the woman who had been raped did not receive the empathy and understanding usually extended to people in crisis.[28]

Not only is the view held for the adult female, but the female child victim as well. Clinicians are noted for making their own judgments regarding the sexual provocativeness of children. In a study by Lauretta Bender and Abram Blau of sixteen children (eleven females and six males) the following summary was made:

> The child was either a passive or active partner in the sex relations with the adult, and in some instances seemed to be the initiator or seducer. Nearly all of the children had conspicuously charming and attractive personalities.... Their emotional reactions were remarkably devoid of guilt, fear or anxiety regarding the sexual experience. There was evidence that the child derived some emotional satisfaction from the experience.[29]

False Accusation

Sir Matthew Hale (1609–1676) assumed a key role in the history of witchcraft and rape trials. Presiding at the notorious seventeenth-century English witch trial, Hale sentenced to death Amy Duny and Rose Cullender after they were convicted of witchcraft. Fifty years following his death, Hale's cautionary rule on rape—"it must be remembered . . . that it is an accusation easily to be made and hard to be proved, and harder to be defended by the party accused, tho never so innocent"—were published in his volume *Historia Placitorum Coronae*.[30] This ruling—although totally inaccurate—enjoyed wide acceptance in the male-dominated courts and significantly influenced American medical and law texts until the mid-1970s.

Physicians were especially warned about women and children who lie: In 1886, "Brazen-faced children whose stories are manifestly false," and later in 1913, "Many girls will use every means possible to mislead, and their endeavor to evade the trust is at times surprising, even wonderful."[31] G. Williams, a district police surgeon, suggested that physicians be guided by their observations of physical conditions and to forget what they hear:

> As a matter of fact, the girls' statements often amount to nothing. . . many of these girls lie as easily as a morphine fiend[32]

Various reasons were given as to why women and children lie. In 1895, "She may be after blackmail; she may be self-deceived, insane, or coached by others"; In 1962, "The woman invents the story to shock the doctor or to accentuate her own feeling of importance."[33] Physicians were encouraged to carefully check for personality problems of the victims in cases where "the force used in obtaining intercourse might have been brought on by the provocativeness of the victim."[34]

Perhaps the identification component rested uneasily with the physician. In a 1913 article, one reason given for examining a woman in the presence of a witness was stated as "physicians are in constant danger of having this charge brought against them."[35] And, of course, rape did not happen with certain females as Williams states:

> This may appear to be a bold statement, but it must be remembered that the mere crossing of the knees absolutely prevents penetration, and, taking into consideration the tremendous power of the pelvis and abductor thigh muscles, a man must struggle desperately to penetrate the vagina of a vigorous, virtue-protecting girl.[36]

Feminine Masochism

One of the most controversial themes in the rape and battering literature is masochism which Freud described as follows: (1) as a condition under which sexual excitation may be roused (erotogenic); (2) as an expression of feminine nature (feminine); and (3) as a norm of behavior (moral). Freud stated that feminine masochism was based on the "lust of pain" and that the impulse of the ego as a rule remains hidden from the person and must be inferred from his behavior.[37] From this interpretation has derived the implications that rape victims "ask for it" or "want it" even though it is not in their conscious awareness.

Freud admitted to his difficulty in convincing patients about this unconscious sense of guilt feelings that they could not observe in themselves. Therefore, he suggested using the term "need for punishment" as a substitute for unconscious feelings of guilt.[38]

Helena Deutsch continued writing on feminine psychology and identified the central concepts of womanhood as passivity and female masochism.[39] Deutsch's theory—based on a phylogenic hypothesis—purports that when man stood upright he freed himself from sexual dependence on woman and could not take sexual possession without her consent. Therefore, Deutsch asserts, only man (of all living creatures) is capable of rape. Deutsch speculates that the sexual act, originally an act of violence, wherein the woman, weaker and more taxed by her reproductive function, could not resist, was gradually transformed into an act of pleasure. In discussing anxieties, Deutsch further writes that the center of all anxieties in man is castration; the center of woman's anxieties is gradually transformed from genital fear through fear of defloration and rape into the fear of childbirth or death. This process, as the discussion continues, follows biologically determined paths placing emphasis on the close relationship between pain and sexual pleasure. Intercourse, to the female, is closely associated with the act of defloration, and defloration with rape and a painful penetration of the body.

In 1938, Karen Horney, a highly respected neo-Freudian analyst, concluded that Deutsch was saying "What woman ultimately wants in intercourse is to be raped and violated; what she wants in mental life is to be humiliated."[40] Deutsch defended this statement by writing, ". . . it is true that I consider masochism 'an elemental power in feminine life,' but . . . I have tried to show that one of women's tasks is to govern this masochism, to steer it into the right paths, and thus to protect herself against those dangers that Horney thinks I consider woman's 'normal lot.'"[41]

One might question why women have so readily accepted the interpretation of others—especially men—and not asserted their own theories on the explanation of their life and behavior. Fortunately, contemporary female scholars are beginning to do just that. The new work in the psychology of women should begin to combat the old theories of masochism, sexual provocation, and false accusation so that they can no longer be used to blame female victims of sexual abuse.

Incest

Incest—illegal sexual behavior by an adult with a child related through kinship—is described by Sgroi as a "crime that our society abhors in the abstract, but tolerates in reality."[42] In defense of that intentionally provocative statement she challenges people to examine the ways in which child protection issues regarding incest are addressed in the various states. Sgroi suggests that we tolerate sexual assault on children because it is the last component of the maltreatment syndrome in youths that has yet to be faced squarely. The issue for many may be too distressing, "too close to home," too Freudian, or "too dirty." Archaic laws exist which subordinate the best interests of children to the property rights of adults.[43]

Traditional Views of Causation

Sociological and anthropological theory has traditionally dealt with the subject of incest in terms of the taboo characteristics in the culture. The purpose of the incest taboo is generally believed to be the maintenance of kinship structure.[44]

Incest cuts across class status as well as history and geography.[45] Incest, we are told, was practiced by some of the rich and powerful royal families in Egypt as well as the ancient Greeks and Romans.[46] Other countries reporting on incest include Australia, Sweden, Japan, as well as Indian tribes and primitive cultures.[47]

It is a bit paradoxical that the incest issue—upon which the foundation of psychodynamic formulations originated—has been so neglected in terms of psychiatric research. The scant literature that existed prior to the 1960s viewed overt incest as an exotic but negligible phenomenon occurring between inadequate sociopathic fathers and seductive, retarded daughters.[48] The psychiatric literature does discuss incest in terms of object choice such as parent, child, sibling, or other blood relative; frequency of occurrence; genealogy; and sexual orientation. Motivation themes in the literature include revenge, penis envy, family affair, family group survival, response to loss, types of sexual activity, and the offender.[49]

A major issue in incest, from a clinical perspective, is the magnitude of emotional impact of a childhood sexual trauma for adulthood. Early writings by Freud (1895) on hysteria stated that hysterical symptoms could be understood when traced to an early traumatic experience, and that the trauma was always related to the patient's sexual life.[50] He said that the trauma manifested itself when revived later, usually after puberty, as a memory.

However, Freud later reversed his belief and said that the sexual seductions his patients reported were not all reports of real events, and this created a major shift in the priorities of psychological investigation. The external realistic trauma was replaced in importance by infantile sexual wishes and fantasies. Clinicians, as they understood the universality of those wishes and fantasies, began to focus attention on the person's reaction to the wishes and fantasies.

Freud's essay on the sexual theories of children cites three observations which have major importance in the psychoanalytic world:

1. The issue of sex-differentiation (penis envy),

2. Cloaca theory (anal eroticism), and

3. The sadistic conception of coitus in which the stronger person inflicts on the weaker by force.

It is perhaps this last observation that has relevance to incest and rape behavior. Freud says, "...this sadistic conception itself gives the impression of a reappearance of that obscure impulse toward cruel activity...linked up with penis-excitation."[51]

In 1932, Sandor Ferenczi presented a paper at the Viennese Psychoanalytic Society on the occasion of Freud's seventy-fifth birthday titled, "The Passions of Adults and Their Influence on the Sexual and Character Development of Children."[52] This paper presented his belief that childhood trauma had been unjustly neglected over the years and that insufficient depth was afforded the exploration of external factors resulting in premature interpretations and explanations. Ferenczi noted this in his patients who were exhibiting symptoms ranging from attacks of anxiety, nightmares, and flashbacks—"almost hallucinatory repetitions of traumatic experiences." Ferenczi said:

> I had to give free rein to self-criticism. I started to listen to my patients, when, in their attacks, they called me insensitive, cold, even hard and cruel, when they reproached me with being selfish, heartless, conceited. ...I began to test my own conscience...for most of my patients energetically refused to accept such an interpretive demand although it was well supported by analytic material.[53]

This paper was later retitled and published as "Confusion of Tongues between the Adult and the Child" with a subtitle of "The Language of Tenderness and of Passion." The main message that apparently was lost through the years in the literature provided the corroborative evidence for Ferenczi's premise that the "trauma," especially sexual trauma, as the pathogenic factor cannot be valued highly enough. Ferenczi documented the following outcomes of early childhood trauma as:

1. The introjection of the guilt feelings of the adult;

2. The child's sexual life remains undeveloped or assumes perverted forms;

3. A traumatic progression of a precocious maturity;

4. The terrorism of suffering.[54]

The misinterpreted version of Ferenczi's work that incest is not traumatic to the child is also being challenged by contemporary clinicians.[55] Diane H. Browning and Bonny Boatman note that the "sequelae to incest were overwhelming in all 14 cases...including repeated rape and incest... moves and changes of school."[56] Other disruptive events, such as, father's hospitalization or imprisonment, divorce, loss of financial support, and destructive behaviors, were noted in families of incest victims. In a descriptive report on patterns of incest, Roland Summit and JoAnn Kryso cite the social and exploitive components of incest.[57] Elva Poznanski and Peter Blos report from their clinical experience that long-term incest behavior has visible antecedents and visible accompaniments.[58] G. Molnar and P. Cameron report on ten families whose initial psychiatric contact was paternal incest and eight adult women seen for untreated incest and described sample population symptoms as depressive-suicidal or runaway reactions in acute cases and sexual problems in the non-acute adult cases.[59] Judith Herman and Lisa Hirschman analyzed fifteen cases of paternal incest and identified long-term symptoms of sense of distance and isolation, suppression of feelings, conflicts in interpersonal relationships, devaluation of self, and negative identity. In addition, the researchers stated that incest was harmful and left "long lasting scars . . . in adult life they continued to make repeated ineffective attempts to expiate through intense feelings of guilt and shame."[60] And, the results of one of the larger studies of paternal incest in Santa Clara County, California, indicate that most victims, contrary to popular belief, do not enjoy an incestuous relationship.[61]

Vicissitudes of Aggression and Power: Contemporary View

Sexual assault is a serious crime both to a child and to an adult. It is achieving sexual relations with another person against her or his will through physical force or threat of bodily harm. In every act of rape there are three basic psychological components: anger, power, and sexuality. All three factors are present, in varying degrees, in every sexual assault including incest, but distinctive patterns of assault emerge depending on which factor is paramount or dominant in the dynamics of the offender. These themes will be discussed in terms of anger rape, power rape, and sadistic rape.[62]

Anger Rape. In some cases of sexual assault, it is very apparent that sexuality becomes a means of expressing and discharging feelings of pent-up anger and rage. The assault is characterized by physical brutality. Far more actual force is used in the commission of the offense than would be necessary if the intent were simply to overpower the victim and achieve sexual penetration. Sex becomes the weapon by which the offender can degrade his victim. It is a weapon he uses to express his anger and rage. It is his means of retaliation for what he perceives or what he has experienced to be wrongs suffered at the hands of important women in his life and he is seeking to hurt, punish, degrade, and humiliate his victim.

Power Rape. In another pattern of rape, power appears to be the dominant factor motivating the offender. Incest cases are more likely to fall in this category. In these assaults, it is not the offender's intent to harm his victim but to possess him or her sexually. Sexuality becomes the means of compensating for underlying feelings of inadequacy and serves to express issues of mastery, strength, control, authority, and identity. There is a desperate need on the part of the offender to reassure himself about his adequacy and competency as a man. Rape here allows him to feel strong, powerful, and in control of someone else. He hopes his victim will welcome and be impressed by his sexual embrace, in order to feel reassured that he is a desirable person. It is through sexual assault that the offender seeks to assert his mastery and potency and to reaffirm his identity. It is through rape that he hopes to deny any deep-seated feelings of inadequacy, worthlessness, and vulnerability, and to shut out disturbing doubts about his masculinity.

Sadistic Rape. In a third pattern of rape, both sexuality and aggression become fused into a single psychological experience known as sadism. Aggression itself is eroticized, and this offender finds the deliberate and intentional sexual abuse of his victim intensely exciting and gratifying. Such assaults usually involve bondage and torture, ritualistic behaviors, and symbolic victims (that is, victims seem to share some common characteristics in regard to their appearance or profession). In some cases the offender is an individual who cannot achieve sexual satisfaction unless his victim physically resists him. He becomes aroused or excited only when aggression is present. He finds pleasure in taking a victim against his or her will, and, in extreme cases the sadistic rapist may murder his victim and mutilate her body. In some cases, rather than have actual intercourse with the victim, he may use some type of object or instrument with which to rape, such as a stick or bottle.

Child Molestation

Incest can also be examined within a further contemporary view of sexual abuse. From this perspective, the dynamics of pressured sexuality become important since they are often used in adult and child sexual activity. This view is that dominance by authority is a way to insure sexual control over a child. This offense is characterized by a relative lack of physical force in the commission of the offense; in fact, the offender generally behaves in counter aggressive ways. His typical *modus operandi* is either one of enticement in which he attempts to sexually engage the child through persuasion or cajolement, or one of entrapment in which he takes advantage of having put the child in a situation where the victim feels indebted or obligated in some way to the offender. This offender makes efforts to persuade his victim to cooperate and to acquiesce or consent to the sexual relationship, often times by bribing or rewarding the child with attention, affection, approval, money, gifts, treats, and good times. But he is usually dissuaded if the child actively refuses or resists, and he does not resort to physical force. His aim is to gain sexual control of the child by developing a willing or consenting sexual relationship. At some level, he cares for the child and is emotionally identified and involved with him or her. In sex pressure situations, sexuality appears to be in the service of dependency needs for physical contact and affection. Such offenders appear to desire the child as a love-object and typically describe the victim as innocent, loving, open, affectionate, attractive, and undemanding. They feel safer and more comfortable with a child.[63]

Children are prime victim targets. They are trained to do what adults tell them to do. Many of the same qualities that make a child a "good" child also make him or her an "easy" victim. Very often victim and offender know each other prior to their sexual involvement and sometimes they are related. This involvement can be continuing and fairly consistent over time.[64]

In pressuring the child into sexual activity the offender often uses a combination of material rewards (candy, money, toys), psychological rewards (attention, interest, affection), and misrepresentation of moral standards ("It's OK to do."). Once sexual contact is achieved the child may find it pleasant, unpleasant, or neither. Victims reporting a pleasurable reaction typically described hand-genital contact rather than penetration.

Having achieved sexual contact, the offender now must avoid detection; to do so he will attempt to pledge his victim to silence. The offender may say it is something secret between them, or in the entrapment cases, he may threaten to harm the child if she or he does tell. In most situations, the burden to keep the secret is psychologically experienced as fear. Victims have spontaneously described these fears which bind them to the secret as fear of punishment, fear of repercussions from telling, fear of abandonment or rejection, and not knowing how to describe what has happened.[65]

PATTERNS OF VICTIM RESPONSE

Intra-family Rape

In the 1970s, several publications appeared in the psychiatric literature presenting a more contemporary view of rape—from the victim's perspective and as an external stress for the victim. Rather than discussing rape so exclusively in terms of intrapsychic concepts, the new view began to portray rape as an event imposed upon the woman from the outside. This new perspective is useful in examining victim responses to sexual abuse within the family.

Clinical research from a study of 109 child, adolescent, and adult rape victims in 1974 described the act of being raped generating an enormous amount of anxiety to the victim. This finding was the basis of describing an acute traumatic reaction following rape called the rape trauma syndrome in which the nucleus of the anxiety is the life-threatening and/or highly stressful impact of the experience on the victim.[66]

Rape Trauma Syndrome

Rape trauma syndrome is the acute phase and long-term reorganization process that occurs as a result of a forcible rape or attempted forcible rape.[67] This syndrome of behavioral, somatic, and psychological reactions is an acute stress reaction to a life-threatening situation. The syndrome is usually a two-phase reaction. The first is the acute phase, a period in which there is a great deal of disorganization in the woman's life-style as a result of the rape. Physical symptoms are especially noticeable and one prominent feeling noted is fear. The second phase begins when the woman begins to reorganize her life-style. Although the time of onset varies from victim to victim, the second phase often begins about two to three weeks after the attack. Motor activity changes and nightmares and phobias are especially likely during this phase.

The impact reactions occur in the immediate hours following the rape and the woman may experience an extremely wide range of emotions. The impact of the rape may be so severe that feelings of shock or disbelief are expressed. When interviewed within a few hours of the rape, the victims mainly show two emotional styles: the expressed style, in which feelings of fear, anger, and anxiety were shown through such behavior as crying, sobbing, smiling, restlessness, and tenseness; and the controlled style, in which feelings were masked or hidden and a calm, composed, or subdued affect was seen.

Somatic Reactions. During the first several weeks following a rape, many of the acute somatic manifestations described below were evident.

1. Physical trauma. This includes general soreness and bruising from the physical attack in various parts of the body such as the throat, neck, breasts, thighs, legs, and arms. Irritation and trauma to throat are especially a problem in victims forced to have oral sex.

2. Skeletal muscle tension. Tension headaches and fatigue, as well as sleep pattern disturbances, are common symptoms. Women were either not able to sleep or would fall asleep only to wake and not be able to go back to sleep.

3. Gastrointestinal irritability. Victims might complain of stomach pains. The appetite might be affected and the victim might state that she could not eat, food had no taste, or she felt nauseated from thinking about the rape.

4. Genitourinary disturbance. Gynecological symptoms such as vaginal discharge, itching, a burning sensation on urination, and generalized pain were common. A number of women developed chronic vaginal infections following the rape. Rectal bleeding and pain were reported by women who had been forced to have anal sex.

Emotional Reactions. Victims expressed a wide gamut of feelings as they began to deal with the aftereffects of the rape. These feelings ranged from rage, humiliation, and embarrassment to anger, revenge, and self-blame. Fear of physical violence and death was the primary feeling described. Self-blame was another reaction described—partly because of their socialization to the attitude of "blame the victim."

Long-Term Effects. Various factors affected the coping behavior regarding the trauma experienced by the victim, that is, ego strength, social network support, and the way people treat them as victims. This coping and reorganization process began at different times for the individual victims. There were various long-term effects including an increase in motor activity; dreams and nightmares; the development of fears and phobias, especially in the area of sexual fears.

There were two noted variations of rape trauma syndrome: a compounded reaction in which victims had either a past or current history of physical, psychiatric, or social difficulties. It was noted in this group that victims developed additional symptoms such as depression, psychotic behavior, psychosomatic disorders, suicidal behavior, and acting-out behavior associated with alcoholism, drug use, and sexual activity. The second variation was silent rape reaction. Since a significant proportion of women still do not report a rape, especially spouse rape, nurses should be alert to this syndrome. This reaction occurs in the victim who has not told anyone of the rape, who has not settled her feelings and reactions on the issue, and who is carrying a tremendous psychological burden.

Incest Victim Response

In 1932, Ferenczi stated his belief that the "real rape of girls who have hardly grown out of the age of infants, similar acts of mature women with boys, and also enforced homosexual acts, are more frequent occurrences than has hitherto been assumed."[68] This observation led Ferenczi to further elaborate on the theory of identification or introjection of the aggressor as a major component of his hypothesis on the etiology of sexual trauma. This view is reviewed for contemporary consideration.

Ferenczi believed that in the incestuous seductions, the child is psychologically paralyzed with anxiety. Children feel physically and morally helpless. Their personalities are not adequately organized in order to be able to protest, even if only in thought for the overriding powerful force and authority of the adult makes them unaware of their senses. Ferenczi continues: "the same anxiety, however, if it reaches a certain maximum, compels them to subordinate themselves like automata to the will of the aggressor, to devine each one of his desires and to gratify these; completely oblivious of themselves they identify themselves with the aggressor."[69]

It is through this identification or introjection of the aggressor that the aggressor disappears as part of the external reality, and becomes intrapsychic instead of extrapsychic. The intrapsychic is then subjected, in a dreamlike state as in the traumatic trance, to the primary process, that is, according to the pleasure principle, it can be modified or changed by the use of positive or negative hallucinations. In any case, the attack as a rigid external reality ceases to exist and in the traumatic trance the child succeeds in maintaining the previous situation of tenderness. The misused child changes into a mechanical, obedient automaton or becomes defiant, but is unable to account for the reasons of her defiance. The sexual life of the child remains undeveloped or assumes perverted forms. Ferenczi states his underlying assumption that the child's underdeveloped personality reacts to sudden distress not by defense but by anxiety-ridden identification and by introjection of the menacing person or aggressor.

The cultural constructs of society must also be considered in the issue of incest. Herman and Hirschman comment on incest in a patriarchal society as follows:

> A patriarchal society, then, most abhors the idea of incest between mother and son, because this is an affront to the father's prerogatives. Though incest between father and daughter is also forbidden, the prohibition carries considerably less weight and is, therefore, more frequently violated . . . . This is in fact the case. Incest offenders are frequently described as "family tyrants": These fathers, who are often quite incapable of relating their despotic claim to leadership to their social efforts for the family, tend toward abuses of authority of every conceivable kind, and they not infrequently endeavor to secure their dominant position by socially isolating the members of the family from the world outside[70]

These authors conclude and predict that the greater the degree of a male-oriented and male-dominated society, the greater the likelihood of father-daughter incest.

The literature cites two major dilemmas that the incest victim faces: role confusion and divided loyalty. In terms of the role confusion, Herman and Hirschman describe the situation as follows: A woman who has been raped by a nonfamily member can cope with the experience by reacting to it as an intentionally cruel and harmful attack. She is free to hate the rapist because she is not socially or psychologically dependent upon him. But the daughter-victim of incest is dependent on her perpetrator-father for additional parental tasks such as protection and care. Her mother frequently is not an ally and thus she has no recourse. To quote the authors,

> She does not dare express, or even feel, the depths of her anger at being used. She must comply with her father's demands or risk losing the parental love that she needs. She is not an adult. She cannot walk out of the situation (though she may try to run away). She must endure it, and find in it what compensation she can.[71]

The second issue of divided family loyalty arises if the incest is exposed.[72] The child takes the risk of pressuring the family to place its loyalty either with her and against the perpetrator (another family member) or with the perpetrator and against her. It is highly improbable that a family can remain equally divided between the two family members. Obviously, the closer the family relationship, the more difficult the family decision.

Long-Term Effects of Incest

There are adult women who are making courageous efforts to break through the barriers of childhood silence on incest. One outstanding survivor, as incest victims prefer to be called, is the author of the opening poem to this chapter as well as the author to a collection of poems entitled, *Betrayal.*[73] This thirty-one-year-old woman began facing her "fourteen-year ghost" after recovering from an adult rape experience with the assistance of her psychologist-therapist. As is often noticed in cases of chronic and/or multiple incest victims, this woman had to be hypnotized to recall the past. The following is her memory and experiences.

> It started when I was 4 years old. He put his fingers inside me; I went into the closet and stayed there. All I remember is bleeding on my sister's blue shoes. Had vaginal pain until this incident was totally recalled and also woke in the night sitting in the closet. Then I remembered being deprived of water at night because I was a bed wetter. Mother would hang the sheets outside my window for people to see; couldn't drink anything after supper; was beaten with a belt. She assumed I did it on purpose and she was punishing me (I stopped bed wetting when I moved away from home at 17). My brother offered me water if he could touch me. One night, mom caught him coming out of my room (I was 8) and she beat me severely with a belt because I was a wicked, sinful little girl. She used hot water enemas and douches to cleanse the devil out. After that, I *never* said anything. If my parents didn't help me, who would? So, the fondling went on till I was 14. Then my brother went away to college. I was wild and sexually active as a teenager. I just didn't care about sex. Sex was a way of getting what I wanted: as a child: water, food, peace from my mother. As a teenager: gifts, learned how to drive a car, money and most important, freedom to be by myself. Another problem I had as a child: I was very hard to wake—so much so that my parents took me to many doctors. I always felt something was wrong with me. The night before my high school graduation, my brother and his new wife came home for the

Intra-familial Sexual Abuse

ceremonies. That night while I was sleeping, he came into my room and raped me. I remember mother's good wash cloth stuffed in my mouth but nothing else till a few hypnosis sessions. I didn't move or cry out—why would anyone help me now? I moved out of the home then, but two months later found out I was pregnant and had to have an abortion. Under hypnosis I went through the labor and delivery for 45 minutes. Psychosomatic pain *always* starts before the actual memory of a trauma. Back to the abortion. There were no sedatives. I was made to look at the fetus. I've lost nearly 25 pounds through all this memory and the sadness is so overwhelming it almost suffocates me. The anger is so intense, I'm afraid of it. Revenge is what I feel the most and loneliness. My poetry is my outlet and provider of some peace of mind. The reason I am writing this is because I wish more people, especially professionals, knew or understood what it can feel like when a child realizes that he/she was not protected by their parents; and, how it feels when there does not seem to be a safe place anywhere. Some people knew about my brother and didn't do anything because my father was rich and influential and they were afraid. I found this out a few months ago by asking old neighbors, friends, and relatives. Right now, I feel I'll never forgive them and I'm so angry and hurt and most of all wonder why I wasn't *worth* it! My parents were both alcoholics. Mother died on my birthday in 1977 and father is still alive but ill. My older brother and I have no communication except I sent him my poetry on incest a few weeks ago, but no reply yet.

One of the poems sent to her brother follows.

MEMORIES OF THE RAIN
Older brother, oldest lover,
like a blackened banana I
feel rotted through and through.
How it started I don't recall.
Concealing feelings of helplessness,
dreaming of daylight freedom
that never came; only the rain.
So often I'm thrown into the past.
Night after night he'd call my name,
so I'd stare out the window
counting the rain.
I still wake in the night hoping
he won't be there, and I'm surrounded
alone wrapped in me; no torment there.
Remembering years ago possessed
by pain, always staring out the
window at the rain. Now, he's out
of reach and I sleep so peacefully.
Putting the past and distance behind me
he no longer is the enemy, just sad memories
of the rain.
    K. Amanda Vaden
    Reprinted with permission of *Up the Wall*
    (Alexandria, Va.) forthcoming

This personal recollection poignantly illustrates the trauma of incest to a victim. To further give a picture of the effects of intrafamilial sexual abuse, the following description of a therapeutic group of incest victims is presented. The description highlights not only the experiences of the women, but it also underscores the need for intervention, sometimes long after the acts of violence have occurred. (Additional specific nursing interventions for intrafamily sexual abuse are presented in Chapters 8 and 10.)

Group Therapy with Incest Victims*

Clinical experience has shown that certain group processes provide corrective necessary developmental experiences

---

*This section is written by June Johnson, R.N., M.S., and Jane Jacobs, M.S.W.

which many women who have had early incest episodes have been deprived of by virtue of the complex psychological trauma involved. Because of their guilt and shame, these women had concealed the history of their incest even from those with whom they relate most closely. The incest secret became a symbol of profound difference from other people. Interpersonal relating was seriously impeded by fears of exposing the secret. The consequence was pervasive difficulty both in forming intimate relationships with men and other women and in developing a coherent identity.

It seems that fear of intimate sharing and defective identity formation are intensified for women who were exposed to incest during latency or earlier because their social isolation has interfered with important latency tasks. The mutual relatively uninhibited sharing of secrets, fantasies, and significant experiences with friends of the same sex provides a variety of self-validation functions that will be discussed in more detail later.

For women who participated in this psychotherapy group, incest episodes had begun prior to adolescence, and they were not able to use latency relationships to gain peer and self-acceptance. They used the group in part as an opportunity to experience peer relationships in the growth-productive ways that they could not manage earlier. The emotional difficulties associated with incest and the specific ways in which group processes facilitated these specific areas of emotional growth through a period of one year of group psychotherapy will be discussed.

The childhood incest experiences of these women were creating major interpersonal problems in their lives, especially with men but also with other women. All of them had been or were in individual psychotherapy and they along with their therapists, felt that individual treatment had done little to help them understand, resolve, and constructively integrate the experience in a way that could permit intimate and committed relationships with others. The women's sharing of the incest experience with only the therapist seemed simply to remain an insulated dyadic matter that made them less inclined to chance the risks and rewards of trusting others with their secret.

All the women joined the group knowing it was for incest victims only. All were fearful of disclosure and questioned both group leaders closely about confidentiality and the leaders' trustworthiness. Their fears centered around the leaders' capacity to be helpful in understanding them and preventing any emotional decompensation which might ensue after the disclosure of long-unexpressed traumatic experiences.

In the beginning, six women formed the group, but within six weeks two of them dropped out. Three more were then added following a great deal of discussion about lack of trust in and fear of new members. The group's composition remained constant until one of the original members moved to another part of the state.

All the women were Caucasian, ranging in age from twenty-one to thirty-two and of varying socioeconomic and educational backgrounds. Two were married, each with one child. One woman was separated from her husband and had two children. Four were single and lived apart from their families. None of these women had severe character disorders, were borderline, or psychotic. However, all had major interpersonal and identity difficulties, and it seemed that their incest experiences were the central organizing factor in these sectors of their personalities.

Five of the women were victims of their

Intra-familial Sexual Abuse

fathers; four of these state that their siblings also suffered the same fate. Another woman's experience was with her older brother, and the other, with her great-uncle. The experiences ranged from genital fondling to full intercourse. For all of them, incest began between ages six and eight and stopped at early adolescence. None had ever shared the experience with peers, but all except one had tried to tell their mothers or other family members. Their childhood attempts were met with anger, denial, admonishments about talking dirty, or worse, being accused of initiating the contact and hence being responsible for their own victimization. These family responses engendered rage in them, which served then only to intensify their feelings of self-devaluation, guilt, shame, low self-esteem, and intense feelings of being different from other girls their own age. This mortifying feeling of being different appears to have prevented them from being intimate with same sex peers especially during their latency period, but also to a substantial degree throughout their lives.

Their inability to develop close friendships during latency was reflected by the absence of several key capacities. Henry Stack Sullivan discusses major functions of "chum" relationships during the preadolescent period.[74] He describes latency friendships as the first example of genuine enduring concern for another person. Through a process which Sullivan refers to as "consensual validation," chums confirm for each other the inherent worthiness of one another's views of themselves and their worlds. This involves long intimate conversations during which participants tell each other their deepest secrets as well as strategies for concealing such information from certain others. Chums provide each other vital appraisals, both positive and negative. They validate "good" traits of which the other was not aware. On the other hand, they correct distortions in the way a friend sees herself and her relationships. Character tendencies such as egocentricity and the expectation of unmitigated sympathy can be modified through peer feedback before they become enduring character traits. For Sullivan the correction and such "parataxic distortions" are the cornerstone of sound interpersonal functioning. Moreover, the intensity of the latency friendship provides the model for successful heterosexual intimacy in adolescence and adulthood, when the individual shifts this ability to share and love from a same-sexed to an opposite-sexed person.

Each group member began with a conviction that her incest experience was unique rather than an experience similar to and shared by others. At first, it was as if they had repressed the central factor in the group's formation and they feared such disclosure. Nevertheless, in contrast with their work in individual therapy, they soon acknowledged that they shared much in common as a result of their early incest experiences. They were able, relatively quickly, to risk sharing intimate information with each other without overwhelming fear of mortification. As they experienced validation and support from each other, they began increasingly to use the group in just the way Sullivan describes preadolescent chum relationships.

The few who had at some time tentatively attempted to share their experience with female friends had been met by blank responses as if their story was incomprehensible, frightening, and certainly not one of the treasured and shared experiences of childhood. For all of them, a sense of themselves as dirty, defiled, perverse, and generally set apart from other women was quite striking. It formed a sector of negative identity.[75] The negative identity had to be concealed even though it formed so much of the core of their self-experience. As a result, lifelong relationships remained relatively superficial, and the yearning for a full closeness was thwarted by dread of disclosure. They felt a tremendous need for the relief which could only be obtained through sharing their story with others. This pressure, this yearning for validation, could be accomplished only by risking exposure of the long-held secret and secret self which had separated them from their peers and their childhood from their adulthood. Irving D. Yalom indicates that the individual's sense of uniqueness is heightened in the early stages of a group and requires relief. He states,

> It is not the sheer process of validation which is important, it is not only the disclosure of others' problems similar to our own and the ensuing disconformation of our wretched uniqueness that is important, it is the affective sharing of one's inner world and then the acceptance by others that seems of paramount importance.[76]

These remarks of Yalom and our references to Sullivan and Erikson highlight the aberrant developmental experiences of these women and their consequences. Thus, these women were significantly limited in the experience of interpersonal intimacy during latency which allows one to see oneself through another's eyes, to correct one's distortions of self, to have one's goodness confirmed, and to dispel one's illusions of being different from others. This developmental impoverishment seriously thwarted self-acceptance with painful and superficial relationships with both men and women as the current consequence.

Despite this dread of disclosure, the need for and pressure toward sharing became paramount during the initial phase of the group. Most of the women soon felt the group could not progress until each individual's story was told. Together they took the leap and accomplished this. Painful sobbing and anguish were expressed by all. At the same time each woman was able to listen, to encourage, and to support the member whose turn it was to tell her story. Some needed actively to be held and comforted while telling of their devastating childhood exploitation at the hands of those they most trusted, needed, and loved. Some ashamedly stated they had experienced pleasurable physical sensations, had even at times waited for their fathers to come to them. Their guilt was exceedingly strong, accompanied by shame, and readily mobilized in the present as a major impediment to their achieving adult sexual pleasure.

Most of them have been able to have only fleeting, impersonal, exploitive sexual contacts with men—the kind referred to as "one-night stands." They are frightened of sex, inorgasmic, and only manage to endure sexual contact. They find it almost impossible as adult women to take control of their sexuality somewhat as they were unable to do as children. Many report that the only way they can experience sexual pleasure during sexual play with men or in intercourse is through fantasies about their original incestuous sexual partner.

As these sad, uncomfortable stories were shared, all the participants, for the first time in their lives, felt the full intimacy and validation with another human being that normally is a part of latency, the "best friend" period of our lives which we remember as one of unconditional acceptance of ourselves by another human being and vice versa—that is, the consensual validation of personal worth that Sullivan described.

This intimacy, validation, sharing, acceptance of one another, and evolving positive identity as women has led to increased self-esteem and feelings of self-worth, as evidenced by the changes in the interactions of these women with others, both in and outside the group. For example, two of the single women who had not dated in over two years reported accepting dates with men approximately four months after the group had been formed. Both informed the members of their anxiety about their impending dates, and one agreed to role play the anticipated encounter. Both members subsequently discussed the dates with the group, focusing on their initial discomfort and eventual relaxation once they realized they could influence the quality of the evening as much as the men could.

The two married women indicated that the interpersonal sharing within the group was developing within them a greater capacity for intimacy with their husbands, with whom they previously shared little or nothing about their incestuous past and its bearing on their sexual inhibitions.

One of these two women entered the group six months after the birth of her first child, a boy. She had become seriously depressed after his birth. His birth had resurrected her childhood memories of sexual abuse by her father and had also stimulated fear that she might sexually abuse her male child in years to come.

When first seen in the group, the disorganization of her thought processes, her blunted affective expression, and certain peculiar yawnlike speech mannerisms which interrupted her flow of talk altogether suggested that her ego-functioning might be borderline. She swallowed her words and spoke very softly so that it was as difficult to hear her as it was to understand the point she was trying to make. These problems were frequently called to her attention by other group members, which surprised her because she claimed she did not realize that her ways of communicating presented any problems.

After six months in the group she related a poignant encounter with her mother following her brother's wedding. During the wedding she was flooded with sexual memories of her father. She tried to discuss this with her mother who responded in an aloof, withdrawn fashion. As she sobbingly related the story, she blurted out how much she wanted her mother to hold, soothe, and comfort her during this time. The members of the group quickly and naturally responded to supply that which her mother could not. They physically held, rocked, and comforted her until her sobbing subsided. The group then role played a scene with her in which she was able to tell her mother she needed to be soothed and held. A few weeks later during a visit to her mother's she was actually able to do this. Her mother was able to respond in an intimate emotional encounter which the patient described to the group. It was striking to hear the quality of her description. Now her speech was direct, coherent, with none of the mannerisms described previously, and her affective expression was full, not blunted. Her improvement has continued, as has her increasing intimacy with both her mother and her husband. She is very much aware of the difference now in her thought and speech patterns, to the point that she was able to tell the group that she wonders how anyone could have listened to or understood her during the early phases of the group. She said she had often felt her thoughts were a jumbled mess, frequently unrelated to each other, and this along with her speech pattern was a way she had for preventing herself from being overwhelmed and out of control. She has made remarkable progress.

Consensual validation is a key developmental experience during the preadolescent phase. The importance of this phase is emphasized by Sullivan.[77] These confirmatory relations were evidenced in the group when one of the members, a twenty-five-year-old single woman named Sarah, received a letter from her father, whom she hadn't seen for a year, that is, not since she had confronted him with their incestuous relations, which had consisted of full intercourse when she was eight to twelve. In the letter he begged her to rectify his loss of his family and his home through her disclosure of the incest. Although he asserted that he loved her, he inferred that it was her fault that his life had been disrupted.

As she read the letter to the group, Sarah was overwhelmed by guilt and began to sob. The group firmly and caringly reminded her that she had not done anything wrong; her father was responsible for his plight as a result of his actions. For many months after the confrontation at age twenty-four, Sarah had felt profoundly destructive because her parents had split up after her disclosure. The group on this occasion confirmed Sarah's courage in having confronted her father. Their repeated valuing of her actions gradually helped soothe her. As they each confirmed the worthiness of her behavior, and lent force to the modification of her guilt, they were also implicitly valuing their own attempts to confront their incest experiences openly and honestly.

We have described the deprivation of these women in latency of the "seeing oneself through the other's eyes" that is so essential to the correction of the disturbed self-perceptions and to actual behavioral corrections that can be effected and molded into one's identity. An interaction of this nature which took place in the group involved Debbie, a twenty-eight-year-old married woman who used bodily and facial expressions to call attention to herself and to monopolize the group's attention. On one occasion she told the group a complicated story in which her in-laws were pressuring her to take care of a sick member of the family. She accepted this burden despite feeling ill-equipped, rageful, and regressively helpless. The group was supportive, but also clearly related to Debbie that she needed to learn to set realistic limits on others' demands of her rather than following her old compliant pattern based in self-devaluation and anger.

After part of another session was monopolized with Debbie's problem, the group began to assert one of its norms, that is, that everyone needed access to the limited "air time" of the group meeting. Members agreed that sometimes one had to wait one's turn so everyone could have a chance to talk. Since this discussion about sharing Debbie has been better able to contain her needs without withdrawing from the group. In accepting the group's limits, she seems to be developing a greater capacity for setting limits on others' demands on her and on making unrealistic demands herself on others. The interaction of the group with Debbie promises change in her sense of herself because in its respectful correctiveness it promotes a positive sense of her belonging, one which nudges her toward replacing a negative sector of identity with a positive one.

These vignettes illustrate some specific ways in which group therapy experience has provided crucial validation functions which under normal circumstances are experienced as inherent in the preadolescent friendship network. Such functions include:

1. Confirmation that others' perceive one as one perceives oneself;
2. The correction of inaccurate perceptions of oneself;
3. The recognition that one possesses and is valued for some of the same traits that one esteems in others;
4. The capacity to value the traits in oneself that others affirm.

The intensity and personal meaning of the incest secret is such that it imparts the quality of integration of self that is achieved in part by the knowledge that one is thoroughly known and valued by other persons. Through members' consensual validation of one another's personal qualities and worth, the group therapy process seems particularly suited to the correction of self images, the building of self-esteem, and the solidification of self-structure.

Summary

In summary, the purpose of this chapter has been to help establish a climate of belief for intrafamilial sexual abuse. Every nurse has the capacity to make a difference in the equilibrium of silence. Familiarity with the manifestations of this sexual violence in families will help alert nurses to the possibility of incest, other forms of sexual abuse against children, and marital rape in their practice.

The discovery of child sexual abuse and spouse rape at first will seem overwhelming in the stigmatic context in which they exist. Prejudicial thinking about women has been shown to have greatly influenced the traditional theoretical frameworks of causation offered to explain intrafamilial sexual abuse and the subsequent treatment of victims. Nursing research and other contemporary investigations have emphasized the power and violence factors inherent in sexual victimization of family members. The responses of victims include both physical and psychological difficulties which can persist long after the events when there are no effective interventions. Yet nursing practice can be crucial in the prevention of long-term trauma as shown in the example of group therapy with victims. The problem of intrafamilial sexual abuse challenges myths about families and violent sexual acts and can be disquieting. Fortunately, there are now systems of investigation, description, and resolution to reduce the problem to human dimensions.

Chapter 7

1. Suzanne M. Sgroi, "Sexual Molestation of Children: The Last Frontier in Child Abuse," *Children Today* 4, no. 44 (1975): 18-21.
2. Benjamin DeMott, "Criminal Intimacies," *Psychology Today* 16, no. 8 (1977): 72-74.
3. Joseph Peters, "Child Rape: Defusing a Psychological Time Bomb," *Hospital Physician* 9, no. 46 (1973).

4. Roland Summit, "Recognition and Treatment of Child Sexual Abuse," in *Providing for the Emotional Health of the Pediatric Patient*, ed. C. E. Hollingsworth (New York: Spectrum, 1981).

5. A. Nicholas Groth, Robert E. Longo, and J. Bradley McFadin, "Undetected Recidivism among Rapists and Child Molesters," *Crime and Delinquency* 28, no. 3 (1982): 450-58.

6. Judith Herman and Lisa Hirschman, "Families at Risk for Father-Daughter Incest," *American Journal of Psychiatry* 138, no. 7 (July 1981): 967-70.

7. David Finkelhor and Kristi Yllo, "Forced Sex in Marriage," *Crime and Delinquency* 28, no. 3 (July 1982): 459-78.

8. R. Summitt, "Recognition and Treatment."

9. Suzanne M. Sgroi, "A National Needs Assessment for Protecting Victims of Child Sexual Assault," in *Sexual Assault of Children and Adolescents*, ed. Ann W. Burgess, A. Nicholas Groth, Lynda L. Holstrom, and S. M. Sgori (Lexington, Mass.: D.C. Heath & Co., 1978), p. xv.

10. Louise Armstrong, *Kiss Daddy Goodnight: A Speakout on Incest* (New York: Hawthorn Books, 1978).

11. Doris Stevens and Lucy Berliner, "Special Techniques for Child Witnesses," in *The Sexual Victimology of Youth*, ed. L. G. Schultz (Springfield, Ill.: Charles C. Thomas, 1979), pp. 246-56.

12. Herman and Hirschman, "Families at Risk."

13. D. J. Henderson, "Incest," in *Comprehensive Textbook of Psychiatry*, ed. A. M. Freedman, H. I. Kaplan, and B. J. Sadock (Baltimore: Williams & Wilkins Co., 1975).

14. J. Landis, "Experiences of 500 Children with Adult Sexual Deviants," *Psychiatric Quarterly Supplement* 30 (1956): 91-109; John H. Gagnon, "Female Child Victims of Sex Offenses," *Social Problems* 13 (1965): 176-92; David Finkelhor, *Sexually Victimized Children* (New York: Free Press, 1979).

15. David Finkelhor, "What's Wrong with Sex between Adults and Children?" *American Journal of Orthopsychiatry* 49, no. 4 (1979): 629-97.

16. Roland Summit, "Beyond Belief: The Reluctant Discovery of Incest," in *Women in Context*, ed. M. Kirkpatrick (New York: Plenum, 1981).

17. Finkelhor, "What's Wrong?"

18. Summit, "Beyond Belief."

19. A. Nicholas Groth, *Men Who Rape* (New York: Plenum, 1979); Ann W. Burgess, "The Prevalence of Child Pornography," *Change* (1982).

20. Ann W. Burgess, A. Nicholas Groth, and Maureen P. McCausland, "Child Sex Initiation Rings," *American Journal of Orthopsychiatry* 51 (January 1981): 110-19.

21. Peggy Spektor, Testimony delivered to the Law Enforcement Subcommittee of the Minnesota House of Representatives, 29 February 1980; Mildred D. Pagelow, "Does the Law Help Battered Wives? Some Research Notes," (Paper presented at the Annual Meeting of the Law and Society Association, Madison, Wisconsin, 1980.

22. Diana H. Russell, *Rape in Marriage* (New York: MacMillan, 1982).

23. D. Finkelhor and K. Yllo, "Forced Sex."

24. J. Schulman, "Expansion of the Marital Rape Exemption," *National Center on Women and Family Law Newsletter* (July, 1980), 3-4.

25. Finkelhor and Yllo, "Forced Sex in Marriage."

26. Gilbert Geis, "Rape in Marriage: Law and Law Reform in England, the United States, and Sweden," *Adelaide Law Review* (June 1978): 284-302.

27. William Ryan, *Blaming the Victim* (New York: Random House, Pantheon Books, 1971).

28. Malhah T. Notman and Carol C. Nadelson, "The Rape Victim: Psychodynamic Considerations," *American Journal of Psychiatry* 133, no. 4 (1976): 412.

29. Lauretta Bender and Abram Blau, "The Reaction of Children to Sexual Relations with Adults," *American Journal of Orthopsychiatry* 7 (1937): 517.

30. Matthew Hale, *Historica Placitorum Coronae* (London: Nutt & Gosling, 1734), p. 635.

31. J. Walker, "Reports with Comments of Twenty-One Cases of Indecent Assault and Rape upon Children," *Archives of Pediatrics* 3 (1886); G. Williams, "Rape in Children and Young Girls," *International Clinics* 2 (1913).

32. Williams, "Rape in Children," p. 247.

33. R. W. Anthony, "Rape," *Boston Medical and Surgical Journal* 123, no. 2 (1895): 31; Seymour Halleck,"The Physician's Role in the Management of Victims of Sex Offenders," *JAMA* 180 (1962).

34. Halleck, "Physician's Role."

35. Williams, "Rape in Children," p. 259.

36. Ibid.

37. Sigmund Freud, "The Economic Problem in Masochism" (1924), *Collected Papers*, 2, J. Strachey, ed. (London: Hogarth Press, 1955), pp. 257, 266.

38. Ibid., p. 263.

39. Helena Deutsch, *The Psychology of Women* (New York: Grune & Stratton, 1944), p. 1.

40. Karen Horney, *New Ways in Psychology* (New York: Norton, 1938), p. 110.

41. Ibid., p. 278.

42. Sgroi, "National Needs Assessment," p. 1.

43. Ibid., pp. 1-12.

44. Claude Levi-Strauss, *The Elementary Structures of Kinship* (Boston: Beacon Press, 1969).

45. Henry Giarretto, Anna Giarretto and Suzanne Sgroi, "Coordinated Community Treatment of Incest," in Ann W. Burgess et. al. *Sexual Abuse of Children and Adolescents* (Lexington, Mass.: D.C. Heath & Co., 1978).

46. Russell Middleton, "Brother-Sister and Father-Daughter Marriage in Ancient Egypt," *American Sociological Review* 27, no. 5 (1962): 603-11; Elva Poznanski and Peter Blos, Jr., "Incest," *Medical Aspects of Human Sexuality* (October 1975).

47. T. Sonden, "Incest Crimes in Sweden and Their Causes," *Acta Psychiatric Neurology* 11 (1936); S. Kubo, "Researches and Studies on Incest in Japan," *Hiroshima Journal of Medical Science* 8 (1862); George Devereaux, "The Social and Cultural Implications of Incest among the Mahave Indians," *Psychoanalytic Quarterly* 8 (1939); J. Cooper, "Incest Prohibitions in Primitive Culture," *Primitive Man* 5 (1932).

48. Roland Summit and JoAnn Kryso, "Sexual Abuse of Children: A Clinical Spectrum," *American Journal of Orthopsychiatry* 48 (1978).

49. Nancy Lukianowicz, "Incest I: Paternal Incest," *International Journal of Psychiatry* 120 (1972): 301-318; Noel Lustig, John W. Dresser, Seth W. Spellman, and Thomas B. Murray, "Incest," *Archives of General Psychiatry* 14, no. 1 (1966); Donald J. Langsley, Michael N. Schwartz, and Robert H. Fairbain, "Father-Son Incest," *Comparative Psychiatry* 9 (1968); Pavel Machotka, Frank S. Pittman, and Kalman Flomenhaft, "Incest as a Family Affair," *Family Process* 6 (1967); S. Kubo, "Researches and Studies on Incest in Japan," *Hiroshima Journal of Medical Science* 8, no 1 (1959); George A. Awad, "Father-Son Incest: A Case Report," *Journal of Nervous and Mental Disease* 162, no. 2 (1976): 135-39; Hector Cavallin, "Incestuous Fathers: A Clinical Report," *American Journal of Psychiatry* 122 (1966); Bruno M. Cormier, Miriam Kennedy, and Jadwiga Sangowicz, "Psychodynamics of Father-Daughter Incest," *Canadian Psychiatric Association* 7, no. 5 (1962); Lillian

Gordon, "Incest as Revenge against the Pre-oedipal Mother," *Psychoanalytic Review* 42 (1955); Thomas G. Gutheil and Nicholas C. Avery, "Multiple Overt Incest as Family Defense against Loss," *Family Process* 16, no. 1 (1977): 105-116; H. S. Howard, "Incest—the Revenge Motive," *Delaware State Medical Journal* 31, no. 8 (1959); Joseph Peters, "Children Who Are Victims of Sexual Assault and the Psychology of Offenders," *American Journal of Psychotherapy* 30, no. 3 (1976), 398-421; David L. Raphling, Bob L. Carpenter, and Allan Davis, "Incest: A Genealogical Study," *Archives of General Psychiatry* 16 (1967); James B. Raybin, "Homosexual Incest," *Journal of Nervous and Mental Disease* 148, no. 2 (1969); Matilde W. Rascovsky and Arnaldo Rascovsky, "On Consummated Incest," *International Journal of Psychoanalysis* 30 (1950); J. B. Thompkins, "Penis Envy and Incest," *Psychoanalytic Review* 27 (1940); S. K. Weinberg, *Incest Behavior* (New York: Citadel, 1955); Irving B. Weiner, "Father-Daughter Incest: A Clinical Report," *Psychiatric Quarterly* 36 (1962).

50. Freud, "Studies on Hysteria," (1895), in *Collected Papers*, 2.

51. Freud, "On the Sexual Theories of Children," (1908), in *Collected Papers*, 2; 70.

52. Sandor Ferenczi, "Confusion of Tongues between Adult and the Child," *International Journal of Psychoanalysis* 30 (1949).

53. Ibid., p. 227.

54. Ibid., pp. 228-29.

55. L. Abraham, "The Experiencing of a Sexual Trauma as a Form of Sexual Activity" (1907), in *Selected Papers*, trans. by D. Bryon and A. Strachey (London: Hogarth Press, 1927); Atalay Yorukoglu and John P. Kemph, "Children Not Severely Damaged by Incest with a Parent," *Journal of the American Association of Childhood Psychiatry* 5 (1966): 111-24.

56. Diane H. Browning and Bonny Boatman, "Incest: Children at Risk," *American Journal of Psychiatry* 134 (1977): 69-72.

57. Summit and Kryso, "Sexual Abuse of Children," p. 248.

58. E. Poznanski and P. Blos, "Incest," p. 54.

59. G. Molnar and P. Cameron, "Incest Syndromes: Observations in a General Hospital Psychiatric Unit," *Canadian Psychiatric Association Journal* 20 (1975): 373.

60. Judith Herman and Lisa Hirschman, "Father-Daughter Incest," *Signs: Journal of Culture and Society* 2, no. 4 (1977): 749-753.

61. Giarretto, Giarretto, and Sgroi, "Coordinated Community Treatment," p. 236.

62. A. Nicholas Groth, Ann E. Burgess and Lynda L. Holmstrom, "Power, Anger, and Sexuality," *American Journal of Psychiatry* 134 (1977): 1239-43.

63. A. Nicholas Groth and Ann W. Burgess, "Motivational Intent in the Sexual Assault of Children," *Criminal Justice and Behavior* 4 (1977): 253-64.

64. Ann W. Burgess and Lynda L. Holmstrom, "Sexual Trauma of Children and Adolescents," *Nursing Clinics of North America* 10 (September 1975): 551-63.

65. Ibid.

66. Ann W. Burgess and Lynda L. Holmstrom, "Rape Trauma Syndrome," *American Journal of Psychiatry* 131 (1974): 981-86.

67. Ibid.

68. Ferenczi, "Confusion of Tongues," p. 227.

69. Ibid., p. 228.

70. Herman and Hirschman, "Father-Daughter Incest," p. 741.

71. Ibid., p. 748.

72. Ann W. Burgess, Lynda L. Holmstrom, and Maureen P. McCausland, "Child Sexual Assault by a Family Member: Decisions Following Disclosure," *Victimology* 2 (1977): 236-50.

73. K. Amanda Vaden, *Betrayal* (Montgomery, Ala.: Preferred Healthstyles, 1982).

74. Henry Stack Sullivan, *The Interpersonal Theory of Psychiatry* (New York: Norton, 1953).

75. Erik Erikson, *Childhood and Society* (New York: Norton, 1950). Erikson's failure to adequately study the female developmental process is acknowledged.

76. Irving D. Yalom, *The Theory and Practice of Group Psychotherapy* (New York: Basic Books, 1975).

77. Sullivan, *Interpersonal Theory of Psychiatry*.

Nursing Care of Families Using Violence

Jacquelyn Campbell

"Breaking away"

I have to escape from beneath this dark cloud
cold, ominous, easy to hide in

Need to let sunshine into my life

I'll be blinded by the sudden burst of light
Like a child taking first steps
Falling down sometimes
Get up and try again

Raising my children not to hide beneath the cloud

Laughing and free, we'll grow together
getting our strength from warmth
of the light

    Linda Strawder

Reprinted from *Every Twelve Seconds*, compiled by Susan Venters (Hillsboro, Oregon: Shelter, 1981) by permission of the author.

A violent family is in pain. Without understanding the underlying dynamics nor necessarily labeling the violent behavior as a problem, violent family members are hurting each other, emotionally and physically. Even those members not directly involved as victim or perpetrator are learning that violence is acceptable and are highly at risk to use it themselves, either in the family or outside of it. They are also hurt by the destructive family dynamics. The homes of these families are academies where the children in them learn to become violent adults. Nurses see these families in hospitals, clinics, homes, and mental health settings. Their effective nursing care can be crucial in preventing further violence and in helping specific violent families to end the pain they are causing in each other.

A violent family is considered to be one in which at least one family member is using physical force against another, resulting in physical and/or emotional destructive injury. The issue of when physical discipline of children becomes destructive is important, but is discussed in Chapter 5. In most cases there is also intent to injure on the part of the violent family member, although this is frequently difficult to determine. Thus, a violent family can be one in which there is child abuse, wife abuse, abuse of elderly members, severe physical aggression between siblings, violence by adolescents against parents, or any combination thereof. A family in which there is incest is also considered to be violent, since even if physical force is not actually used, it is implied, and destructive injury is a consequence.

The nursing care section of this book begins with this chapter describing the nursing care of violent or potentially violent families in which the family as a whole is considered the focus of intervention. The suggested interventions are based upon the theoretical frameworks of families, violence, and kinds of family abuse described in previous sections. This chapter will also suggest nursing measures for decreasing violence in our society generally, which will have the effect of decreasing the legitimacy of violence within families. Specific nursing interventions for victims of elder abuse, abuse of female partners, and child abuse are described in Chapters 6, 9 and 10.

Three areas of theoretical background are important in setting the stage for nursing care of violent families. It is necessary to understand:

1. Why the family seems especially prone to use violence as a conflict resolution strategy,

2. The evidence suggesting the intergenerational transmission of violence,

3. The connections between wife abuse and child abuse.

THE FAMILY AS A VIOLENCE-PRODUCING INSTITUTION

The national survey done by Murray Straus and his associates showed that 33 percent of 2,143 conjugal pairs used some form of physical aggression toward a spouse during 1975 and 72 percent of 1,146 couples with children in the home used some form of violence toward them.[1] In addition, there is the growing evidence that elderly family members are being abused (see Chapter 6). These kinds of data explode the myth that the American family is a nonviolent institution. Richard J. Gelles and Murray Straus have suggested several factors that they feel contribute to the family in general using violence.[2]

The first characteristic of families is that there is a great deal of "time at risk" for violence between family members. They spend many hours of every day interacting with each other, time which has the potential of becoming violent. Closely related is the idea that the wide range of activities and interests that a family is involved in affords many possible areas of conflict.

The intensity of involvement in families is another potentiating factor. What may be a minor irritation in a relationship with a friend or coworker may be seriously upsetting between family members. The activities of family members may also impinge on each other's privacy, usage of family equipment, and ability to engage in activities of their own. The many different ages and the difference in sex among family members is also a conflict generating factor.[3]

In addition, there is the concept that family members have the right to try and influence the behavior and values of each other which sets the stage for disagreements. Children have no choice about belonging to this particular group of people, so that solving problems by leaving the group is usually impossible for them. Major life stressors, inherent in the development of the family, also contribute to the possibilities of physical aggression, yet the nuclear family of today is frequently isolated from the support systems of relatives. Finally, the American culture sanctions a certain amount of violence within families both overtly, as in approval of physical punishment for children, and covertly, as in the widespread approval of hitting wives by men.[4]

The cumulative effect of these characteristics of families is that the family can become a very stressful, conflict producing arena where people spend a great deal of time. The family is expected to "absorb emotional tension from external situations as well as internally generated family stresses."[5] Adults also may have been taught in their childhood that violence is an acceptable way to solve problems and therefore be more apt to use physical aggression in response to stresses experienced in normal family life.

THE INTERGENERATIONAL TRANSMISSION OF VIOLENCE

Social learning theory (see Chapter 2) provides the background for understanding the evidence that there is an intergenerational transmission of violence within families. When children are hit by their parents, even as a disciplinary measure, the child learns a powerful message. First of all the parents are demonstrating that violence is an acceptable way to deal with conflict, and second, that love and violence are intertwined. As Gelles explains, "The child learns that those who love him or her the most are also those who hit and have the right to hit."[6]

Suzanne K. Steinmetz, in a study of fifty-seven demographically varied families, found that families primarily used one of three methods of conflict resolution, discussion, verbal aggression (screaming, yelling, threatening), or physical aggression. Whichever form the husband and wife were primarily exposed to in their families of orientation was most likely to be used in their family of procreation. This was true of husband-wife conflicts, parent-child disagreements, and sibling to sibling problems.[7]

The national survey done by Straus, Gelles, and Steinmetz also indicated that "the people who had been hit as teen-agers tended to be the most violent to their own husbands or wives and to their own children."[8] They also found that the siblings who had experienced the most violence at the hands of their parents were most likely to be severely physically aggressive toward each other. Children also hit parents in violent families. Eighteen percent of the children Straus and his colleagues studied had hit one of their parents during the survey year. Not surprisingly, these children had also been frequently and often severely the victims of parental violence. Finally, the survey showed that, "When a child grows up in a home where parents use lots of physical punishment and also hit each other, the chances of becoming a violent husband, wife, or parent are the greatest of all."

THE CONNECTIONS BETWEEN WIFE ABUSE AND CHILD ABUSE

The data summarized in the previous section would suggest that families who are being abusive toward each other at the spousal level or toward children would be prone to be involved in the other form of abuse also. The information available is not conclusive in this regard. Most studies have surveyed samples of abused wives or child abusers for evidence of the other kind of abuse so that a generalizable picture is difficult to obtain. However, the same national survey cited earlier found that couples who did not use physical aggression toward each other at all were the least likely to be abusive toward their children. At the other end of the spectrum, "28% of the children of these high violence couples had been abused during the year."[9]

The studies of samples of abused women and children have also pointed to the interrelationship between spouse and child abuse. Estimates vary as to how much overlap there is, but most research indicates a higher rate of child abuse for violent couples and a higher rate of wife abuse in parents documented as child abusers than in the normal population.[10] This evidence makes sense in terms of the idea that certain families tend to be violent in all of their resolution attempts of serious conflicts.

The factors associated with the family as a violence-prone institution, the intergenerational transmission of violence, and the connections between wife abuse and child abuse suggest that there are families that are violent or prone to being violent which need interventions as a total unit. Nursing interventions with these families are based on the nursing process and begin with assessment.

ASSESSMENT

Before the nurse can make an effective assessment of violence in a family, she must first examine her own feelings about the subject and be committed to the idea that violence is an important health problem and within the scope of nursing. Violence is not an easy area to explore with families, and it is usually much easier to just not get into it. Strong feelings may be aroused, of anger and despair in family members, and of justifiable fear in the nurse. Before she begins routinely to explore violence in family nursing care, it is useful for the nurse to attend workshops on the issue and/or arrange for group discussions with her colleagues. In such settings, role play can be used to help nurses anticipate dealing with confrontations within families. Once a family member has been identified as violent or potentially violent, that information colors the nurse's interactions with him or her. Nurses need to be able to share their fear with peers and explore ways of handling it through discussion.

The incidence of physical injury and death from violence outside and especially within the home indicates the seriousness of the problem. Nurses are probably in people's homes more than any other professionals. If nursing care of families does not include assessing and intervening with violence, it will probably not be identified as a problem until someone has been seriously injured or killed. Rather than waiting for that to occur and letting the police or courts or social worker intervene at that point, with demonstrably poor results, nursing can work for early identification and prevention as with any other serious health problem. After examining her feelings and working to gain knowledge and expertise, the nurse is in a prime position to make a significant impact in the prevention of morbidity and mortality from violence.

The other aspect of feeling exploration to be noted is the idea that family conflict resolution is a private matter and nobody's business but the family's. These feelings can also be discussed in workshops or nursing conferences in the agency involved. The families may also feel this way and perceive their privacy as being invaded by questions in this area. If the nurse handles her questions in this realm as a routine area of assessment with a matter-of-fact demeanor, the inquiry will seem more comfortable. If the family questions the need for such exploration, the nurse can share the facts about the prevalence of abuse and injuries from violence. This is valuable not only in making the family feel more at ease, but also in educating the public about the problem of violence. The first few times the nurse includes a detailed assessment about violence may be uncomfortable for her, but just as nursing has learned to include sexual functioning assessment without discomfort, violence in the family can also be learned to be handled easily with practice.

An important area to consider in any family assessment is family strengths. The healthy areas of family functioning need to be explored with the family, both in order to see the total picture and to identify areas that can be built upon in nursing interventions. The model of family well-being as presented in Chapter 3 can be used as a framework for identification of family strengths. Using this framework, the nurse would include in the assessment looking for areas of family functioning, both past and present, where needs of individual members are met by the family and the family has adequate physical and affective resources. An inventory of social supports both within and outside the family, providing direct aid, emotional support, and/or affirmation to members or the total family unit will indicate relationships that can be strengthened and utilized further. Healthy coping mechanisms used to deal with normative life changes and developmental issues would be identified. Areas where the family feels a sense of accomplishment and problems felt to be effectively solved need as thorough an exploration as areas of difficulty. Family actions that foster appropriate help seeking and utilization behavior can be identified as actions to be encouraged for future referrals. As a general indication of family well-being, each individual member can be asked about their personal sense of their own life as a whole and their perception of their family. Family functions which have enhanced individual and total unit perceptions of well-being in the past would be identified as important family mechanisms to be encouraged by nursing care.

Assessment of a total family is usually done in primary care health settings, in community nursing, and in mental health settings when a whole family has been referred. Whenever a family history is being taken, it is important that patterns of family conflict resolution be explored. Questions about this area of concern should also be included in the social/personal section of the history of individuals. Physical assessment of family members will, of course, include watching for signs of trauma. Observation of intrafamilial interactions are also important in family assessment. Taken together, the history, physical exam and nursing observations, done with an awareness of the possibility of violence in the family, will bring to light potential and actual problems the family is having with violence.

History

There are several areas of the history of families that can indicate that the family may be having or is prone to having, problems with violence. These areas, along with at-risk findings, have been outlined in Table 8-1. In addition, as part of the data collection, the nurse should use direct questions about physical aggression. Questions about methods of disciplining children, including physical punishment, are usually routinely asked in the nursing history of families, but in the past direct inquiry about other forms of violence have often been neglected. The nurse needs to ask whether hitting is ever done between any family members.

Nursing judgment is required in assessing how many of the at-risk findings constitute a real problem with physical aggression in the family. Physical punishment of children is usually considered normal with little follow-up questioning. On initial assessment the nurse needs to inquire more about such childrearing practices, how often physical punishment is used, whether or not such implements as

Table 8-1 *Indicators of Potential or Actual Violence in a Family from Nursing History*

Area of Assessment	At-Risk Responses
I. Information from Genogram	Severe physical punishment or husband-wife violence in parental families of origin
	Violent death or serious injury from violence in genogram
	Family members incarcerated for violent crime
	Family members in parental families of origin using violence outside the home
	Wife abuse in husband's previous marital relationship
II. Family Structure	Single-parent home
	Dependent grandparent in home
	Blended family (involving stepparents and/or stepchildren)
III. Family Resources	Unemployment; poverty
	Inadequate housing
	Elderly member with controlled resources
	Financial problems
	Total control of monetary resources by male head of household
	Perception of inadequate "fit" of family resources to family demands
IV. Family Roles	Rigid traditional sex roles
	Individual or family dissatisfaction with roles family expects individuals to fulfill
	Roles incompatible
	Roles rigid, unchangeable
V. Family Boundaries	Boundaries rigid; mistrust of all outsiders
VI. Family Communication Patterns	Family communications nonnurturing; destructive to some members
	Communications ambiguous
	Lack of communications among family members
VII. Family Conflict Resolution Patterns	Extensive use of verbal aggression; many threats of violence
	Evidence of physical aggression used in husband-wife, parent-child, sibling-sibling or parent-grandparent conflict resolution
	Conflicts seldom resolved to everyone's satisfaction
VIII. Family Power Distribution	Autocratic decision-making by father
	Children have no power
	Grandparent in home who is powerless
	Frequent power struggles

Nursing Care of Families Using Violence

Table 8-1 (Cont.)

Area of Assessment	At-Risk Responses
IX. Family Values	Violence considered acceptable or valued
	Great incongruence of values amongst family members or between family and society
	Differing values amongst family members considered intolerable
X. Emotional Climate	High tension in home
	Lack of visible affection
	Scapegoating
	High anxiety in family member(s)
	Lack of support between family members
	Frequent disparagement between family members
XI. Division of Labor	Rigid division of labor according to sex
	Members highly dissatisfied with division of labor
XII. Support Systems	Family isolation
	Family inhibitions to help seeking
	Children not forming close, supportive peer relationships (especially same-sex peer relationships)
	Lack of support systems considered useful for direct aid, emotional support, and/or affirmation
	Relatives are highly critical; tension among extended family
	Sudden withdrawal by adolescent from social activity and peers
	Violence in extended family
XIII. Developmental Stages	More than one family member facing difficult developmental crisis
	Lack of knowledge in parents of what to expect at various developmental stages in children, selves, and grandparents
XIV. Stressors	At-risk scores on stress scale
	Lack of successful coping mechanisms to deal with stress in past
	Situational crises
	Stress-related physical symptoms in family members
XV. Socialization of Children	Physical punishment used
	Only one parent disciplines children
	Lack of nurturance of children
	Children displaying aggressive behavior, at home or outside of home
	Juvenile delinquency or sexual promiscuity in children

(continued)

Table 8-1 (Cont.)

Area of Assessment	At-Risk Responses
XVI. Intrafamily Relationships	Sexual dissatisfaction between parents
	High dependency between family members; autonomy in children not allowed; symbiotic relationships
	Rigid triangulation
	Frequent threats of divorce or separation between parents
	Violence between family members
	Extramarital affairs
	Poor school performance or truancy in children
	Family never has times that they enjoy being together
	Problems between stepparent and stepchildren
	Problems between parents and in-laws when living in the home or close by
	Children running away
XVII. Perception of Family Well-Being	Persistent feelings of dissatisfaction with family life as a whole in one or more family members
	Perception of family as unable to deal effectively with problems
	Perception of family as accomplishing little or nothing
	Perception of family not fulfilling the most important family functions
	Individual needs exceeding family ability to meet on a regular basis
XVIII. Health History	Frequent trauma injuries to family members
	Adolescent suicide attempts
	Serious illness in a family member
	History of treatment for mental illness or vaginal trauma
	History of venereal disease or genital trauma in children
	Drug or alcohol abuse
	Substance abuse in adolescents

(Also include responses from Tables 9-1 and 10-2).

belts are ever used, whether the form of such punishment is spanking or slapping or hitting with fists. After a relationship with the family is established, this area can be returned to and the nurse can discuss the implications of even the mildest forms of physical punishment.

Another area which is infrequently explored fully is sibling fighting. Keeping in mind the Steinmetz findings that sibling conflict resolution mirrors adult and parent-child methods in both form and severity, the full picture of sibling fights and how they are handled needs to be carefully assessed.[11] Children often learn how to handle anger in their relationships with brothers and sisters and how the parents guide such interactions. When brothers and sisters are allowed to use unrestricted physical aggression against each other, they also learn that violence is endorsed as a way to solve problems. The potential for severity in such conflicts is also frequently overlooked. Extrapolating from their findings in the large national survey of family violence, Straus, Gelles, and Steinmetz estimate that "2.3 million children in the United States have at some time used a knife or gun on a brother or sister."[12] Siblings using physical aggression against each other can no longer be considered necessarily normal, nor can this be considered an area not needing intervention.

Sexual abuse within the family is difficult to assess and may only come to light after intense involvement with the family. It is important that nurses be aware of the possibility of incest and try to elicit information about its occurrence when there are indications that it may be a possibility. Taking an individual history on each family member prior to, during, or after conducting the physical exam in private may be an avenue to use for uncovering sexual abuse. Victims of incest are usually able to disclose the activity to helping professionals when directly asked about it.[13] Changes in the behavior of the child or indications of vaginal irritation and/or trauma are important suggestions that incestuous activities have taken place. It is also important to assess the relationship, by observation and history, of female children to adult males who are in and around the home frequently. It must be remembered that sexual abuse is frequently carried out by uncles, cousins, and close family friends as well as by fathers and stepfathers. The mother of the child may have knowledge or suspicions of the incest, and as the relationship with the nurse develops, she may ask oblique questions concerning "normal" sexual activity or make general references to problems in the sexual relationship between herself and her spouse. It is important that these questions be followed up, and if there is any indication of possible sexual abuse, direct queries should be made about it.

The incestuous family is often very closed and isolates itself from helping professionals if possible. An aura of secrecy in the general family feeling tone and a closed attitude toward the nurse's questions during the history-taking phase may alert her to the possibility of incest. It is important to keep the lines of communication open with these families and delay closing the case until further assessment can be made. It may take a great deal of time before trust can be engendered in these families, and the nurse must be patient. Another way to obtain the needed information is to elicit the help of another adult who the child trusts; often a teacher or school nurse can be extremely helpful in this regard. The nurse can share her uneasiness about the possibility of sexual abuse in the family and ask the other professional to approach the child if she herself has not yet formed a trusting relationship with the girl. If the suspicions of incest are strong, Protective Services must be informed as with any other case of child abuse. There is no such thing as consensual sex between an adult family member and a child. As Judith Herman states,

> Because a child is powerless in relation to an adult, she is not free to refuse a sexual advance. Therefore, any sexual relationship between the two must necessarily take on some of the coercive characteristics of a rape, even if, as is usually the case, the adult uses positive enticements rather than force to establish the relationship.[14]

Assessment Tools

The genogram or kinship diagram is an important tool of family assessment. The genogram can fruitfully include questions on violence as well as other health problems. This will have to be asked about specifically or it will not come to light. Keeping in mind the intergenerational transmission of violence, the genogram should include inquiries about wife and child abuse, violent injury and death, histories of incarceration for violent crime, and family members' use of violence in interpersonal relationships outside the home. Cultural sensitivity and an awareness of differential treatment by the law according to race and class is necessary when assessing this information, however. Questions that start with asking about people ever having been hit and followed up with asking about how often the hitting occurred and how severe it was are more useful than using the word abuse. Many people do not recognize a history of significant violence as abuse when it has happened to them or a family member.

Nursing assessment of families may include more formal assessment tools which tap areas of concern especially for determining potential for violence. The Feetham Family Functioning Survey (FFFS) has been shown to be a reliable and concurrently valid nursing measure which can quickly indicate perceptions of dissatisfaction with family functioning.[15] The instrument is designed to be self-administered and can be completed in ten minutes. When scores on this instrument indicate perception of problems in family functioning, it provides a useful beginning point for discussion about the areas indicated as problematic (for example, the FFFS indicator, "Disagreement with Spouse") which would include questions about possible violence.

Physical Assessment

As well as physical exam of individual family members, an important part of the objective portion of assessment is observations of family interactions. Physical exam at-risk findings for abuse of individuals can be found in Tables 9-2 and 10-2 in the chapters on nursing care of abused children and abused wives. Table 8-2 in this chapter instead focuses on important areas of observation that the nurse needs to make in order to assess the possibility of violence in the family. Objective observation of family members interacting with each other is very important in highlighting discrepancies between what actually happens and what has been described. Home visits when as much of the family as possible is home are extremely valuable in this regard. Community health nursing home visits often take place when only the mother and preschool children and/or a grandparent are at home, and the nurse may miss important elements. Creativity is needed to insure a total assessment of the family, and interventions for family problems with violence are almost impossible if the nurse only has a relationship with the mother. The nurse should attempt to have fairly lengthy visits of initial assessment. Children may be able to maintain their "best behavior" for a short time, but a longer visit will often allow interactions to become more nearly what they are without a stranger in the home.

The nurse will also often find that complete assessment with relation to observa-

Table 8-2 Indicators of Potential or Actual Violence in a Family from Nursing Observation

Area of Assessment	At-Risk Observations
I. General Considerations	Observations differ significantly from information gathered on history
II. Family Resources	Family members inadequately clothed and groomed
	One family member inadequately clothed and/or groomed, but the rest are not
	Household totally disorganized and family members indicate displeasure with the lack of organization
III. Family Roles	One parent looks to the other to hold major interaction with children
	One parent answers all questions
	One parent looks to other for approval before answering questions
IV. Family Communication Patterns	Members continually interrupt each other
	Members answer questions for each other; one member never talks for him or herself
	Negative nonverbal behavior in other members when one family member is speaking
	Members frequently misunderstand each other
	Members do not listen to each other
V. Family Conflict Resolution	Verbal aggression used in front of nurse
VI. Family Power Distribution	Members act afraid of another member
	One person makes all decisions
	Power struggles
VII. Emotional Climate	Nonverbals unhappy, anxious, fearful
	Excessive physical distance maintained between members
	Members never touch each other
	Tense atmosphere
	Secretive atmosphere
	Voice tones sharp, nonaffectionate, disparaging

(Also include observations from Table 9-2 and 10-3.)

tions about possible violence comes over time. As the relationship with the family develops and the members become more comfortable with the nurse, more normal interactions will be conducted in her presence. The family may also reveal more about the nature of their relationships verbally as the helping relationship is formed. The nurse can return to areas of the history that she feels the family was reticent or uncomfortable about in the working stage of the relationship. It is often useful to have shown the family that the nurse is empathetic, knowledgeable, and helpful in other more concrete or traditionally nursing areas of family concern before attempting to fully assess and intervene with potential or actual violence.

Nursing Diagnosis

Family assessment data are now synthesized into family nursing diagnoses. As with an individual, the nurse must work with the family in the identification of problems and concerns. The first priority of this final stage of assessment is a listing of family strengths as both the nurse and the family perceive them. This starts diagnosis in a positive note and identifies areas of competence that can be built upon. Even the family badly disintegrated by violence has strengths that need to be recognized by all as a basis for confidence that problems can be worked out. Problems with violence may well not be the primary concern of the family at first. If the nurse's judgment does not indicate serious danger to any of the family members or suspicion of child or other dependent person abuse, which must be immediately reported, she can indicate her observations concerning potential violence but wait to work on the problem until the family is ready or has had their more immediate health problems dealt with. It is often useful to state the concerns about violence in terms of ways of solving disagreements or methods of disciplining children rather than using the words violence or abuse which can appear judgmental and threatening to the family.

The sample nursing process at the end of the chapter (Table 8-3) indicates several possible nursing diagnoses which may be used for a family experiencing potential of actual violence. These are of course only hypothetical diagnoses, but they may be helpful in working or providing a base for modification according to each particular family.

PLANNING

The first portion of the planning process is setting goals with the family. This can be difficult when working with an entire family, because goals for one member may not match those of another. The process is best carried out with the entire family group and can provide a form of intervention as the family discusses what they really want in terms of conflict resolution. Frequently, members are encouraged in such a setting to express desires for the future that no one else realized they had. Parents are often surprised at how much fighting between each other assumed to be "in private," is actually known and of concern to children. Children are almost always aware of parental verbal and physical aggression towards each other, and open discussion with the nurse acting as role model and referee if necessary, is very helpful, both as clarification to parents and children as to what is happening and as a starting point of goal setting.

If it cannot be arranged for the whole family to work together with the nurse to identify goals, a family meeting can be suggested before the next session with the nurse. It is extremely important that every member of the family, no matter how young, have input into the planning process. A group process of learning how to have whole family discussions and family problem-solving sessions, can be a new experience for a family and an important intervention in and of itself. Goal setting is an excellent place to start because it focuses on ideas for the future, often less conflict generating than problems in the past. It is useful for the problem identification, goal setting, and planning to be done on paper with a copy for the family. They can then work on reformulations during time when the nurse is not present. If the whole family cannot be persuaded to work together, at the very least, room should be left on the sheets for input from absent family members.

The family must be helped to set concrete and easily achievable short-term goals as well as more idealistic long-term goals. They can be encouraged to see that the short-term goals are steps toward the long-term solutions and therefore more easily achievable but important to set and evaluate in terms of marking progress toward the future goals. Goal setting, when done correctly, can serve as an important motivator for all the family members. Achievement of short-term goals is a valuable reinforcer of the effort being expended.

When the whole family has been involved with goal setting and planning interventions, there is much more likelihood of successful nursing care. The family is also better equipped to decide what is actually feasible for them than the nurse. The nurse can make suggestions, make sure that each family member has a say, and can encourage exploration of alternatives, but she must be very careful not to impose solutions on the family. The inclusion of children in the planning process is a good way to get some very creative suggestions for interventions. It also helps their sense of being important to the family and models a truly democratic way of solving family problems. The whole family may be very uncomfortable with this mode of group interaction at first, especially if they have been used to an autocratic method of family decision making. It is extremely important that the nurse try to arrange a total family interaction time when she can be present for the planning process. Absent family members may sabotage the interventions if they have not had input. The nurse should also be there to guide the interaction and teach the family how it can be done if they are not used to such a process. This is the basis for continued interventions.

NURSING INTERVENTION

Nursing interventions with families experiencing violence can be taken at the societal and community level as well as with individual families. Nursing care is directed toward the prevention of violence in families as well as the identification and treatment of families who are already involved with the problem. From incidence statistics and the aspects of family life that make violence a possibility, it is readily apparent that much work needs to be done. The first task is to prevent the seeds of violence from being planted in this, unfortunately fertile ground, the family.

Primary Prevention

Primary prevention of violent families is a task to be undertaken by many segments of our society, including nurses. To prevent families from becoming violent, nursing must promote nonviolence in family interactions and in society in general, take specific measures to try to eliminate physical aggression from the family arena, and identify and intervene with families who are at risk to become violent.

Promotion of Nonviolence

Elimination of violence from our society is an awesome undertaking. However, there are some specific measures that nurses can advocate for on a societal level which can make a difference. The first of these is to decrease the amount of violence in the media. Based on social learning theory, less violence on television, in children's books, and in movies will decrease the amount of modeling for violence that is needed for learning.

Measures have been instituted to rate movies for violence (and sex) so that young children may be prevented from seeing films that are problematic for them. These ratings are unclear guidelines for parents concerned about violence. The PG (Parental Guidance) rating is the most troublesome in terms of violence. It takes diligent reading of movie reviews and asking other parents to determine if a movie rated PG contains a great deal of violence. The raters seem to be more concerned with graphic sex than with the murder and mayhem being shown in some PG films. The context of the violence is also very important. For children old enough to distinguish fantasy from reality, an obviously unrealistic movie containing violence may have less of an aggression producing result.[16] When the hero of the film uses force to achieve laudable aims or violent characters are not punished for their acts, a message of the legitimacy of using violence is conveyed. Nurses need to advocate a rating system that differentiates PG films on the basis of violence.

Violence on television continues to be a problem for parents. In spite of the laudable efforts of the PTA and AMA, children's television programming continues to be violent and evening programs, even in the so-called family hour, are filled with physical aggression. Parental supervision of children's TV viewing is only part of the answer. As soon as public outcry efforts run out of momentum, the networks seem to return to violence. Nurses need to help in maintaining pressure on the programmers to decrease the violence being shown.

Another aspect of societal advocacy that nurses can join, is the fight for gun control legislation. Sixty-two percent of Americans surveyed in the most recent Gallup poll favor some form of more stringent gun laws, yet the National Rifle Association's powerful lobby has kept this from becoming a reality. The connections between unrestricted gun ownership and homicide rates seem clear. The United States has a yearly homicide rate of 9.7 per 100,000 compared to the strict handgun law countries of Japan, Britain, and West Germany which have homicide rates of 1.6, 1.3, and 1.3, respectively.[17] Advocating for gun control is not the only answer to violence, but it is a start. It would not only prevent some arguments from becoming lethal, it would also create more of a climate of negative sanction toward violence.

Most nurses have not been involved in political advocacy in the past. However, the ANA and state nurses' associations are beginning to lead the profession in using the potential political power that nurses have. Individual nurses can be effective by writing their legislators, but this impact can be magnified many times by working through the local and state units of the ANA. Linkages can be formed with other organizations concerned about these issues, and nurses can spearhead national campaigns which would have considerable power. There is considerable support for decreasing media violence and gun control legislation. What remains is mobilization and effective political action.

The other arena where nurses can have considerable impact is in childrearing. Whole cultures are totally nonviolent, and their way of living can be mainly traced to the way their children are raised and the strong sanctions against aggression in their cultures. High school parenting classes and childbirth education classes are the places to start with strong messages about raising children without using physical punishment. Both laboratory studies of aggression and anthropological research on nonviolent cultures suggest that cooperation, empathy, nurturance, tenderness, sensitivity to feelings, and an abhorrence to violence need to be taught as primary values to young children of both sexes. In other words, boys need to be socialized more like girls are. Nurses can also be useful in supporting the teaching of nonaggressive problem solving to children in preschools. The use of physical punishment in schools must be abolished wherever it is found. When schools use physical aggression to discipline students they are only teaching that our society sanctions the use of violence, and they are teaching it not only to the children being punished, but to the rest of the students in that school system as well. Wherever nurses have contact with parents, in clinics, in school nursing, in community health nursing, in inpatient and outpatient pediatric settings, the message of nonviolence can be spread.

Another important societal and community intervention is for nurses to advocate for and teach special classes to schoolchildren on sex and violence. Important gains can be made in the prevention and early detection of incest if children know what is inappropriate sexual contact and who they should tell if any such occurs. A full discussion of incest with children, including the invariable threats to not tell and protestations of normalcy and affection by the offender, arms children with the knowledge necessary to get help immediately before serious physical and emotional damage has been done. Such discussions can best be held within the context of a general health curriculum. This kind of curriculum would include general sex education, health promotion, and emotional health content incorporating how to deal with violence and the promotion of nonviolence values and problem-solving methods. The curriculum would be taught at every grade level, with age-appropriate teaching methodologies. Nurses can advocate for the establishment of such curricula both as school nurses and community health professionals and as concerned citizens and parents.

A final area of broad nursing intervention is the promotion of healthy attitudes toward the elderly and advocacy of programs which allow older Americans independence and useful functioning as long as possible. Nurses can be in the forefront in helping the young respect the aging process, rather than dread and fear it. Learning institutions and social service agencies need to take advantage of the potential participation of older adults. Programs which provide home health care or daycare to the elderly must be advocated. It is unrealistic to expect that all dependent elderly can be totally cared for in their children's homes. Nurses are ideal to begin and administer such programs. Promotion of third-party payments for nurse-administered daycare centers is also needed.

Families at Risk

The identification of families at risk to become violent includes both performing assessment in one's own professional practice and advocating for its inclusion by other health professionals. Any family which uses physical punishment or any form of physical aggression can be considered at risk to become violent, because violence tends to escalate under stress. Families under a great deal of stress, from poverty, unemployment, recent divorce or death in the family, severe illness in a family member, developmental crises in family members, remarriage, and changes in location or job can be considered to be at risk also. This is especially true if their methods of conflict resolution are problematic to any of the family members. In addition, families where communications are unclear or discordant or at a very low level can be identified as at risk to become violent. An absence of emotional nurturance or psychological abuse can also be considered as at-risk indicators. A final category of families at risk for violence are those with a dependent elderly person in the home, especially if there is a history of verbal and/or physical aggression in the family and/or the elderly family member is adding considerable financial or emotional stress to the home (see Chapter 6). An overall framework to identify families at risk is to evaluate the "fit" of family resources to demand (see Chapter 3).

Interventions with these families consist of primarily helping them to develop democratic ways of solving problems in the family. Steinmetz's study showed that the more democratic the family was, in power relationships and in conflict resolution, the less likely they were to use physical aggression.[18] She also found that the most effective outcomes of conflict, in family members' perceptions, were those that were treated as a shared problem that could be solved with mutual benefits. Destructive resolutions were those that became adversary contests, power struggles between family members. Nurses need to help families evolve more constructive ways to deal with the inevitable disagreements that characterize family life. It is useful to sit down with the whole family and help them work through a relatively minor conflict that has come up amongst them. One that is not rife with deep emotions or a long-standing history of arguments about it is best. Once the family has seen how this kind of disagreement can be solved without it becoming a power struggle or aggressive argument, they can start to practice the same kind of thing with more difficult problems.

Effective means of disciplining children, besides the use of physical punishment, need to be discussed and modeled by the nurse. This idea may seem very foreign to the parents, and a careful laying of groundwork is necessary before any suggested alternatives will be heard. It is frequently useful to explore with the parents how they themselves were punished as children and how they perceived hitting by their parents. The perceptions of the physical aggression can also be explored with the children. If the nurse can show how effective her use of positive reinforcement can be with the family's children, this is a powerful teaching method. Getting the parents to at least try other methods of correction and carefully evaluating their results is also useful. Children who are becoming aggressive themselves both outside the home and within it are a good example for the nurse to tie with the use of physical punishment in the home. This is a tricky area of intervention, and the development of a firm trusting relationship is necessary before parents will listen to the nurse on the subject of discipline.

Another aspect of intervention is to help the family develop and use more fully various support systems. Today's nuclear family has become more isolated from relatives, the church, and neighbors. It is more likely to move frequently than the families of the past. Community agencies and groups may be able to take the place of some of the more traditional support systems, but the family may need help in finding groups that are suitable and of interest to them. They also may want someone to attend such a group with them for the first time. The nurse may be that person, or she may be able to suggest another family in the area who could go also.

Other interventions with families at risk may include helping to alleviate some of the stressors the family is facing. The nurse may be able to work with social services in helping family members to obtain jobs, further education, or work training. Anticipatory guidance for developmental crises, such as adolescence, birth of the first child, and retirement can be very helpful for families. Part of the intervention is to help the family assess how much stress they are under and the normalcy of tension in the home in particularly stressful times. Ways the family members can help each other with stress, including helping to arrange for times and places of privacy for the individuals, can be useful.

Problems with family communications and/or a lack of nurturance of family members can best be addressed through sessions conducted with the whole family to improve communications. The professional nurse can easily conduct this kind of family intervention with the extensive background in therapeutic communications provided in most nursing education. The principles are the same; the family is helped to see blocks that the members are presently using in communication with each other, and members are taught to use active listening and therapeutic techniques of exploration of feelings. The most widely used block in family interactions is giving advice, and modeling of shared problem solving can be done by the nurse to provide an alternative. Family members can be taught to make their messages clear and unambiguous. They need to be helped to respond to each other in ways that are nurturant and self-worth enhancing rather than destructive. Almost all families at risk can benefit from at least a few sessions of this kind of family intervention.

A final possible intervention is referral to agencies directed toward the prevention of child abuse or other agencies offering classes in parenting or other such services. Some of these programs offer respite care of children for families under a great deal of stress and a variety of groups for parents to help them deal with stress. These kinds of alternatives are useful as an adjunct to nursing care. Daycare programs for the elderly or home health agencies that offer help with household management as well as health care for dependent elderly persons can offer the same kind of assistance to families hard pressed to deal with an ill grandparent or one who has more needs than the family can provide on a daily basis without inordinant stress.

Secondary Prevention Interventions

Secondary prevention level interventions include identification of families that are beginning to use violence beyond the physical punishment of children. Such families may be referred because of possibilities of abuse or because a child is becoming violent in school. Nurses may identify incestuous families secondary to the diagnosis of venereal disease in young children. This may be considered a definite sign of sexual abuse, and almost definitely incest, because the child would have told of the sexual contact unless it was with a relative or close family friend. Adolescent female runaways are also frequently incest victims; one estimate is that 70 percent of the children who run away from home are sexually abused.[19] Male and female runaways may also be fleeing other forms of violence in the home. Juvenile delinquents often also are reflecting the violence in their families, and sexually promiscuous teenage girls are frequently the victims of incest and other forms of violence. When a child (or adolescent) is identified as a problem because of aggression toward his or her parents, it must be remembered that the child may be retaliating for abuse received or he or she may be intervening to protect the mother from wife abuse. These families are starting to use violence toward each other in a variety of ways and must be intervened with as quickly as possible to prevent further physical and emotional damage.

Immediate intervention may frequently take the form of crisis intervention. If a particularly violent episode resulting in serious physical injury has occurred, or a son or daughter has run away or been arrested, or incest has just been discovered, the family may well be in a situation for which they have no previously learned coping mechanisms. In such a state, the family is extremely open to assistance offered by the nurse, but may not be able to participate as fully in mutual assessment and planning as has been suggested previously because of high anxiety. The nurse may need to make a quick assessment, mainly based on the crisis situation, and offer concrete assistance that will decrease the anxiety.

Crisis intervention also includes helping the family members define what the situation means for each of them in terms of their feelings about it and their intellectual understanding of what has happened. The nurse may be able to clarify for family members exactly what is likely to happen next, because a great deal of the anxiety generated in a crisis is fear of the unknown. Supportive networks need to be established, for instance relatives, friends, or clergy called, so that the family will have continued support and people to whom to express feelings after the nurse has gone. It is important that family members themselves indicate who they perceive as supportive; it may not be traditional sources.[20]

The healthy coping mechanisms that the nurse sees being used should be encouraged and family members helped to understand that strong feelings are normal in the situation and may not always be handled nicely. The family may use a great deal of denial in the crisis situation, especially at first, while they gather their resources. They may deny the seriousness of the situation or blame it on irrelevant external factors. The denial must be allowed although not encouraged and insight supported as it begins to appear. Family members are often very good at helping each other begin to see the ramifications of the crisis situation and should be encouraged to interact together as much as possible.

The total family is affected by violence and thus needs to be considered the focus of intervention. Younger children may misunderstand or be frightened by what has happened, and the first impulse of parents is often to send them away to a friend or relative. This may be useful for infants and toddlers, and the nurse can help to arrange it, but older children are better served if they are allowed to stay and participate in discussion. The nurse can make sure that the children understand what is going on, reassure them that they are not to blame in some way, and find out whether they themselves would rather stay or go.

The final part of crisis intervention is to make sure that the family will be followed up by concerned professionals. This may be done by the nurse herself, depending on her professional role, or by another nurse or professional to whom the family is referred. During the four to six weeks immediately following the crisis-precipitating event, the family is particularly open to learning new coping mechanisms and working on eliminating the violence from the home. It is imperative that this time of crisis be used to full advantage in terms of promotion of growth. This may be the only time in which violent family members are willing to accept help, and referral must be swift and appropriate. This may be the most important nursing intervention of the crisis period, and the nurse must be sure that the referred to agency or person is acceptable to the family and will see them immediately.

Nursing intervention at the secondary prevention level will frequently involve working with protective services. If the violence is directed toward children, either physically or sexually, a report to protective services is mandatory. They can also be helpful in working with the families by providing counseling and a variety of social services. The same is true of adult branches of protective services that operate in most cities. Although not as strongly mandated by law, reporting of elderly or spouse abuse to adult protective services may be appropriate, especially if the family is resistive to other interventions. An investigation by the agency will ensue which impresses on the family the seriousness of the problem and may prompt their seeking help through protective services or other agencies. The nurse may have the advantage of being able to work with the family through and after adult or child protective service investigation. Even when there has not been enough evidence to warrant abuse or assault charges, the nurse can continue to work with the family in preventing further violence. Nurses need to be aware, in advance of referral, exactly how protective services operate in the particular community in which they practice. They need to be able to explain to families precisely what will ensue and how much time will be involved. It is extremely helpful if the nurse is on personal terms with the professionals at the local protective services so that coordination and continuity efforts are successful and the nurse is current on agent protocal and policy.

Other agencies may be used as referrals by the nurse. Community mental health clinics and private psychiatrists, psychologists, and social workers knowledgeable about violence in families may be helpful. Nurse-to-nurse referrals are often preferable, when the identifying nurse's professional role does not include the kind of long-term home visitation or therapy sessions required by such families. Psychiatric mental health clinical nurse specialists, nurse family therapists, and family nurse practitioners are often available as consultants in community health agencies or as part of community mental health centers or primary care clinics. Nurses practicing in other settings need to search out these nurse specialists and make sure they are knowledgeable about violence. Then linkages can be formed so that the nurse-to-nurse referrals are conducted with a minimum of red tape and waiting for the families.

The identifying nurse may continue to work with the family on some of their other health concerns and in reinforcing and supporting the therapy being conducted by other professionals. It is beyond the scope of this book to actually teach the basics of family therapy with a seriously dysfunctional family.[21] However, some descriptions of aspects of family therapy specific to families experiencing violence will be described.

Family therapy with violent families necessitates the nurse having a firm personal support system of colleagues with which she can discuss the progression of therapy. Violent families, including those who are incestuous, engender strong feelings in the nurse and can be extremely draining. In addition, the intrafamily dynamics are very strong and the nurse can easily become caught up in them. The Minuchen model of "joining" the family can be helpful in gaining a true appreciation for the values of the family and engendering trust, but enmeshment with a severely violent family can cloud judgment if careful self-awareness is not maintained.[22] Frequent discussions with a supervisor or colleague can help the nurse stay objective. It also must be kept in mind that these families have usually taken several years to get to such a destructive juncture, and the roots of the violence may have preceded the present situation by several generations. Therefore, progress in eliminating the violence will take a great deal of time and hard work on the part of all the participants.

A behavioral family therapy model is frequently suggested for working with violent families.[23] This is helpful in assisting the family with understanding how violent interaction patterns are learned, and in keeping the interactions focused in the here and now, thereby escaping a pattern of blaming individual members for past parts in the violence. At the same time, it is imperative for individual members to take responsibility for their own violent behavior. No matter what model of family therapy is used, it may be necessary for the nurse to use considerable confrontation in making sure that this occurs. The therapy would then focus on the extinction of violent behavior on the part of all family members by setting up enforceable, definite, and undesirable consequences for further violence, coupled with reinforcement of nonviolent behaviors and the teaching of new ways to deal with stress and arguments. Contracts with the nurse and among family members may be helpful in specifically delineating the consequences of physically aggressive behavior. The family members will have to monitor the behavior of each other between therapy sessions, and it is imperative that everyone understand exactly what will happen. It is not enough that the violent relationship of primary concern (such as wife abuse) be the subject of behavior elimination or reinforcing; all the physical aggression in the household must be stopped and new methods of dealing with anger instituted.

As well as using behavioral techniques, it is important that the communication patterns between family members be analyzed and improved. Family members should also have a chance to express their feelings and learn how to accept positive as well as negative feelings from their kin. The power distribution among family members also needs to be analyzed and equalized in most violent families. All these types of intervention are very difficult and demanding.

If at all possible, especially if the family is large and includes several adolescents, a co-therapist arrangement is ideal. There is so much going on in a violent family that two therapists are much more likely to be able to pick up all the underlying dynamics. They can also support each other in confrontation and prevent triangulation attempts that frequently occur with just one therapist in a violent family. If the therapists are male and female, this is also very helpful as many of the family problems may stem from sex role difficulties.

Homework assignments are a useful methodology of intervention with violent family therapy. This allows work to be continued on problems between sessions which is valuable in light of the difficulty of the problems being addressed. Assignments can be in the form of monitoring conflicts and how they were resolved and how constructive the resolution was. Members of the family can also be assigned to spend specific periods of time with other members with whom communication has been strained. Activities designed to enhance communication and which both members have decided would be fun can be decided on for these periods. Whole family activities can also be assigned with input from the members as to what would be enjoyable. Violent families are often so caught up in conflict that they have forgotten how to have fun together. It is valuable if the nurse can at least once accompany the family on an outing. This helps to cement the therapeutic relationship and allows the nurse to observe the family away from home or office.

Secondary prevention measures may also include working with the criminal justice system. The nurse may be called upon to testify in court and/or to create liaisons between the enforcement agencies or lawyers and the family and other professionals involved. She may also be of help by being a supportive and knowledgeable person for the family in the courtroom and during the court proceedings. All of these activities necessitate a working knowledge of the law (as it applies to family violence) and of the criminal justice system. The beginnings of such information can be found in Chapters 14 and 15 of this book. In addition, the nurse needs to advocate for the education and sensitization of judges, district attorneys, police, and defense lawyers to the issues surrounding family violence and the plight of the victims. With such background, the court experience can be therapeutic and of practical assistance for the family, rather than a traumatizing experience.[24]

Secondary prevention of violence in families can thus be seen as a potential area for nursing to make considerable impact. Identification of families using violence in conflict resolution may take place in many nursing settings, including inpatient areas, when this is routinely assessed. Nurses in community health settings, mental health agencies, and primary care facilities may be in a prime position to provide effective interventions, case coordination, and important referrals. Nurse specialists in family therapy and family functioning may continue the interventions in the form of family therapy and long-term case management and follow-up.

Tertiary Prevention

Tertiary level nursing interventions for violence are usually carried out with families who have been broken up because of violence. This may include working with parents who have had a child or children placed in foster homes because of abuse; families who have a member incarcerated because of sexual, elderly, wife, sibling, or child assault or intrafamilial homicide; and families who have gone through a divorce or have a child who has run away permanently because of violence. Some significant emotional and perhaps physical damage has been done, and the nurse is mainly concerned with helping the family return to as healthy functioning as possible and to grieve for their losses.

Part of intervention on the tertiary level is to work with the children. They need to have the emotional effects of the violence assessed and dealt with and to be involved with the learning of different ways to cope with anger to counteract the learning of violent means which has already occurred. More detailed means of working with the children are outlined specifically in Chapter 11.

The adolescents of violent families may be acting out their disturbances in school, by running away, and in engaging in sexual or delinquent activities, as mentioned previously. Coordination efforts are needed with the professionals working directly with these teenagers as a result of their behavior. Nurses can play a significant role in runaway programs for adolescents. It would be extremely helpful for a nurse to be part of the paid staff of such agencies, where teenagers who have run away from home are frequently housed temporarily. These adolescents may have a variety of health problems, including the sexual abuse, other sexual concerns, drug abuse, and alcohol misuse which can effectively be intervened with by a nurse. Group sessions on health matters are an extremely useful mode of intervention with these young people. If a full- or part-time nurse cannot be hired for the program, community health nurses or volunteer nurses can involve themselves in such agencies on the planning level as well as in direct services.

All the family members need concerned, empathetic family sessions with the nurse concerning the effects of the violence on them. The family needs to grieve for the lost family member and the loss of the family as a total unit. The nurse can support them through their stages of mourning and encourage expression of feelings about the events. The family should also examine the impact of violence on their lives and work to eliminate any remaining physical aggression between members. Identification of serious psychological or physical aftereffects is also needed, and appropriate referrals should be made where indicated.

EVALUATION

The evaluation of nursing care of violent families is based upon achievement of the goals set with the family during the planning stage of intervention. Evaluation is an ongoing process starting with the short-term goals with revisions of the plans and long-term goals as needed. As part of evaluation, it is also important to reassess with the family periodically. It is important to conduct evaluation with the entire family so that extensive praise can be given for progress achieved and so that no family member feels judged in his or her absence. Ongoing evaluation also includes frequent contacts with other professionals and/or agencies involved to maintain continuity.

Self-evaluation is also done by the nurse on the basis of the goals. When working with violent or potentially violent families, it is important that the nurse continually look at herself and reevaluate her perceptions and feelings. It may well be that the problems are more extensive than was originally assessed. The full extent of the violence often does not become clear until the nurse has worked with the family for quite some time. Long-term interventions with such families can become draining, and the nurse may decide that her effectiveness as primary therapist or case manager has eroded over time. In such cases it is best to discuss her feelings with the family as well as with a supervisor. If the nurse transfers the family to another professional without a full airing of the dilemma with the family, they may feel abandoned or fear that their case is hopeless.

Final evaluation is the time that the family is encouraged to make realistic plans for the future. If nursing intervention is ending before the problems with violence have been completely resolved, the family needs to have names of people who can be contacted for future interventions. These contacts can also be made if the family experiences a period of particular stress when the physical aggression is apt to exacerbate. If the family can anticipate problems and seek help early, another round of violent interaction may be prevented.

SAMPLE NURSING PROCESS

A sample nursing process for a hypothetical case has been included (Table 8-3). This illustration of nursing care is meant to be helpful in showing how nursing care can be given to victims of family violence. The sample is not meant to be all-inclusive of possible nursing diagnoses or interventions for the problems of violence, but to serve to illustrate what might be used in a hypothetical case. The background given is very brief, and the history and observations only indicate findings related to the violence. In actual nursing care, a much more detailed and holistic history and physical assessment would be conducted.

Summary

Nursing care of violent or potentially violent families is based on theoretical framework that the nature of family interaction is such that violence can easily develop, that physically aggressive interaction modes are transmitted through family socialization from one generation to the next, and that families who are found to be abusive in one form may well be abusive in another as well. Thus, nursing care based on the total family unit is frequently indicated. The nature of the suggested nursing practice is of necessity based upon clinical experience and family nursing principles because of the paucity of nursing research specific to family violence.

Assessment of families for possible violence includes direct questioning about forms of conflict resolution. Other indications that the family may be at risk for or actually experiencing violence were summarized in Tables 8-1 and 8-2. The assessment for violence ends with nursing diagnoses being formulated with the family, a process which should include identification of family strengths. On the basis of the problems listed, the family works together with the nurse to formulate short- and long-term goals and interventions. This process of planning together can be a form of intervention in itself. Interventions are based on the three levels of prevention and include interventions of societal and community advocacy for nonviolence as well as measures taken with individual families. The nurse is in an excellent position to work with the entire family, as well as to be a liaison between the family and other professionals and agencies. Nursing care is finally evaluated with the family on the basis of the goals set. The nursing care of violent families is both challenging and rewarding and has the potential for being an arena where nurses can make a significant impact on decreasing the violent nature of American society.

Table 8-3 Sample Nursing Process

Brief Background

The Smith family is a white middle-class family consisting of the mother, Dora; her second husband, Bill; Patty, a 14-year-old daughter from Dora's first marriage; and Billy, a 10-year-old son of this marriage. Dora's mother, Eileen, also lives with the family and is incapacitated by chronic arthritis. Patty has approached the school nurse with a "twisted" arm which also has several elongated bruises around the wrist. Patty admits to the school nurse that her stepfather has twisted her arm. Upon direct questioning, Patty indicates that the incident occurred when her stepfather approached her sexually and he grabbed and twisted her arm after she refused his advances. The school nurse obtains permission from Patty and her mother to make a home visit. The stepfather is not present when she arrives, but Patty, Dora, Eileen, and Billy are there.

The nurse's observations and history of the family include, but are not limited to the following:

Significant History	Dora states that she and Bill have a satisfactory sexual life. Bill is under a great deal of stress because of a new boss and being "behind" with the bills, and he is extremely irritable toward Dora and she does not feel as "close" to him as she would like. Bill makes all of the decisions in the family and believes in "taking a belt to the kids" when they don't behave. She expresses horror at the news that Bill has tried to have a sexual relationship with Patty. Eileen is totally quiet during the interview and Dora talks for her, even when a question is directly asked of Eileen. Dora says that Eileen is becoming very difficult to care for as her arthritis worsens. Billy has been in trouble in school because of frequent fights with other children and cursing at teachers. Dora expresses a high degree of commitment to "making this marriage work."
Significant Observations	Nonverbals are highly anxious and Eileen looks afraid of Dora. Patty sits very close to Dora and they occasionally touch. Affectionate tones of voice and glances are used between them. Both Eileen and Billy sit apart from the other two. Billy has a sullen expression and answers questions abruptly and without elaboration. Dora's tone of voice is disparaging when she talks about Eileen.

Table 8-3 (Cont.)

Three of the family nursing diagnoses identified are listed in order of priority:

I. Potential for violence (incest) related to spousal marital problems, family stress, inadequate family and individual (father) coping mechanisms, unequal power relationships, and dysfunctional communication patterns.
II. Potential for violence (elderly) related to family stress, dysfunctional communication patterns, chronic illness in grandmother, increased role responsibilities (mother), and inadequate family and individual (mother) coping mechanisms.
III. Aggressive behavior patterns (father and son) related to corporal punishment, observations of aggressive behavior, family stress, and destructive conflict resolution patterns.

I. Potential for subsequent violence (incest)

Family Goals	Nursing Intervention
Overall: No further sexual advances toward Patty as evidenced by: 1. Patty reporting no further advances 2. Protective Service investigation showing no further advances 3. Patty's fear of stepfather diminishing	I. The nurse will: A. Report incident to Protective Services after discussion of such with family on first home visit. B. Initiate and maintain contact with Protective Services to coordinate care. C. Refer family for family therapy with a Family Nurse Practitioner working in a community mental health center. D. Initiate and maintain contact with Family Nurse Practitioner to reinforce and support therapy. E. See Patty regularly in school to discuss the progress being made in the family, monitor events in the home according to her perceptions, and help her express feelings about what is happening and has happened. F. Make regular home visits when all family members are present to obtain the perceptions of other family members and to make continued assessments. G. Build on observed strength of closeness between Patty and Dora by encouraging mother/daughter interactions.
Long-Term: Increased satisfaction with marital relationship at the end of three months as evidenced by:	II. Form therapeutic relationship with family: A. Discuss fully the marital relationship with mother and father.

(continued)

Table 8-3 (Cont.)

Family Goals	Nursing Intervention
1. Signs of decreased tension in the home 2. Dora reporting feeling "closer" to husband	B. Help parents see the relationship of the stress in home with their relationship. C. Build on mother's commitment to marriage as a motivator to improve relationship. D. Support expression of feelings to nurse and of partners to each other. E. Help partners develop more effective coping mechanisms to deal with stress and to help each other cope. F. Suggest regular times for partners to be together alone, including weekends away. Help to arrange for babysitting and suggest Patty learn to care for grandmother at times. G. Teach family how to listen effectively to each other and communicate with respect for the other person. H. Teach parents how to encourage feeling expression to each other as a coping mechanism for dealing with stress and as a relationship-enhancing strategy.

Evaluation is based on achievement of goals as perceived by family and as indicated by criteria met.

II. Potential for subsequent violence (elderly)

Family Goals	Nursing Intervention
Short-term: Increased family sharing of responsibilities of physical care of grandmother at the end of two weeks as evidenced by: 1. Mother feeling less tied down 2. Signs of decreased anxiety in grandmother 3. Less disparaging communication patterns toward grandmother by mother 4. Other family members taking care of grandmother's needs when possible	II. The nurse will: A. Refer grandmother to physician for complete medical workup and suggestions of arthritis treatment. B. Encourage contact of mother's siblings for help in caring for grandmother on selected weekends. C. Help family work out a schedule of care for grandmother that all participate in. D. Point out the communication patterns that mother has been using in relationship to grandmother and teach more effective communication skills.

Nursing Care of Families Using Violence

Table 8-3 (Cont.)

II. Potential for subsequent violence (elderly)

Family Goals	**Nursing Intervention**
	E. Help grandmother express feelings about situation.
	F. Help grandmother and mother really communicate with each other by role modeling and pointing out blocks as they occur.
	G. Praise mother's care of grandmother and encourage other family members to express appreciation for it.
Long-term: Demonstration of improved individual and family coping mechanisms at the end of three months as evidenced by:	
1. Mother feeling less tension	A. Support coping mechanisms being developed in family therapy.
2. Family showing less conflict in communications	B. Encourage family to problem solve with health concerns together during regular home visits; praise their efforts.
3. Family holding regular discussions in order to solve problems	C. Teach supportive communication techniques.
	D. Help mother develop individual coping mechanisms such as relaxation techniques, spending time with friends while other family members take care of grandmother, and expressing feelings openly.

Evaluation is based on achievement of goals as perceived by family and as indicated by criteria met.

III. Aggressive behavior problems

Family Goals	**Nursing Intervention**
Short-term: Recognition within family of the connections between aggressive behavior in son and aggressive behavior in father at the end of two weeks as evidenced by:	
1. A decision by father to refrain from physical punishment	A. Discuss the intergenerational transmission of violence with family.
2. Reports from family therapist of constructive conflict resolution	B. Identify with father of how he learned violence in family of origin.
	C. Encourage and praise efforts made.

(continued)

Table 8-3 (Cont.)

III. Aggressive behavior problems
   Family Goals
   3. Reports from Patty of same

   Long-term:
   Less aggressive behavior in Billy at the end of three months as evidenced by:
   1. Less nonverbal negativity in Billy
   2. Fewer reports of aggressive behavior in school

   Nursing Intervention
   D. Suggest family members keeping a log of conflicts, how they were solved, and how effective the solutions were perceived to be. Discuss these logs with the family.

   A. Support interventions being given to Billy through his school; maintain coordination with professionals there and provide communication between Billy's school and family.
   B. Encourage father to spend at least half hour every day in some kind of one-to-one activity.
   C. Encourage feeling expression between Billy and father.
   D. Praise Billy for nonaggressive behavior and efforts to change. Encourage family to use a great deal of praise with Billy also.

Evaluation is based on achievement of goals as perceived by family and as indicated by criteria met.

Chapter 8

1. Ursula Dibble and Murray Straus, "Some Social Structure Determinants of Inconsistency between Attitudes and Behavior: The Case of Family Violence," *Journal of Marriage and the Family* 42 (February 1980): 73.

2. Richard J. Gelles and Murray A. Straus, "Determinants of Violence in the Family," *Contemporary Theories About the Family* (Vol. I) Wesley Burr, Reuben Hill, F. Ivan Nye and Ira Reiss, eds. (New York: The Free Press, 1979) pp. 549-77, pp. 552-53.

3. Ibid., p. 553.

4. Ibid., p. 553.

5. Suzanne K. Steinmetz, *Cycle of Violence* (New York: Praeger Publishers, 1977), p. 1.

6. Gelles and Straus, "Determinants of Violence in the Family," p. 554.

7. Steinmetz, *Cycle of Violence*, p. 108.

8. Murray A. Straus, Richard J. Gelles, and Suzanne K. Steinmetz, *Behind Closed Doors* (Garden City, N.Y.: Doubleday, 1980), pp. 116, 113, 119, 122.

9. Ibid., p. 115.

10. Karen Coleman, "Conjugal Violence: What Thirty-Three Men Report," *Journal of Marital and Family Therapy* 6 (April 1980): 210; J. J. Gayford, "The Aetiology of Repeated Serious Physical Assaults by Husbands on Wives," *Medicine, Science, and the Law* 19 (January 1979): 23; Jean Renvoize, *Web of Violence* (London:

Routledge and Kegan Paul, 1978) p. 55; Bruce J. Rounsaville and Myrna A. Weissman, "Battered Women: A Medical Problem Requiring Detection," *International Journal of Psychiatry in Medicine* 8 (1977-78): 191-202.

11. Steinmetz, *Cycle of Violence*, p. 116.

12. Straus, Gelles and Steinmetz, *Behind Closed Doors*, p. 117.

13. Ann W. Burgess and Lynda L. Holmstrom, *Rape: Crisis and Recovery* (Bowie, Md.: Robert J. Brady Co., 1979), p. 69.

14. Judith Herman, *Father-Daughter Incest* (Cambridge: Harvard University Press, 1981), p. 27.

15. Carolyn S. Roberts and Suzanne L. Feetham, "Assessing Family Functioning across Three Areas of Relationships," *Nursing Research* 31 (July/August 1982): 231-35.

16. Douglas Sawin, "The Fantasy-Reality Distinction in Televised Violence: Modifying Influences on Children's Aggression," *Journal of Research in Personality* 15 (September 1981): 329.

17. "The Duel over Gun Control," *Time* (23 March 1981), 33.

18. Steinmetz, *Cycle of Violence*, p. 12.

19. Ellen Dunwoody, "Sexual Abuse of Children: A Serious, Widespread Problem," *Response* 5 (July/August 1982): 1-2, 13-14, 2.

20. See Chapter 3.

21. It is suggested that nurses whose roles and credentials include family therapy base their approach on traditional family therapy models reformulated according to nursing conceptual frameworks. Examples of such reformation are given in Ann A. Whall, "Family System Theory: Relationship to Nursing Conceptual Models," in Joyce Fitzpatrick et. al. *Nursing Models and Their Psychiatric Mental Health Applications* (Bowie, Md.: Robert J. Brady Co., 1982), pp. 69-94.

22. Salvadore Minuchin, *Families and Family Therapy* (Cambridge: Harvard University Press, 1974), p. 127.

23. Deborah Watts and Christine Courtis, "Trends in the Treatment of Men Who Commit Violence Against Women," *Personnel and Guidance Journal* 60 (December 1981): 246.

24. Dunwoody, "Sexual Abuse of Children," p. 13.

Nursing Care of Abused Women

Jacquelyn Campbell

scared frightened and
all alone
cant go back to my home
left with only the clothes
on my back
wondering if I'll make it
on the right track
all i have is my daughter and me
made it to the shelter
we are free
now all i have to do is make
a life for katie and me
you gave me hope, courage
and most of all love
and so now i can spread my wings
take off again and go on

    N.L.

I am writing a poem
and it is one of thanks
to the women who've come seeking shelter
to those who have given me strength
its easy to share all your laughter
its harder to share your own tears
so
thank you my sisters, my neighbors
for helping me deal with my fears
its you who have given me courage
to face my own life as it is
and its you who have taken the 1st step
so your children can grow up and live
there are some who can't work in a shelter
and your right it's not all peaches and cream
But its worth all the petty displeasures
just to watch someone learning to dream

    (we grow from each other's growing)
    Kathy Clair

Both poems reprinted from *Every Twelve Seconds*, compiled by Susan Venters (Hillsboro, Oregon: Shelter, 1981) by permission of the authors.

Professional nursing care of battered women is based on theoretical foundations (see Chapter 4) and individualized to women encountered in a variety of settings. Routine assessment for battering, especially in situations identified as being highly conducive to its occurrence, is a necessity in nursing. With awareness of the scope of the problem and a working knowledge of possible indications, nurses can be alert to the possibility of abuse. At-risk findings suggestive of abuse are identified in addition to nursing interventions at all levels of prevention. The starting point is a discussion of how to approach the battered woman so that she feels free to discuss the problem.

APPROACHING THE BATTERED WOMAN

The nurse is especially likely to encounter abused women in the emergency room, in prenatal and maternal care settings, in community health, in primary care settings, in occupational health, and in the mental health field. In addition, she may identify battered women in any inpatient setting. It is not enough to question women about abuse only if there are overt injuries or signs of unhappiness in the marital or cohabiting relationship. A routine question like, "Does your husband or boyfriend ever hit you?" should be included in the history of any woman who indicates a close relationship with a man. Violet Ramonaitis Lichtenstein recommends asking, "Have you ever been physically hurt by anyone?" while inquiring "about past trauma or injuries," or dealing with physical aggression as part of the psychosocial history when inquiring about methods of conflict resolution.[1] The incidence of wife abuse is widespread enough to warrant this. The indications of how few battered women are identified by anyone as such and their reported desire to tell of abuse if asked are especially important reasons to routinely include such questions. The question can be prefaced by an acknowledgment of the sensitivity of the issue and both the nurse's and woman's probable embarrassment with it. The nurse can also explain a bit about the widespread and hidden nature of the problem, since even if the woman is not abused, the information is important public education.

It is extremely important that questioning about battering be conducted in private and with assurances of confidentiality. Battered women are frequently ashamed of the abuse and justifiably frightened of their spouse's power. They are also terribly afraid that he will be told. They have usually had previous experience with the health care system which has not engendered trust. Careful attention to the nurse's own nonverbal cues and proxemics (use of space) is warranted. Some indication of familiarity with the problem is usually helpful in allaying the abused woman's feelings that she is alone in this predicament. It is sometimes difficult in a busy emergency room to take the time to get the woman alone and actually sit down to talk to her. Yet if there is any kind of physical injury, no matter how plausible the explanation or how solicitous the spouse may seem, a few minutes of exploration of possible abuse is definitely justified in light of documented frequent failures in proper diagnosis.

In a study of 481 females entering a hospital emergency room, only 13 of the 197 probable battered women identified were recognized as such by the attending physician.[2] Virginia Koch Drake reports that none of her sample of 12 abused women were asked specifically if they had been abused when they sought help from the medical system. She goes on to say:

> No woman reported positive feelings about the health care received. They felt they were treated impersonally, insensitively, and received minimal to no support from the providers.

One of Drake's subjects said "I just wish somebody would of come right out and asked me. I always hope they'll do that."[3] Nurses must find a secluded place and do just that, ask.

The community health nurse also finds privacy at a premium. The battered woman is usually loath to discuss the problem in front of the children, and the abusive spouse will frequently find a reason to be present when any helping professional is in the home. Suggesting a short walk with the wife, using the reason that the weather is fine or the nurse is restless, may be an effective way to get the woman alone. A battered woman will sometimes be resistant to the idea of home visitation at all; she has usually been warned to keep strangers out of the house. Meeting her at other locations, a restaurant, a social service agency, or a childcare center, may be useful.

When privacy has been obtained and a nonauthoritarian atmosphere created, gentleness is mandatory. At the same time, direct questions are the most useful; the nurse cannot expect the abused woman to respond to oblique references. It must also be kept in mind that the woman may well deny abuse and even if she admits to violence in the relationship, will probably minimize its occurrence at first. If violence is denied but the nurse has valid indications that it is occurring, it is imperative that the door be left open for discussion in the future. Battered women have frequently recounted being handed the name and phone number of a helping person with personal assurances that the person mentioned is trustworthy and knowledgeable about battering. They may not have acted on the referral immediately, but they stress how important the gesture was to them. Some say they kept the card or paper for months, sometimes even years, until they were ready to reach out. In a denial situation, it is also important to document the indications and questions and answers carefully, so that other nurses and professionals can add that piece to data gathered subsequently. Sometimes a presentation of accumulated evidence can help the woman see a pattern of increasing severity and frequency which may tip the scales in favor of seeking help.

There is frustration inherent in situations where the nurse suspects abuse, but only sees the woman once and battering is denied. Such frustration may be

Nursing Care of Abused Women

easily transmitted into anger at the abused woman. It is helpful to recognize the denial as a normal response to battering and allow the abused woman that defense, just as the nurse allows a dying client to deny the knowledge of death until he or she is able to deal with it. However, allowing denial does not mean agreeing with it, and it is easy to convey the impression that the negative answer to queries about violence is the "right" response, the one the nurse was hoping to hear. As with all responses to battered women, the nurse is better prepared to deal with denial effectively if she has thoroughly examined her own attitudes about wife abuse. She must carefully sort out her own reactions to all the myths about battering and look at her general responses to victims of violence. It is extremely helpful to slowly think through a scenario where oneself is the victim of wife abuse at the hands of a man deeply loved, as impossible as that may seem, and place that scene at a time when one's own self-esteem was at the very lowest ebb. Once the nurse has realized that abuse could have or could in the future happen to her, she can better identify with the woman and understand her reactions. Clinical discussion groups and role play with other nurses will also help develop the necessary sensitivity.

The abused woman may admit to being hit, but she may use a variety of mechanisms to minimize the seriousness of the problem. This may take the form of blaming herself for the incidents, blaming alcohol use in her husband, asserting that the violence is permanently over, attributing its occurrence to a period of family stress or other forms of rationalization or intellectualization. Again this is useful to view as partial denial as a reaction to a devastating situation. Gentle exploration of the history of abuse helps the nurse gather data as part of the nursing process. It also helps the woman look at the patterns that have evolved and the magnitude of abuse and thereby be better equipped to make decisions about the future. As Wendy Goldberg and Anne Carey suggest, assessment of the battered woman can be made "an integral part of the therapeutic plan."[4] This is especially important in settings where she may not be seen again.

ASSESSMENT

As indicated, the thorough assessment of any woman in an intimate relationship with a man will include a question in the history about the presence of violence in that relationship. The findings in the history and physical that should alert the professional nurse to the possibility of wife abuse are presented in Tables 9-1 and 9-2. No single at-risk finding in the tables would necessarily indicate abuse, but several such findings would warrant at least an at-risk diagnosis. As with all assessments, the nurse must exercise considerable professional judgment in coming to conclusions, and the client must be apprised of the interpretation, however uncomfortable that may be in the case of battering. When being hit or abuse is confirmed or significantly pointed to, there are several areas of assessment specific to battered women that need to be carefully explored.

History

When violence has been indicated, the most effective means of getting the history of abuse is to use the Kinlein model and allow the woman to talk about the problem from her perspective, "not interrupted," and "given time for full scope, emphasis and even repetition."[5] This can be initiated with a request to "tell me about the hitting," or some such open-ended statement. If the woman asks where to begin, telling her "anywhere you would like" works well. If the information about abuse has come up in the middle of a systematic history, the nurse can indicate her interest in pursuing the topic further and in detail with the woman. The woman would be given the choice of talking about it then or returning to the issue at the end of the more formal history.

The nurse's role during the narration is to listen empathetically and if she follows the Kinlein model completely, writing down every word that is said. This serves to underscore the perception of importance the nurse is imparting to what is being said and is a useful record to refer to later. M. Lucille Kinlein is able to write, listen, and keep eye contact simultaneously which takes practice, but whether the record is kept verbatim or not, documentation of the specifics is extremely important. The nurse may be called upon to testify in court about the abuse, and as previously mentioned, both the abused woman and the nurse need to be able to evaluate the history for patterns. The purpose of the record and limited confidentiality must of course be explained to the woman. Her greatest fear will probably be that the record will somehow be available to her spouse.

After the narration, the nurse may need to clarify certain aspects of the story. Kinlein suggests only clarifying what has been previously said, not going into new areas of concern. This will probably be the most useful approach if the nurse is going to see the woman again or is sure that her total health needs will be addressed elsewhere. However, certain aspects of the situation need to be explored in order for the woman herself to make a complete assessment. If follow-up is assured, these areas may be assessed in subsequent sessions, but they should not be forgotten.

The woman's feelings about the beatings need to be talked about. She may be using a process of intellectualization or disassociation of feelings and describe the situation without affect. Again, this is a common protective mechanism in severe loss situations and if gentle query into her feelings is not responded to, the protection can be assumed to be necessary, at least temporarily. However, the woman may not be describing feelings because she has assumed that her emotions are somehow unacceptable. She may be especially afraid of anger and sometimes feel the desire to hurt or even kill in return. Barbara Star's sample of forty-six battered women were significantly less able to express anger than her control group of twelve not physically abused women.[6] (It should be noted that both groups in the Star study reported emotional abuse.) Whatever the feelings are, the abused woman needs reassurance that it is normal for her to have strong and frequently socially undesirable emotions. It often also is helpful to describe to the woman the whole gamut of feelings that abused women frequently feel, from feeling angry, trapped, despairing, and hopeless to feeling great love for the man and confidence that violence will not reoccur. The nurse should also stress that these feelings may be held simultaneously and that the woman may frequently vacillate between them. Even if the woman does not "own" her emotions at the time of as-

Nursing Care of Abused Women

sessment, it will be helpful to her to remember their normalcy and acceptability given the situation when she does become aware of these reactions.

Another important aspect to get a picture of is the pattern of abuse. The nurse needs to carefully assess with the woman exactly how much danger she is in. Beatings that are escalating over time or following Walker's cycle of abuse pattern with each "acute battering incident" increasing in severity need to be looked at carefully.[7] It is sometimes helpful to make a rough calendar with the woman, especially if the abuse is of long duration, indicating the incidents of abuse and how severely they can be rated. The use of a weapon or the presence of a gun in the house is important to note. Threats of using a weapon or killing are also often begun as the violence increases and are a forerunner of actual use. A gun is also a temptation to the woman herself. Advice to get rid of the firearm is usually impractical, because the woman is not in control of such matters, and the man may equate its possession with his manhood, a common sign of machismo. Some abused women, however, are able to be creative with ways to make the gun inoperable, and this can be suggested. When the nurse, with knowledge of the danger of homicide inherent in abusive relationships, assesses there to be severe danger to the woman, she must take assertive action. The facts about the connection of homicide and abuse can be presented to the woman, and she will frequently admit to fear of this eventuality. Alternatives can be discussed, but the possibility that the woman will be able to avoid further abuse when it has escalated to this extent, must be discounted. The woman changing her own behavior within the relationship has been found to be basically irrelevant in severe abuse. If the woman is unable to take action to otherwise significantly change the situation, the nurse may need to call in Protective Services and/or the police. There is usually sufficient evidence of physical injury, old if not current, in such situations to warrant such actions. Immediate removal to a wife abuse shelter is another possibility.

After current danger has been assessed, and if it is not found to be paramount, the pattern of abuse can be looked at to determine what has triggered the incidents. It is important not to end this part of the assessment with the woman feeling that she must just change her behavior towards the spouse in order to avoid further violence. This hints that she is somehow to blame. Instead, this assessment can focus on the stressors that are occurring within the relationship to help the woman understand the mechanisms that are operating. It may also be useful to determine the amount of violence that occurred in the spouse's family of origin to help the woman connect his childhood learning with her present beatings and thereby understand his behavior and how deeply it may be rooted.

The patterns of psychological abuse and controlling behavior, including jealousy and enforced isolation, need to be investigated with the woman. This is important to her ability to see the battering as part of the total picture of the relationship and also useful for her identification of where her possible feelings of entrapment, low self-esteem, and depression may originate. Her support systems are also important to evaluate.

The woman's dependency on the marriage is important to assess, both in light of the amount of loss she can be expected to be confronting and in terms of her potential ability to leave. Debra Kalmuss and Murray Straus have identified two distinct areas of dependency on marriage: objective, dependence, conditions which tie the woman to marriage in terms of economic survival such as young children or few financial resources or potential resources; and subjective dependence, how tied she perceives herself to be in terms of emotional investment.[8] Using data from the Murray A. Straus, Richard J. Gelles, and Suzanne K. Steinmetz nationally representative survey of 2,143 couples, the authors found subjective dependence significantly correlated by multivariate analysis with less severe physical aggression while objective dependence was strongly related to abuse. Lisa Mahon also found an "internalized . . . total commitment to marriage" present in her extremely small sample (N=11) of battered women in long-term relationships.[9] Strong indications of both objective and subjective dependence on the marriage and heavy commitment to it would predict intense grieving reaction in the woman and less ability to contemplate leaving the relationship without interventions.

The woman's perceptions about her children are also an important part of the history. Children of abused women are also frequently abused, although the extent of that phenomena and who is actually doing the beatings is not yet well documented in the literature.[10] However, this is an important aspect, and indications of child abuse must be reported as they would be in any other situation. The woman is also frequently and justifiably concerned about the effect of the violence on the children, and the facts as they are known about intergenerational transmission of violence need to be shared. Conversely, the battered wife may describe her children as the reason that she stays in the relationship and this needs to be carefully considered with her. She may be able to outline, with the help of the nurse, the pros and cons of the relationship in terms of the children which can be helpful in her assessment of the ramifications of the abuse.

Finally, the area of sexual abuse needs to be explored with the woman. Both clinical experience and literature review indicate this as a prevalent aspect of battering, but a topic that will seldom be inititiated by the woman. Again, an introduction about the frequency of the dilemma can be useful in bringing up sexual abuse. The woman may not see being forced into sex or unusual sexual activities as abuse, but she may be able to acknowledge discomfort in the sexual relationship which can be talked about in general.

Thus, the history-taking part of assessment with an abused woman will include all the normal areas of questioning, but will also incorporate some areas specific to battering. The first narration of the woman may include at least some of the areas spontaneously, but when they are not covered, the nurse must use judgement as to what additional areas need to be explored in light of time restrictions, possibilities of continued contact, and priorities suggested by the woman's verbal and nonverbal description. The areas postponed in terms of history should be noted for further follow-up or passed on as topics to be covered in subsequent assessment by the professional to whom the woman is referred.

Physical Examination

The physical examination of the battered or suspected abused woman should be conducted as any other physical assess-

Nursing Care of Abused Women

Table 9-1 *Indicators of Potential or Actual Wife Abuse from History*

Area of Assessment	At-Risk Responses*
I. Primary Concern/Reason for Visit	Unwarranted delay between time of injury and seeking treatment
	Inappropriate spouse reactions (lack of concern, overconcern, threatening demeanor, reluctance to leave wife, etc.)
	Vague information about cause of injury or problem; discrepancy between physical findings and verbal description of cause; obviously incongruous cause of injury given
	Minimizing serious injury
	Seeking emergency room treatment for vague stress-related symptoms and minor injuries
II. Family Health History	
A. Home of Origin	Traditional values about women's role taught
	Spouse abuse or child abuse (may not be significant for wife but should be noted)
B. Children	Children abused
	Physical punishment used routinely and severely with children
	Children are hostile toward or fearful of father
	Father perceives children as an additional burden
	Father demands unquestioning obedience from children
C. Spouse	Alcohol or drug abuse
	Holds machismo values
	Experience with violence outside of home, including violence against women in previous relationships
	Low self-esteem; lack of power in workplace or other arenas outside of home
	Uses force in sexual activities
	Unemployment
	Extreme jealousy of female friendships, work, and children as well as other men; jealousy frequently unfounded
	Stressors such as death in family, moving, change of jobs, trouble at work, etc.
	Abused as a child or witnessed father abusing mother
D. Household	Poverty
	Conflicts solved by aggression or violence
	Isolated from neighbors, relatives; few friends; lack of support systems
III. Past Health History	Fractures and trauma injuries
	Depression, anxiety symptoms, substance abuse
	Injuries while pregnant
	Spontaneous abortions
	Psychophysiological complaints

(continued)

Table 9-1 (Cont.)

Area of Assessment	At-Risk Responses*
IV. Nutrition	Evidence of experiencing overeating or anorexia as reactions to stress Sudden changes in weight
V. Personal/Social	Low self-esteem, evaluates self poorly in relation to others and ideal self, has trouble listing strengths, makes negative comments about self frequently, doubts own abilities Expresses feelings of being trapped, powerlessness, that situation is hopeless, that it is futile to make future plans Chronic fatigue, apathy Feels responsible for spouse's behavior Holds traditional values about the home, a wife's prescribed role, the husband's prerogatives, strong commitment to marriage External locus of control orientation, feels no control over situation, believes fate or other forces determine events Major decisions in household made by spouse, indicates far less power than he has in relationship, activities controlled by spouse, money controlled by spouse Few support systems, few friends, little outside home activity, outside relationships have been discouraged by spouse Physical aggression in courtship
VI. Sleep	Sleep disturbances, insomnia, sleeping more than 10-12 hours per day
VII. Elimination	Chronic constipation or diarrhea or elimination disturbances related to stress
VIII. Illness	Frequent psychophysiological illnesses Treatment for mental illness Use of tranquilizers and/or mood elevators and/or antidepressants
IX. Operations/Hospitalizations	Hospitalizations for trauma injuries Suicide attempts Hospitalization for depression Refusals of hospitalization when suggested by physician
X. Personal Safety	Handgun(s) in home History of frequent accidents Does not take safety precautions
XI. Health Care Utilization	No regular provider Indicates mistrust of health care system
XII. Review of Systems	Headaches, undiagnosed GI symptoms, palpitations, other possible psychophysiological complaints

Table 9-1 (Cont.)

Area of Assessment	At-Risk Responses*
	Sexual difficulties, feels husband is "rough" in sexual activities, lack of sexual desire, pain with intercourse
	Joint pain and/or other areas of tenderness especially at the extremities
	Chronic pain

*At-risk responses are derived from clinical experience plus extensive review of literature. Especially useful was Violet Ramonaitis Lichtenstein, "The Battered Woman: Guidelines for Effective Nursing Intervention," *Issues in Mental Health Nursing* 3 (1981): pp. 237-450) and Wendy Goldberg and Anne L. Carey, "Domestic Violence Victims in the Emergency Setting," *Topics in Emergency Medicine* 3 (January 1982), pp. 65-75.

ment of an adult female. Careful attention must be paid to any signs of injury, past and present, with exact measurement of even the most insignificant-looking bruise. Pictures drawn in the chart and/or photographs are important means of documentation. Since there is evidence that the predominance of injuries to the battered woman are to the face, chest, breasts and abdomen, special attention would be paid to these areas.[11] The incidence of accompanying sexual abuse would also indicate careful examination of the genitalia for physical signs of such. Extreme gentleness is important in light of the body image damage that has been done.

The general appearance of the woman should include observations about her behavior as well as physical appearance. Nonverbal behavior that indicates a sense of shame about her body is fairly common in battered women and understandable in terms of body image insult. Other affective behaviors can give clues as to how the woman deals with feelings.

The mental status examination is an extremely important part of physical assessment with battered women. Signs of depression should be carefully noted and suicidal intent considered as a real possibility. An assessment of self-esteem is important as part of the mental status examination. Some indication of such will be apparent in the history, but in light of the prevalence of low self-esteem in battered women, a more objective measure is called for. Asking the woman to list her strengths and weaknesses is one way to assess self-esteem more carefully. Other ways are inquiring as to how nearly she feels she approximates the person she would like to be or asking her to evaluate herself in comparison to her friends.

Nursing Diagnosis

The diagnosing part of assessment is best begun with sharing with the abused woman her strengths as the nurse sees them. This is extremely important in terms of the potential low self-esteem and the generally prevailing attitude of battered women that they will be condemned for their behavior—if not in terms of inciting the beatings in some way, at least for not ending the relationship. Abused women are frequently extremely creative in finding ways to deal with a violent spouse and in bringing up their children with a minimum of damage. They need recognition

Table 9-2 Indicators of Potential or Actual Wife Abuse from Physical Exam

Area of Assessment	At-Risk Findings
I. General Appearance	Increased anxiety in presence of spouse
	Watching spouse for approval of answers to questions
	Signs of fatigue
	Inappropriate or anxious nonverbal behavior
	Nonverbal communication suggesting shame about body
	Flinches when touched
	Poor grooming, inappropriate attire
II. Vital Statistics	Overweight or underweight
	Hypertension
III. Skin	Bruises, welts, edema, or scars especially on breasts, upper arms, abdomen, chest, face, and genitalia
	Burns
IV. Head	Subdural hematoma
V. Eyes	Swelling
	Subconjunctival hemorrhage
VI. Genital/Urinary	Edema, bruises, tenderness, external bleeding
VII. Rectal	Bruising, bleeding, edema, irritation
VIII. Musculoskeletal	Fractures, especially of facial bones, spiral fractures of radius or ulna, ribs
	Shoulder dislocation
	Limited motion of an extremity
	Old fractures in various stages of healing
IX. Abdomen	Abdominal injuries in pregnant women
	Intra-abdominal injury
X. Neurological	Hyperactive reflex responses
	Areas of numbness from old injuries
	Inappropriate or flat affect
	Depression
	Anxiety, fear
	Suicidal ideation
	Problems with recall of some events
	Low self-esteem

and support for those efforts. At this point it is also helpful to explain how normal her reactions (such as depression) and behavior are in light of the impact of being beaten in a marriage. It is important for the nurse to remember how much blame and suggestions of pathology the woman usually receives and to "bend over backwards" to give the woman praise in terms of specific strengths that she possesses. Clinical experience has shown it useful to actually record these strengths and show the woman that they are part of the record and therefore felt to be as important as any problems she may have.

The next part of the diagnosing process is to ask the woman to list any concerns she has and what priority she places on them. To the surprise of the nurse, the woman may focus on a problem that seems peripheral to abuse. This may be part of a testing process for the woman and/or may be what seems central to her existence at that moment. These feelings must be respected in deciding the course of nursing interventions. When the woman has listed the areas that she feels need attention, the nurse can add others asking if the woman agrees that they also need inclusion. This is a point where the nurse may need to explain the holistic nature of nursing; some women may feel that the nurse is primarily interested in physical injury.

Another important aspect of the nurse's contribution to the diagnostic process is to help the woman look at any patterns of stress-related symptoms. Battered women frequently report problems such as headaches, gastrointestinal symptoms, heart palpitations, and so forth. The woman may not see these complaints as related to the almost constant stress that she is experiencing and may need help in connecting their occurrence to patterns of beating. Again the emphasis should be on the normalcy of these symptoms appearing in her situation, although the possibility of further medical diagnosis and intervention should also be discussed.

Nursing diagnoses in the case of battered women may cover a wide range of concerns. To help the reader in formulating some possible appropriate diagnostic statements, a sample nursing process has been included at the end of the chapter (Table 9-3).

PLANNING

The planning stage of the nursing process requires working with the battered woman to develop goals and interventions that seem appropriate to her. Short-term goals need to be fairly simple and concrete. Achievement of these first goals will be of immeasurable value in showing the woman that some of her problems can be solved, that she is capable of achieving solutions even in her restricted situation, and that working for long-term goals is also feasible. The battered woman may seem very passive in the goal-setting phase, because of her feelings of being trapped generally, her mistrust of helping professionals, and/or the protective mechanism of not looking toward the future, trying to deal only with each day as it comes. The nurse needs to recognize this behavior as normal and work very hard to help the woman formulate her own goals. This may be considered as partially an intervention; it is helping the woman develop problem-solving techniques.

Long-term goals may be even more difficult for the abused woman to develop. The nurse must be careful not to prematurely impose a goal of leaving the abuser during this process. The battered woman may take months or years to get to this point, and she may never reach it. She may, however, inquire whether the nurse feels like this *should* be a goal, because she is often used to this advice. Needless to say, the nurse may need to explore her own thinking on the subject. If the woman is not yet ready to contemplate the future, long-term goals may need to be set later in the course of the relationship.

The process of planning should be left in the hands of the abused woman. Support and suggested alternatives can be offered by the nurse. It is very difficult for nurses to really imagine what the battering situation is like, especially if there is unemployment, several young children, and a dearth of support systems accompanying the problem. Clinical experience has shown that abused women have often thought of anything that traditional nursing has to suggest. The women themselves, with encouragement to think as widely and fancifully as they can, usually discover the germs of effective solutions that can be refined and explored and expanded with the nurse. Such a process can often be a great deal of fun for both the woman and the nurse. There is nothing more useful for raising self-esteem for the woman than coming up with her own solutions and being praised effusively for them.

NURSING INTERVENTION

Professional nursing interventions for the problem of wife abuse are based on the three levels of prevention. It is not enough for nurses to identify and give care to the individual battered woman; they must look to the societal causes and work to eliminate their influence.

Primary Prevention

Primary prevention involves:

1. Interventions at the societal level,
2. Identification of women at risk to become abused,
3. Implementation of nursing care both with those women at risk and with their potential abusers.

Because wife abuse originates in sexism and the patriarchal social structure, prevention must start at this point. As Lichenstein asserts, "To prevent abuse, social attitudes toward women must be changed. Dependency of women must be eliminated. This means economic, social, and psychological dependency."[12]

Health Promotion: Interventions at the Societal Level

Political activism is a mandatory role for nurses in changing the social structure so that women are no longer so dependent. Melva Jo Hendrix states, "the day has long since passed when health care professionals can afford to be apolitical."[13] Each individual nurse cannot be expected to take on every political cause that has impact on these issues. However, each nurse can make one such issue something that she becomes truly involved in, and then at least vote and write to elected officials about the rest. Support for the reintroduced Equal Rights Amendment (ERA) is an obvious place to start, and the issue of equal compensation for work of comparable worth is an area of immense implication for the profession of nursing as well as for the economic dependence of all women. The lack of affordable, responsible childcare for working mothers also remains a significant block to economic independence for women. Private industry and government need constant prodding to make daycare a reality for every woman who needs it. Nurses can join with other women in fighting for these issues and can thereby realize the enormous strength of women working together which is necessary when one is taking on deeply embedded values and structures.

To eliminate sexism, the childrearing

patterns of our culture need to be radically altered. Problems with male identification leading to machismo attitudes can be assuaged by full participation of fathers in all aspects of parenting. Boys can be encouraged toward this in parenting classes in high school, and prenatal classes are also important in this regard. Fathers involved in labor and delivery may be more likely to be involved in childrearing later. Nurses can also participate in public education to promote male participation in childrearing; the proliferation of cable television health programs presents excellent opportunities.

The sexism, male dominance, and violence portrayed on televison and in children's books must be protested frequently and vehemently. On an adult level, pornography, especially that depicting violence against women, has to be curtailed. Recent laboratory and field studies suggest that viewing erotic films that show women being the victims of violence increases men's aggression and acceptance of interpersonal violence against women.[14] Erotica and pornography can be differentiated by mutuality and reciprocity in the sexual acts portrayed in the former while the latter depicts the humiliation and domination of women, if not actual violence.[15] With these differentiations in mind, one can argue effectively against pornography without getting caught in the issues of freedom of speech and open attitudes toward sex. Feminists advocate women banding together against pornography, demonstrating against movies depicting violent sex, confronting men who buy pornographic materials, and educating the public as to the dangers of such media.[16]

The adult male in today's society feels threatened. The feminist movement is challenging his traditional prerogatives, and economic malaise is eroding his chances of attaining power and prestige in the work environment. He gets mixed messages in the media and from women as to whether strength and macho characteristics or gentleness and advocating sexual equality are preferable. Activities for health promotion for men should include supporting men's groups for discussion of the evolving male role and for helping men to get in touch with their feelings and learn to express them without using aggression. Nursing assessment of individual men, including boys and adolescent males, should include a discussion of these issues and how the man is dealing with them. This is fully as important as assessing for physical problems.

Women also need help in overcoming psychological dependence on men. This need has been addressed quite well in women's support groups and consciousness-raising groups that have been an outgrowth of the women's movement. However, these groups remain predominantly organized and used by middle-class women. Poorer women generally do not perceive themselves as having the leisure time, the childcare, or the transportation to take advantage of such groups and are not sure of their welcome. They are often overwhelmed by the problems of everyday living. Yet discussions of women's roles and gaining support from each other can be part of groups organized around more "practical" aims, groups that can be held in poor neighborhoods with childcare provided. Waiting rooms of hospital and/or public health clinics can be used to engage men and women in meaningful conversations on all kinds of issues. Professionals often complain that people "do not take advantage" of educational programs and discussion groups offered and yet allow the same people they are trying to reach sit for hours in a variety of waiting rooms or stand in endless lines to initiate contact with social and health services. There they are; let's find ways to use this time.

Women who are clients of the mental health system need these kinds of discussions no matter what their presenting symptoms. All women's roles are changing, and all women are dealing with this at some level. The women may not ask for "feminist therapy," but mental health nurses need to lead the struggle to make sure that therapy for women does not further cripple them with reinforcement of traditional psychiatric myths about female dependency. Problems in self-esteem and susceptibility to depression are natural outgrowths of being brought up female in a sexist society. School nurses and community health nurses are in a good position to deal with these issues with adolescent girls. Adolescent mothers can be approached singly or in groups by maternal-child health nurses for discussion of women's issues. These young women are highly at risk to be caught in poverty and external crippling of potentials. Dependence on a man can look extremely attractive as a way to escape, and they need help in growth of the self before they can make wise decisions about intimate relationships with men.

Interventions with Women at Risk

Women at risk to be abused include those in poverty situations; those who believe in the traditional roles and stereotypes of women in marriage; and those intimately involved with men displaying machismo characteristics, especially those macho men who are unemployed, lack power at work, are in highly stressful situations from other causes, abuse alcohol, or were themselves exposed to a violent home as a child. (Other characteristics indicating risk can be found in Table 9-1). A women at risk who has not actually been beaten, may respond affirmatively to questions like, "Has your spouse ever threatened to hit you?" or "Have you ever been afraid that he would hit you?" It is useful to suggest some sort of women's group for these women and to make sure that they realize that increased family stress may begin a cycle of battering; they need to know how to obtain crisis intervention in such a situation. It is also helpful to encourage them to think through a scenario of what they would do if they actually were beaten. This rehearsal usually lends strength if such occurs and does not frighten the woman unnecessarily as might be imagined; she has usually thought of the possibility previously, but without support has not thought it through completely.

Women at risk frequently subscribe to the myth that they can somehow save a man with problems, problems with alcohol or drugs or a violent temper or a rotten childhood, that enough love and patience from her will cure him. They need help in understanding that they cannot be held responsible for a spouse's behavior and that problems like these need professional intervention, not just wifely support. Getting the man to accept help is, of course, a difficult issue. The man who exhibits machismo finds it almost impossible to admit a need for help. Again the individual woman is the best judge of under what conditions the man may be willing to seek help, and the nurse can help her work out ways to make these conditions happen. An authoritarian message that help is necessary from a male physician can sometimes be useful in persuading the man. If the female partner thinks this would be helpful, it can be arranged by the nurse.

Other attitudes frequently displayed by the woman at risk for abuse are that all men are unreasonably jealous, at least occasionally resort to violence, and need to be dominant. Gentleness in male behavior may be woefully absent in her experience and community. A middle class nurse from a different culture may be considered a useless source of information on male behavior in her world. Another nurse or health team member from similar background may be more persuasive on this subject. Even more useful is a group of women who are her peers, some of whom have encountered or successfully demanded different standards of behavior. Such experiences can be difficult to arrange, but the results are worth the trouble.

Assertiveness training is also extremely helpful for both women who are at risk for battering and abused women themselves. Again, assertiveness classes have been much more prevalent for middle-class women than those who are poor. Creativity is needed in making such classes available for the traditionally underserved: at lunch hours in workplaces like factories, office buildings, hospitals, and shopping centers where women are frequently employed; at neighborhood centers; or at Head Start classrooms when the children are occupied. Special care must be taken to be sure that poor women feel invited, that small groups of friends are encouraged to come, and that the relevance to their situation is underscored.

Primary prevention can also take the forms of fighting poverty at the societal level or helping the individual man or woman at risk to find a job. It may also include promoting nonviolence in our culture and in individual families. Preventing wife abuse is certainly an almost overwhelming task, but fortunately others are involved. Nurses need to band together with women and concerned men everywhere. Many groups of professionals can also be included—social workers, psychologists, concerned physicians, feminist lawyers, and some police. Coalitions of nurses with individuals from these groups can be formed. Nurses are welcome on boards of agencies and groups involved with wife abuse and can help set policy in this kind of position. The opportunities for nurses to significantly make an impact on the quest to prevent the battering of women, both in terms of health promotion and identification and intervention for those at risk, are extensive and varied. Nurses can make a difference.

Secondary Prevention

Secondary prevention of wife abuse involves diligent efforts at early case finding and interventions with women in the beginning stages of wife abuse. Drake, basing her conclusions on Walker's cycle of violence theory, suggests that the ideal time for nurses to intervene is between the end of phase two, the acute battering incident, and the beginning of phase three, when the husband may be contrite and re-establish the bonds between the couple.[17] At this point the woman is the most likely to seek medical or nursing care for her injuries and come to the attention of nurses. The woman may be in crisis at this juncture and especially open to help, no matter to what setting she presents herself.

Early Case Finding

The emergency room nurse is extremely important in early case finding. An estimated 18 to 25 percent of all women presented to emergency rooms may be victims of wife abuse.[18] It is appropriate that the professional nurse take responsibility for determining battering since the nurse is more likely to be female and therefore less threatening, and because abuse, with all its psychological and social ramifications, is more logically within the wider scope of nursing than medicine. The woman may come to the emergency room with fairly minor injuries in an attempt to seek help for the primary problem. It is tempting to treat such clients quickly with a lecture about the misuse of emergency rooms. A high index of suspicion for abuse in nurses will prevent these women from going away not truly served. If the injuries are at all serious enough to warrant hospitalization, this should be considered as extremely beneficial in terms of protecting the woman temporarily and giving her a chance to really think away from the batterer and the stresses of home. The emergency room nurse can alert the inpatient staff of the possibility of abuse if it has not been confirmed, so that her nurses can help the woman in this process.

An abused woman may also present herself to mental health facilities with a variety of psychiatric symptoms in an effort to reach out for assistance. In clinical experience with battered women, they have often recounted how the psychiatric staff tended to "dope me up" as a primary intervention, which generally lessened their pain, but also interfered with their resolve to take effective action. As soon as their symptoms abated they were usually released without any interventions to solve the underlying problem. This general course of events did not seem to alter, whether or not they told of the abuse. Battering must be assumed to be a possible cause of or related to depression, anxiety, substance abuse, and marital problems in the mental health arena, and it should receive specific inquiry and intervention.

In a random sample of twenty-six female psychiatric inpatients, 61 percent were identified as battered.[19] The sample is, of course, too small for generalizable conclusions, but the findings do suggest that mental health nurses need to be aware of and be able to intervene with battered women more than is commonly thought. The same nursing study indicated that of the fourteen abused women, eight had reported the abuse to at least one health professional and only four had received a clearly helpful response from one of the health professionals consulted. Other sources have also spoken of the generally detrimental role the mental health care system has played in the past with battered women. They are frequently (71 of 100 abused wives in one study) prescribed tranquilizers or antidepressants.[20] This therapy insinuates that the woman is mentally ill, may mask her discomfort and thereby encourage her to remain in the battering situation, treats the symptoms, not the problem, and certainly does not address the cause, the spouse.

The widespread incidence of battering during pregnancy suggests another important arena where wife abuse can be identified and attended to by nursing. Prenatal clinics, private obstetrical offices, childbirth education classes, and inpatient postpartum floors are all places where nurses practice and can be alert for wife battering. Drake found 100 percent of her sample who had ever been pregnant had been beaten while in that condition.[21] One-half of John Flynn's sample of thirty-three wife abuse victims had been battered while carrying a child.[22] Walker found that most of the women she interviewed reported more severe and more frequent violence during pregnancy.[23] Extrapolating from previous incidence statistics, it can be estimated that one in every fifty pregnant women is being beaten. This is a more common occurrence than placenta previa or diabetes in pregnancy, but questions about abuse are not yet included in routine prenatal histories.

In community health nursing, nurses are in client's homes and deal with families on a regular basis. In such settings, wife abuse may easily come to light if the professional nurse is alert to the possibility and gently asks the right questions. As previously mentioned, many battered women seem anxious to tell if asked empathetically in a safe and private situation. An aspect of community health nursing where nurses may have contact with women in early battering situations is in birth control clinics. This is an excellent setting in which to identify young women who are in relationships that are beginning to be characterized by excessive control by the man and by violence. Descriptions of the spouse making all the decisions about birth control or "forcing" the woman in any way at all are indications that abuse may be present. Follow-up appointments for the woman would therefore be extremely important to arrange even if not absolutely mandatory in terms of the chosen birth control method.

Occupational health is another important case finding setting. Abuse is frequently known by co-workers and friends of the woman in the workplace before it comes to the attention of professionals. A vigorous campaign of distribution of information about wife abuse in the workplace, coupled with suggestions to come to the occupational health nurse if abuse is known, can be useful in early identification. The woman may also be absent recurrently and show evidence of facial bruises, perhaps covered with heavy makeup. She may be defensive about questions regarding her absenteeism and indicate powerlessness in the relationship by saying she is not able to spend her salary according to her own desires or not able to work overtime or rearrange her schedule because of his objections. The workplace is an excellent setting to provide nursing care to a battered woman because of her separation from the spouse.

Primary care settings and physician's offices are other health arenas where abuse can be picked up, especially abuse in middle-class homes. Battered women may often seek medical attention because of stress-related symptoms. Inclusion of questions about abuse in nursing assessment or careful review of physician's findings can be used to identify the battered woman. No matter in what setting abuse is identified, the framework of a grieving response can be used for understanding the battered woman's behavior and as a basis for nursing intervention.

A Framework for Intervention: The Grieving Response

In order to understand the abused woman, it is helpful to look at her behavior in the context of a loss and grieving pattern.[24] Her reaction can thus be seen as an absolutely normal process in a situation of multiple and severe losses. In Western patriarchal society, a successful marriage is usually seen as the single most important achievement for women. This picture is starting to change, but any battered woman is still dealing with a significant loss, that of the idealized version of marriage. The woman is typically thought to be responsible for the success of the marriage, and to face that it is in shambles is to take on considerable loss of self-esteem. Body image loss because of the physical injuries incurred is further a part of the picture. The abused woman has lost a great deal of trust in her mate and in the world as a safe place and has also lost her illusions that the man is basically good for her and an appropriate object of her love and affection. When she contemplates leaving the man she must face the potential losses of status in marriage, financial security or some semblance thereof, a father for her children, her home, and various support systems. The tendency of many abused wives to stay married to their husbands and/or return to them after leaving, and/or drop assault charges against them, and/or idealize them even after leaving has baffled and exasperated the scholars in the field and those working with battered women. This behavior can be perhaps best understood as a reaction to the multiple losses.

The grieving response thus seen can resemble anticipatory grief as outlined by Elizabeth Kubler Ross, but will also contain elements of mourning for the death of a loved one (loss of spouse) and reaction to body image and self-esteem change.[25] The response is also compounded by the fact that the man is not dead even if the woman has left him, and may reappear in her life when she is psychologically vulnerable. If she is still with him, his behavior may complicate the process of anticipatory grief by being sometimes loving and contrite.

Whatever the manifestations and complications, the advantages of using a grieving framework are that it views the response patterns as essentially healthy and as a process to be worked through and supported. As is true with grieving, the process takes considerable time and the behaviors vary in their appearance, sequence, intensity, and length of time required to experience them. For some women, the process may resemble the chronic grieving that individuals with permanent disability and chronic illness frequently display.[26]

All the authors who have traced the grief response have identified an initial period of shock and denial that follows significant loss.[27] The battered woman may deny the importance of the initial battering in a variety of ways. She may admit the violence but blame it on alcohol or a temporary loss of control in her spouse. He generally supports her in this kind of denial. She may also explain away the occurrence as a temporary aberration in an essentially loving relationship, or she may blame the stress that the man is currently undergoing or her own behavior. However, once a man has used violence with his wife, a psychological barrier seems to have been broken, and a pattern of abuse is started. The initial shock and denial of the woman, a perfectly normal response, may be perceived as a form of acquiescence in the wife and/or a sign that the man's goals have been achieved. This may serve to reinforce the behavior.

As the violence reoccurs, the impact and meaning start to become apparent. A variety of strong feelings are subsequently experienced by the woman. However, the intermittent pattern of some abuser's beatings may allow the woman to return to denial during quiescent periods. The feeling that first surfaces is often anger, and the woman may try to fight back, either verbally or physically. Most of the women soon learn that this only worsens the violence directed against them and find it necessary to suppress their anger. The anger may be dealt with by turning it inward, by displacement onto others, by projection, or by developing somatic symptoms.

Guilt is another strong feeling associated with loss and grief, and it has been noted previously that battered women frequently feel guilty. Their guilt is supported by the psychological abuse and blame dealt out by the spouse (frequently a projection on *his* part). Bargaining is a mechanism identified in anticipatory grief which may be used a way to deal with guilt. The battered woman frequently makes a pact with her husband that she will correct whatever behavior he sees as a problem in return for an absence of violence.

The feelings of helplessness, despair, and loss of control so often identified by abused women and clinically seen as depression, are a normal part of grieving. There is extremely painful grief work to be done, which takes considerable time and many tears. The battered woman doubts her ability to cope without the man and may feel totally worthless. She cannot be expected to make the hard decisions and plans necessary for leaving when she is mourning. Idealization of the spouse is often seen during this period which is also characteristic of grieving. This mechanism is often very difficult for professionals dealing with the abused woman to understand, and it may lead to a return to the spouse if she has left or a decision to try to stick it out if she is still with him. When viewed as a normal part of process to be worked through, it is more acceptable.

Acceptance of the loss, along with realistic plans for change, either within the relationship or outside of it, come slowly for most women. Again the degree of loss, in terms of time and energy invested in the relationship, perceived ability to cope without it, and the love felt for the spouse, may prolong the time needed to opt for change. As in anticipatory grief or chronic grieving, some women may never actually work through the grieving process. Progress is seldom direct and without vacillation between stages. Successful adaption to the losses may well depend on the support given to the abused woman through the process. Nursing can be instrumental in providing that support.

Secondary Prevention Nursing Interventions

Interventions at the secondary prevention level would be based on an assessment of where the abused woman is in her grieving process. As previously mentioned, denial and partial denial must be allowed, although not encouraged. The battered woman needs to know the facts about wife abuse, primarily that it generally tends to escalate. During early abuse she will frequently want to know if it isn't possible for the violent spouse to change. This is possible, but the woman needs to be aware that he must want to change and be willing to undergo treatment of some kind. Her efforts need to be directed toward that end, rather than trying to change her behavior so that she can somehow please him more and thus avoid abuse.

A useful approach is to concentrate on assisting the woman to be as healthy as possible in spite of the batterings. This usually seems logical to both abused women and the nurse, and it avoids such pitfalls as encouraging the woman to be more submissive. Areas of concern such as low self-esteem and lack of assertiveness can be approached in a variety of ways. Individual counseling aimed at raising self-esteem and teaching assertiveness skills can be useful as well as groups and classes. Once the abused woman feels better about herself she may be able to set firm limits at home, but without these strengths, suggestions of such may be premature.

Efforts to improve the health of the victim of early abuse can also focus on stress-related symptoms she may be experiencing. Relaxation training, exercise programs, role playing, coping skills development, and teaching the woman to be more in touch with her physiologic self may all be helpful to her. It should also be remembered that battered women are usually being kept socially isolated by the spouse. The nurse can discuss the importance of the woman of having support systems and problem solve with her to try to find and develop new supportive networks or maintain existing ones. Help in alleviating some of the external stressors in the relationship such as lack of childcare or difficulties in finding financial resources may be addressed through referral to social work or other community resources. The woman may need help in finding a job for herself which could be extremely instrumental in improving her self-esteem and decreasing her economic dependence on the spouse. Many batterers find employment in their wife threatening, but alleviation of some of the financial burdens may seem attractive enough to overcome their objections.

A woman in the early stages of battering will frequently seek some way of maintaining the marriage. Marriage counseling is often decried in wife abuse literature as only a palliative measure which may decrease the severity of violence but do nothing to cure the problem and may in fact only delay long-term solutions.[28] However, if marriage counseling is desired by the couple, the nurse can be instrumental in making sure the counseling received is given by someone knowledgeable about abuse, who is not interested in only keeping the couple intact to the detriment of the wife. Rather than traditional marital therapy, models have been developed based on behavioral and social learning theories.[29] The man is encouraged to take responsibility for the violence, using confrontation if necessary, and to learn new ways of dealing with anger. The couple is encouraged to expand their definitions of sex role behavior and helped to learn better ways of communication. The primary goal becomes to stop the violence completely, and if this cannot be done by rebuilding the relationship, the couple is helped with dissolution. Other professionals have found the exchange theory helpful in treatment. As Richard J. Gelles puts it, "If people abuse family members because they can (e.g., costs are low) then a central goal of therapy is to make it so they cannot (raise the costs or lower the rewards)."[30] Nurses can conduct this kind of marital counseling themselves with proper background and training, or they can find out where such counseling is given and work with the woman separately.

As well as providing interventions for individual abused women, the nurse should be concerned with institutional measures at the secondary prevention level. It is not enough that the individual nurse include questions about battering in her own practice; protocols need to be developed officially in all the settings mentioned so that all health professionals are assessing for abuse. An example of such official policy is the Harborview Medical Center's Battered Women Project in Seattle, Washington.[31] This project has developed a "comprehensive, victim-oriented, medical and social work protocol" for abused women similar to those established in many hospitals for rape and child abuse victims. Nurses can form coalitions with groups concerned with battering to approach hospital administrations with the need for such protocols. Nurses also need to support training about abuse for the police, legal professionals, social workers, physicians, and clergy as well as for nurses.[32] Workshops for professionals and interested key people and public education on abuse are needed and can be conducted by nurses.

Tertiary Prevention

Tertiary prevention is aimed at rehabilitation of the severely abused wife. The severely battered woman has been victimized by physical and psychological abuse for a significant amount of time and usually has experienced considerable physical and psychological damage. However, she has usually also developed quite a bit of strength as a result of her ordeal and has many insights into her own nature and that of her husband. Tertiary prevention interventions are often carried out in wife abuse shelters or in mental health settings. The woman is usually experiencing many of the strong emotions associated with grieving and often can be helped at this point to achieve necessary acceptance of the losses and final resolution.

Nursing Roles in Shelters

Shelters for abused women have been established in most major cities in the United States and have been shown to be invaluable to battered women as a haven of physical safety for them and their children and as a setting where effective interventions of many kinds can take place. Most shelters provide individual and group counseling; help with bureaucratic institutions such as the police, legal representation, and social services, childcare, and children's programming; and aid the woman in making future plans, such as employment counseling and linkages with housing authorities. Best of all is the support and knowledge that they are not alone which is gained by the women from each other in the shelter setting.

Unfortunately, many shelters are in desperate financial straits. Funding traditionally has been unstable, and most of the original government and private grants used for initial start-up have expired. Money for battered women's programs has become a very low priority in our present political climate; these programs have become the victims of the same backlash against feminism that has temporarily defeated the ERA. One of the largest and oldest inner-city wife abuse shelters, Women-In-Transition in Detroit, which served up to 650 women and 1,050 children per year, had to close because of lack of funds.[33] Nurses are desperately needed at the policy-making level, on governing boards of shelters, on boards of social service funding agencies, and at the state planning level, in order to advocate for the establishment of more shelters where they are needed and to make sure existing shelters stay open.

Shelters are usually run with a combination of professional and volunteer staff, drawing from social workers, psychologists, occupational therapists, and child-care professionals as paid staff. In addition, many formerly abused women, feminists, nurses, lawyers, and others have been involved in the planning, operations, and volunteer services of shelters. Professional education programs, including nursing programs, have found shelters to be an excellent clinical experience for students.

Health services are usually recognized as a necessary part of shelters, and they are obtained in a variety of ways. It would be ideal to have a professional nurse as part of the paid staff of all shelters, and nurses involved in their planning can advocate for this. When this is not feasible, community health nurses can be contracted for on a part-time basis, or arrangements can be made to refer women and children to nurse clinicians. However, in-house nursing care is preferable considering the dangers involved whenever the woman leaves the shelter, the transportation difficulties, and the traditional mistrust of the health care system held by the poor and underserved in general, and the battered woman specifically. Nurses can fill the gap by volunteering at shelters and performing a variety of roles while there. Shelter staff may need some demonstration of the holistic possibilities of professional nursing; they at first may envision the responsibilities of nurses as only that of monitoring blood pressure, teaching health classes, establishing first aid procedures, or giving advice about the endemic children's diarrhea problems that come with change of diet and new environment. These roles may be important, but there is much more that nurses can do in wife abuse shelters.

The group sessions that most shelters conduct can be successfully led by nurses.

Ellen Hastings Janosik has written about groups for battered wives based on her experience in a shelter.[34] She suggests that the major goals be crisis intervention and giving and getting peer support. The women come and go from the group because of their varying lengths of stay in the shelter, necessitating constant readjustment to differing stages of progress and different faces. The women may also be in a variety of phases of resolution of the grief process. Janosik sees this as an advantage in terms of older group members providing role models for the newer. She suggests a process of "exploring abuse patterns" and "facing problems realistically" as group content, pointing out that the group members represent a "pool of problem-resolving resources to meet the basic survival needs which many of the women face."

Nurses can also lead groups dealing with parenting issues or general health concerns which may include sexual abuse. Clinical experience in shelters suggests that it is generally beneficial to allow the group of women to decide what it is that they want to explore with the nurse, not to have a set agenda. Topics may range from race relations among shelter staff and residents and among residents themselves to breast self-examination. Group sessions can be a lot of fun or deadly serious depending on clients' needs. Flexibility and openness are extremely important when the nurse is acting as group leader.

Women in shelters can also be seen individually for a variety of nursing needs. A shelter is a wonderful place to practice a whole range of nursing skills, from physical assessment to one-to-one counseling. The woman's length of stay in the shelter is extremely variable and the relationship with the nurse may be a single contact or may be of a fairly long-term nature. It is important to have a good community resource network established with actual names and some knowledge of other nurses that women can be referred to for follow-up. Once a battered woman has had a useful contact with a nurse, she is usually enthusiastic about her long-term health care being handled by a nurse unless she has an acute problem needing medical diagnosis. Nursing often provides an excellent avenue through which she can meet her health care needs; battered women frequently express their pleasure with the woman-to-woman contact and the holistic possibilities of nursing care.

Tertiary-level individual interventions ideally start with building on the woman's strengths found in the nursing assessment. It takes a great deal of courage to go to a shelter. One of the most poignant images from this author's clinical experience in shelters, is the sight of the battered woman arriving, usually with several children in tow, at a completely strange place, with all of her hastily gathered belongings in a black plastic garbage bag. How many of us would be willing to leave our home, with few if any financial or material resources, when we have been the victim of wrongdoing, and place our future as a human being in the hands of complete strangers? It is imperative to continually praise the abused woman for that act of courage alone.

Other strengths shown by the woman's appearance at the shelter include the mere fact of physical survival to that point, the successful and often carefully planned escape, and the caring for the children shown by leaving. These need to be recognized as strengths and pointed out to the woman. Additional individual strengths found in assessment are important to stress to help combat the woman's feelings of being trapped and helpless. These also serve as a base for further developing problem-solving strategies. The woman may feel she has used up all her resources in just getting to the shelter and may need to be reminded that if she was able to do that, she can do just about anything with a little help and a little time. The first few days at the shelter may need to be just that, some time to rest and recoup and gather her resources, in safety finally. The newly arrived shelter resident should not be expected to do too much in the way of future planning until she has had a chance just to be relieved. However, it is important that her injuries be carefully documented for future legal proceedings. Since the nurse is often not present upon her arrival, staff can be instructed as to how to measure and describe the physical problems. Photography of injuries is usually desirable. There also may be need for immediate medical intervention, and the nurse can be helpful in setting up protocols within the shelter and making contacts with the nearest emergency room.

Care for physical injuries to battered women can require a great deal of ingenuity on the part of shelter staff and nurse consultants. Examples of women with injuries from clinical experience include a woman with a broken jaw which had been wired internally and set with a metal brace, and a four-day postpartum mother who had been raped by her husband as soon as she got home from the hospital. The latter required hospitalization for hemorrhage and left behind at the shelter her newborn baby and two siblings. It is extremely helpful if the shelter can have a nurse to call in such situations for consultation. Other serious health problems include medication for chronic diseases that has been left behind, dangerously high blood pressure necessitating transportation by ambulance, and severe asthma in a child. The nurse can be helpful in devising a short health history form for the woman and her children which can be filled out upon arrival so that shelter staff members are alerted to health problems needing immediate attention.

Individual nursing assessment can determine other physical health problems that the woman is seeking help with for herself and/or her children. It has been found helpful to announce a specific day and time that the nurse will be at the shelter to see any women who wish to seek care. Staff can also make referrals for such problems as substance abuse or observable poor nutritional status. Communication with staff about health problems is extremely important, and the regular shelter records of the women can be used to enter short nursing entries as to assessment and interventions. With the help of professional nursing care, the women have often found the shelter a good place to begin working on health problems that have been bothering them, which may or may not be directly connected with abuse.

The woman experiencing severe abuse and in a shelter is usually starting to experience the strong emotions of the grieving process. She may need help in combating depression and/or in dealing with her anger. Perhaps the most helpful intervention here is letting the woman know how normal these feelings are in her situation and to help her recognize and accept the ambivalence she often feels about the abuser and her relationship to him. The woman can be helped to recognize her many losses and to grieve for them. Tears can be useful and healing, and the battered woman must not be hurried along into decision-making activities until she has had a chance to mourn. Just as a grieving widow needs to talk and talk about the deceased, the abused woman must be allowed to express herself fully about the man, including the good points and happy memories. Other residents and staff may not encourage this as much as they might; shelter atmosphere sometimes seems very much against all men and this is natural also. However, the individual woman may even need to idealize her man before she moves on, and the nurse can provide and encourage this opportunity.

The anger also needs expression. The shelter, with its close living quarters, many responsibilities, and strong feeling tones, can sometimes be an explosive place. Kids are noisy; people don't always attend to chores; privacy is hard to come by. Anger that has built up over the duration of an abusive relationship without any safe means of expression for fear of further beatings can be released over a minor incident between residents or against staff or against confused and restless children. The battered woman can start to feel resentful if she perceives that she is being judged by staff and other residents for the way she has and is handling the abuse or for the way she mothers her children. The legal system and social services system she has to deal with in order to build a future life can also be frustrating. All these factors can underlie and trigger angry outbursts. These outbursts are best dealt with whenever they come up and the women involved helped to see where the anger comes from and encouraged to express it verbally and assertively. This approach is helpful in both dealing with the situation at hand and in teaching the woman how to deal with anger constructively.

The guilt that the abused woman may feel is also best dealt with by encouragement of expression first. As angry as it may make the nurse to hear the woman blame herself, this is a necessary part of grieving and cutting her off is not helpful. Again, assurance that this is normal is the beginning of intervention. Then the woman can be helped to review events with an emphasis on the batterer's behavior which helps her see that usually what she said and did made no real difference in the final outcome. She also needs to be helped to recognize that no one can take responsibility for another's actions. She may need time to think through events again with this fact in mind and although unable initially to get beyond some measure of guilt, eventually she may report a successful working through of the situation.

The nurse's role in shelters can thus be seen as multifaceted. The nurse works as part of the shelter staff team, and the nature of her interventions is based on the needs of the staff and the residents. There is room for several nurses to work at once at one shelter, either working in a rotating sequence or performing a more specialized role. Nursing roles may evolve over time, as staff and residents recognize what kinds of services are available. There is a definite need for nursing in all shelters, and nurses are urged to become invlolved.

Interventions in Mental Health Settings

The nurse may also give tertiary-level interventions for abused women at both inpatient and outpatient mental health institutions. The middle-class battered woman may be more likely to seek help in these settings or in a private psychiatrist's or psychologist's office area than in a shelter. The abused woman will frequently present with symptoms of depression, including suicidal intent, or be referred for marital difficulties. Getting the abuse out in the open and labeled as such is the first task. The second is to assess her danger, either from herself in terms of suicide or from the batterer and to do crisis intervention if necessary on that basis.

Feminist consciousness-raising groups have been found to be demonstrably useful in helping women increase self-esteem, increase their sense of control, and significantly decrease depression. Rose Weitz defines such groups as

> regular meetings in which women discuss and search for similarities among their personal experiences. Groups then utilize this knowledge of commonalities to develop an understanding of power relations between the sexes and of the role structures and socialization processes which maintain these power relations.[35]

Such groups can be appropriately organized and led by nurses and held in mental health settings. Battered women can be referred to this kind of group consisting of women from all kinds of situations. A similar group can be formed of only abused women which would thereby have elements of the kind of group described as taking place in shelters.

Groups can also be formed of abused women and their spouses. Emphasis is placed on the batterers taking responsibility for the beatings. Interactional therapy as described in the section on marital counseling under "secondary prevention" is considered appropriate. Such a group is difficult to lead, and it may be helpful for the nurse (if female) to have a male co-leader because abusive men are often unwilling to allow confrontation by a female leader. At the same time, such a group can be harmful to the women if there is not a female co-leader to help them be assertive. Having a limited number of couples is also imperative in such a group, because the dynamics are often powerful and can be intimidating.

Individual therapy with abused women in mental health settings will deal with many of the issues discussed under individual interventions with women in shelters. Lenore Walker advocates "feminist psychotherapy" for battered women, being careful to explain that she does not mean therapy which tries to make feminists out of women who hold traditional values in regard to sex roles, but ideally a woman therapist who "believes in the strength of being a woman."[36] Walker goes on to describe therapy which helps the woman explore her own psychological self in relationship to the battering and helps her separate those issues from the ones that are a result of sexist society and her spouse's background and therefore not her fault. Concomitant interventions for the abuser are necessary at the tertiary level. At this point, the battering will only escalate if he does not receive help. If he refuses such intervention, and the confirmed abuser often will, the woman must be helped out of the relationship, if at all possible.

Interventions for Violent Men

It is ironic and terribly aggravating that the abused woman must flee her home or be labeled as sick and receive treatment, while the batterer stays home and is seldom identified as needing interventions. Most abusers do not fit our definitions of mentally ill. Yet surely *their* behavior is what is most in need of change.

Batterers may come to the attention of the mental health system through alcoholic treatment programs, and specific questions about abuse should be included in the histories of such men. Their wives should also be asked about physical violence in the relationship, because the man will frequently deny such occurrences or treat them very lightly. It cannot be assumed that taking care of problems with alcohol will also solve the problems of violence in the relationship; specific interventions for abuse need to be implemented also.

There are beginning to be specific programs for abusive men in a variety of localities. This is certainly a needed development, and some communities are experimenting with mandated counseling for batterers through the law enforcement system. Group treatment seems to be the avenue of choice, based on the Men's Aid program model started in England.[37] Telephone counseling and drop-in services have also been a part of Men's Aid. Confrontation is used to get the abusers to admit their responsibility, and ways of dealing with anger besides hitting are taught. The men are also encouraged to get in touch with their other feelings and learn how to express them and also to deal with changing sex roles and the difficulties in being a man today. Male therapists are generally used in leading such groups, to provide a role model and to better be able to challenge these men.

The Nurse as Advocate

Where such programs for abusive men do not yet exist, the nurse can be instrumental in the community in advocating for their establishment. Once begun, nurses need to encourage this as a useful intervention for battering and to advocate with the police, lawyers, judges, and probation officers to make use of them, as a mandatory alternative to jail or legal proceedings, if necessary. Establishment of these programs should go hand in hand with the formation of shelters for abused wives in all communities.

Advocacy also includes working at the local and state level to make it easier for abused women to find housing if they want to leave the spouse. Linkages can be formed between shelters and other programs for battered women and urban housing programs. Vacant houses can be rehabilitated to provide a home for two abused women and their children in many cases. The women can receive support from each other, build on a friendship started in a shelter or group, and pool their resources to make a home. The housing situation for battered women can also be helped by advocacy with public housing authorities. When these people understand the desperate need and the funding rules which limit the women's stay in shelters, they are often helpful in cutting red tape for battered women.

Advocacy can also take the form of working with the police and the legal profession as outlined in Chapters 13 and 15. In addition, the nurse needs to spread the word about battering in all her professional and social contacts. Shelters always need donations of time, money, supplies, clothing, and food. When talking about abuse, nurses frequently are told of personal battering by acquaintances and fellow professionals. For as battering becomes more of a public issue, individual women feel more comfortable in talking about their own abuse. Advocacy for battered women and demonstration of knowledge on the subject becomes a novel means of case finding and an opportunity for intervention.

EVALUATION

Evaluation of nursing care for abused women is based on achievement of goals set by the individual woman or group being worked with. When the goals are truly formulated by the women themselves, the nurse can avoid the trap of being dissatisfied with interventions that do not necessarily result in the woman leaving the relationship even when the nurse has decided that this course of action would be best. The goals set for nursing care may be quite limited depending on the amount of intervention possible in the particular setting. Achievement of the goals, however modest, can still be a powerful statement of possibilities to the battered wife. Praise for her progress, however small, can be an important reinforcer for the woman to seek further help and to have confidence in her own ability to address the underlying problems.

When working with battered women, the nurse needs to become accustomed to measuring gains in small steps and to deal with the women being in a variety of stages of resolution of this significant health problem. The nurse can begin to recognize that for every abused woman who is still in the throes of denial of the seriousness of abuse, there is another woman who is close to rebuilding a healthy life for herself. It is easy for professionals to become discouraged when working with battered women; similar feelings are expressed by nurses who work with clients with chronic health problems. These feelings can be dealt with by sharing with others who work with abuse and by taking pride in evaluation of what has been achieved when working with the abuse victim. Shelter staffs often need help with this also. Nurses can be of assistance here in pointing out that women who return to the abusive relationship may still have gained a great deal of support and insight by staying in the shelter, feel less alone in dealing with the problem, know where they can go if they are in danger, and be further along in their grieving process than when they first arrived.

During evaluation the nurse may also need to deal with her own feelings of anger against the batterer, especially if the woman has not been experiencing them during the period of nursing intervention. This is again a frequent dilemma of professionals dealing with abused women. If the nurse is working within a shelter situation or with other professionals cognizant of wife abuse, it is appropriate for the nurse to delay her feelings of anger and discuss them later with her colleagues. Even if she does not have a good professional support system, it is important that the nurse not let her own anger show when she is with a woman not feeling anger. However, the feelings must be dealt with constructively, or the nurse will find anger against specific batterers becoming generalized to many men, and this will get in the way of effective nursing practice. Even in shelters, the nurse and staff must be careful to deal with their understandably strong feelings about situations in private or the women will suspect that staff "talks about us" behind their backs. Working with abuse victims engenders many strong feelings, and the nurses and other professionals involved need to set up their own support systems carefully so that they will not become incapacitated by the feelings or "burned out." Evaluation includes the nurse's careful re-evaluation of her own feelings and how they affect her nursing care.

Evaluation of nursing care with the battered woman includes making plans for the future. It is important that the woman who is staying in the relationship have a variety of choices of helpful services that she can call on if she decides to seek further assistance. The nurse must make sure that the individuals to whom she refers the woman are knowledgeable about abuse and immediately can put the woman at ease.

SAMPLE NURSING PROCESS

A sample nursing process has been included to show how each of the four steps might be applied to a hypothetical cause of wife abuse. This is not intended to be applicable to all cases of battered women; instead, it is provided as an illustration of some of the aspects of wife abuse that might be included in nursing care and as a means of suggesting the wording of possible nursing diagnoses. Only a brief description of the case is presented. An in-depth assessment, including a complete history and physical assessment, would be indicated in most actual situations. Evaluation of nursing interventions are based on achievement of goals as perceived by client and as indicated by criteria met.

Summary

Nursing care of abused women is based on thorough assessment, identification of strengths and areas needing nursing intervention, goal setting and making plans with the client, carrying out nursing interventions and working with other professionals in providing services, and evaluating outcomes. Primary prevention includes assertive actions at the societal level directed toward eliminating the sex role patterns that allow and encourage violence against women as well as interventions with women at risk to be battered. Secondary prevention necessitates active case finding. A direct, knowledgeable, and empathetic approach to women suspected of being abused is important in this regard. Nursing interventions at the secondary-prevention level are aimed at eliminating the abuse before the patterns become entrenched. These interventions are carried out in a variety of nursing settings and follow the theoretical framework of accepting the woman where she is in her progress through the grief process, which is a reaction to multiple losses. Tertiary level nursing care may find the nurse providing professional care in wife abuse shelters in a variety of roles or in community or inpatient mental health settings. Nursing care at the secondary and tertiary prevention levels also includes advocacy for better services for both the battered woman and her spouse. Empirical validation of these nursing interventions is needed to document their impact and build practice theory.

Table 9–3 *Sample Nursing Process*

Brief Background

Anne is a 27-year-old black woman, married to John who is 28. They have two children, 5 and 7 years old. Anne is working as a sales clerk; John has been unemployed for two years. Anne was seen in the emergency room of the local hospital when she miscarried in the second month of pregnancy. She also had multiple bruises, 2 fractured ribs, and the emergency room nurse elicited the information that she had been beaten up by her husband, prior to the miscarriage. She has been referred to the local Public Health Department, nursing division, for abuse and follow-up care of her injuries.

The community health nurse's initial assessment (one week later) of Anne includes but is not limited to the following:

Significant History	History of abuse over last 6 years. Says husband is extremely jealous about her work relationships with other men and imagines that she is having affairs. Abuse has escalated over time in frequency and severity. Husband beats her with fists and "shoves her around" at least once a month at current time. He has never used a weapon. Anne feels that being hit "now and then" is a normal part of marriage. She does not attempt to retaliate because the few times she has, she has been beaten more severely. States that she has

(continued)

Table 9-3 (Cont.)

Brief Background

	severe headaches at least once a week. Reports extreme soreness in rib area and generalized fatigue because of "not sleeping well." States wanted baby but does not feel she can talk about it.
General Appearance	Energetic, neatly dressed young woman, average height and weight. Talks quickly with many gestures and smiles.
Skin	5 cm. oval shaped contusion on left arm just above elbow, tender to touch.
Musculoskeletal	Fracture of 9th and 10th right ribs diagnosed by X-ray.
Neurological	Alert, oriented to time, place, person. Uses humor a great deal in describing situation. Does not display sadness over loss of baby. Feels she has no particular strengths.

Nursing diagnoses identified include:

1. Unresolved grieving (using denial and coping with humor) related to miscarriage and wife abuse.
2. Limited mobility and pain related to rib injury from abuse.
3. Stress-related symptoms (headache and insomnia) related to wife abuse and low self-esteem.
4. Potential for subsequent violence related to husband's pathological jealousy and stress in home situation.

Nursing DX	Client Goals	Nursing Intervention
I. Unresolved Grieving	Short Term 1.A. Client will begin to grieve for lost baby by the end of two weeks as evidenced by: Talking about baby Expressing sorrow about loss	1.A.1. Discuss with client what pregnancy meant to her when she indicates readiness. 2. Encourage client to contact her sister whom she has identified as supportive. Form helping relationship with client.
	Short Term 1.B. Client will begin to be in touch with abuse in one month as evidenced by: Expression of ambivalence about husband Expression of ambivalence about marriage	1.B.1. Discuss the general battering problem with client. 2. Encourage expression of feelings about spouse and marriage. 3. Suggest several different support groups for battered women.

Table 9-3 (Cont.)

Nursing DX	Client Goals	Nursing Intervention
II. Limited Mobility	Short Term II.A. Client will be more mobile in one week is evidenced by: Decreased pain in ribs Ability to return to work	II.A.1. Suggest periods of rest. 2. Tape ribs for support and show client how to do herself. 3. Apply heat to area to promote healing (hot showers/baths, heating pad/hot H_2O bottle).
III. Stress-Related Symptoms	Short Term III.A. Client will experience a decrease in stress-related symptoms in 4 weeks as evidenced by: Incidence of headaches decreasing to once every two weeks Client being able to sleep 7 hours per night Client reporting feeling less tension	III.A.1. Teach client relaxation exercises to be used before sleep and one other period per day. 2. Help client choose a regular exercise regimen. 3. Discuss coping mechanisms with client and help her practice in role rehearsal the ones that make sense to her. 4. Discuss sleep patterns with client and encourage sleep enhancing mechanisms that she has used in the past. 5. Help client identify especially stress-producing situations and decide on better ways to deal with them.
	III.B. Client will begin to increase self-awareness and self-exploration by the end of 3 weeks as evidenced by: Being able to discuss own feelings, attitudes, values, and behavior Identifying how women's role in society affects her own situation	B.1. Encourage joining a woman's group. 2. Discuss women's role in society and how this impacts on wife abuse. 3. Identify strengths observed and discuss these with client. 4. Praise efforts at problem solving. 5. Explore feelings, and behaviors with her.

(continued)

Table 9–3 (Cont.)

Nursing DX	Client Goals	Nursing Intervention
		6. Help client identify what she can control and what she cannot.
		7. Provide self as a role model in self-exploration.
	Long Term	
	III.C. Client will increase self-esteem by the end of 6 months as evidenced by: Client being able to list at least 10 significant personal strengths Client being able to identify long-term goals and confidently express realistic plans to achieve them	III.C.1. Continue to explore client's attitudes, feelings, and values with her. 2. Praise problem-solving efforts. 3. Continue to point out special strengths. 4. Help her identify long-term goals and plans.
	Short Term	
IV. Potential for More Serious Injury	IV.A. Client will realistically assess own danger and situation by the end of 4 weeks as evidenced by: Stating realistically the pattern of abuse in the past and making projections for the future based on that Identifying husband's patterns of behavior Identifying effects of violence on children Identifying pros and cons of marriage	IV.A.1. Share facts about wife abuse with client. 2. Help client identify patterns of past abuse with a calendar and encourage realistic projections. 3. Discuss behavior of children in wife abuse homes in general and her children in particular with her. 4. Discuss macho characteristics of abusive men with her and relate to husband's behavior. 5. Make sure she has a place (e.g., a wife abuse shelter or home of a sympathetic relative or friend) to go if in danger. 6. Discuss legal alternatives with her. 7. Help her review the marriage and its effects on her.

Evaluation of nursing interventions are based on achievement of goals as perceived by client and as indicated by criteria met.

Chapter 9

1. Violet Ramonaitis Lichtenstein, "The Battered Woman: Guideline for Effective Nursing Intervention," *Issues in Mental Health Nursing* 3(1981): 244; See also Wendy Goldberg and Ann Carey, "Domestic Violence Victims in the Emergency Setting," *Topics in Emergency Medicine* 3 (January 1982): 65-75, for a list of assessment questions.

2. Evan Stark et al., "Medicine and Patriarchal Violence," *International Journal of Health Services* 9 (1979), p. 465.

3. Virginia Koch Drake, "Battered Women, A Health Care Problem in Disguise," *Image* 14 (June 1982): 45-46.

4. Goldberg and Carey, "Domestic Violence Victims," p. 66.

5. M. Lucille Kinlein, *Independent Nursing Practice with Clients* (Philadelphia: J. B. Lippincott Co., 1977), p. 58.

6. Barbara Star, "Comparing Battered and Non-Battered Women," *Victimology* 3 (1978): 38.

7. Lenore Walker, *The Battered Woman* (New York: Harper & Row, 1979).

8. Debra Kalmuss and Murray Straus, "Wife's Marital Dependency and Wife Abuse," *Journal of Marriage and the Family* 44 (May 1982): 279-80, 283.

9. Lisa Mahon, "Common Characteristics of Abused Women," *Issues in Mental Health Nursing* 3 (January-June 1981): 153.

10. Suzanne Prescott and Carolyn Letko, "Battered Women: A Social Psychological Perspective," in *Battered Women*, ed. Maria Roy (New York: Van Nostrand Reinhold Co., 1977), pp. 72-90, 81; Jean Renvoize, *Web of Violence* (London: Routledge and Kegan Paul, 1978), p. 371.

11. Stark et al., "Medicine and Patriarchal Violence," p. 467.

12. Lichtenstein, "Battered Woman," p. 249.

13. Melva Jo Hendrix, "Home is Where the Hell Is," *Family and Community Health* 4 (August 1981): 58.

14. E. Donnerstein, "Aggressive Erotica and Violence against Women," *Journal of Personality and Social Psychology* 39 (August 1980): 269-277; E. Donnerstein and J. Hallam, "Facilitating Effects of Erotica on Aggression," *Journal of Personality and Social Psychology* 36 (November 1978): 1270-77; Neil Malamuth and James Check, "The Effects of Mass Media Exposure on Acceptance of Violence Against Women: A Field Experiment," *Journal of Research in Personality* 15 (December 1981): 436-46.

15. Margarete Sandelowski, *Women, Health, and Choice* (Englewood Cliffs, N.J.: Prentice-Hall, 1980), 213; Gloria Steinem, "Erotica and Pornography: A Clear and Present Difference," *Ms.*, November 1978, pp. 53-54, 75-78.

16. Martha Gever and Marg Hall, "Fighting Pornography," in *Take Back the Night*, ed. Laura Lederer (New York: William Morrow & Co, 1980), pp. 279-285.

17. Drake, "Battered Women," p. 43.

18. Fleming, *Stopping Wife Abuse*, p. 436; Stark et al., "Medicine and Patriarchal Violence," p. 465.

19. Doreen J. DeBliek "Prevalence of Domestic Violence Reported by Female Psychiatric Inpatients" (unpublished field study, Wayne State University, 1981), pp. 39-40.

20. Gayford, "Wife Battering: A Preliminary Survey of 100 Cases," *British Medical Journal* 1 (January 1975): 195.

21. Drake, "Battered Woman," p. 45.

22. John Flynn, "Recent Findings Related to Wife Abuse," *Social Casework* 63 (January 1977) 13-20, p. 18.

23. Walker, p. 105.

24. This section has been derived from the work of various theorists as well as from the data from the many samples of abused wives previously cited and the author's own experience with battered women. References include: Jean Werner-Beland, *Grief Responses to Long-Term Illness and Disability* (Reston, Va.: Reston Publishing Co., 1980); John Bowlby, *Attachment and Loss*, vol. 1, *Attachment* (New York: Basic Books, 1969); Carolyn E. Carlson and Betty Blackwell, *Behavioral Concepts and Nursing Intervention* (Philadelphia: J. B. Lippincott Co., 1970); George L. Engel, "Grief and Grieving," *American Journal of Nursing* 64 (September 1964): 93-98; Janice B. Flynn and Janice Whitcomb "Unresolved Grief in Battered Women," *Journal of Emergency Nursing* 7 (November/December 1981): 250-54; Rita Weinfourt, "Battered Women: The Grieving Process," *Journal of Psychiatric Nursing and Mental Health Services* vol. 1778 (April 1979): 40-47; Phyllis Silverman, *Helping Women Cope with Grief* (Beverly Hills, Calif.: Sage Publications, 1981), pp. 9-38, 81-99.

25. Elizabeth Kubler-Ross, *On Death and Dying* (New York: Macmillan, 1969).

26. Werner-Beland, *Grief Responses*, pp. 41-61.

27. Carlson and Blackwell, *Behavioral Concepts and Nursing Interventions*, pp. 92-93.

28. Lenore Walker, "How Battering Happens and How to Stop It," in *Battered Women*, ed. Donna Moore (Beverly Hills, Calif.: Sage Publications, 1979), pp. 59-78, 76.

29. Deborah L. Watts and Christine A. Courtois, "Trends in the Treatment of Men Who Commit Violence Against Women," *Personnel and Guidance Journal* 60 (December 1981): 246, 248.

30. Richard J. Gelles, "Applying Research on Family Violence to Clinical Practice." *Journal of Marriage and the Family* 44 (February 1982): 16.

31. John G. Higgins, "Social Services for Abused Wives," *Social Casework* 59 (May 1978): 267.

32. Donna Moore, "Suggestions for Public Policy," in Moore, *Battered Women*, pp. 195, 198.

33. Women-In-Transition, "Second Annual Report" (Detroit: Women-In-Transition, 1980), pp. 5-6.

34. Ellen Hastings Janosik and Lenore Bolling Phipps, *Life Cycle Group Work in Nursing* (Monterey, Calif.: Wadsworth Health Sciences Division, 1982), pp. 208-212.

35. Rose Weitz, "Feminist Consciousness Raising, Self-Concept, and Depression," *Sex Roles* 8 (February 1982): 235-37, 231.

36. Walker, "How Battering Happens," p. 75.

37. Joy Melville, "A Note on Men's Aid," in *Violence and the Family*, J. P. Martin, ed. (Chichester: John Wiley and Sons, 1978), pp. 311-13.

Nursing Care of Abused Children

Janice Humphreys

> i was in pain
> when i was hit by a train
> i was in the hospital for a while
> and it made me smile
> that i was still alive
> i felt dead
> when i hit my head
> but i was still happy
> that i'm going to live
> to twenty five
>
> Eric Willock, age twelve

Reprinted from *Every Twelve Seconds*, compiled by Susan Venters (Hillsboro, Oregon: Shelter, 1981) by permission of the author.

Nursing care of abused and neglected children requires current theory-based knowledge and individualized application. The nurse may become aware of child abuse and neglect at almost any point in her practice with families. The maltreated child may be obvious or may present with less apparent indications of abuse and neglect. Nursing care of families is based upon prevention and therefore does not require evidence of a "problem" for the nurse to intervene. Assessment for potential and actual child abuse and neglect is therefore an integral part of the nursing care of every child and parent. The purpose of this chapter is to assist in the application of the theory and research presented in previous chapters to practice. A nursing process format is used, and a sample nursing process is also included.

SELF-AWARENESS

Care of abusive or potentially abusive families begins with the nurse's examination of her own feelings. A nonjudgmental, helping approach to any client requires awareness and resolution of personal feelings that interfere with giving the highest quality professional nursing care. Kathleen Scharer describes two reactions that can occur when the nurse encounters abuse and neglect. "The first is a horror that a parent could injure his innocent child; as a result the helper [nurse] responds to the parent in an angry, punitive fashion. . . . The second is one of denial."[1] Denial by the nurse that abuse and neglect have occurred may result from the nurse's disbelief that the parent could be responsible. Neither response, anger or denial, is in any way helpful, can impair the safety of the child, and can limit the effectiveness of nursing care.

In a separate article Scharer identifies a third and equally damaging response to child abuse and neglect—rescue fantasy. "Rescue fantasy usually means a form of behavior observed when the nurse or any other helping person appears to feel that she can save or in some way rescue a person for whom she is caring."[2] Rescue fantasies can prevent the nurse from seeing the real needs of the family. An example of a nurse experiencing a rescue fantasy is the staff nurse caring for a neglected infant now gaining weight, who is pleasant but will not use any of the parent's suggestions regarding childcare. Because the child has been neglected, the nurse assumes that only she and the rest of the health care system know what is best for the child. The nurse's feelings thus prevent her from using every interaction with the neglectful family therapeutically. A discussion of how to resolve personal and professional feelings about child abuse and neglect, and the implications for nursing education can be found in Chapter 16.

The nurse must examine the basis for her practice. Does she believe that people who abuse and neglect children are sick? Do parents maltreat their children because they learned to use violence from their parents? The answer is found by first obtaining knowledge of theories of child maltreatment and second by examining her values and feelings in response. Such an examination of feelings is difficult. As was discussed in Chapter 5, part of the reason that no one definition of child abuse and neglect can be identified may have to do with the fear of many that the broader the definition, the closer child maltreatment comes to generally accepted child-rearing practices. Does every adult have the potential to abuse or neglect a child? Concerned professionals may deny that every adult is capable of harming a child. Yet, if the nurse is interested in prevention, it makes sense to acknowledge the possibility that every adult has the potential to be a perpetrator and every child a victim of child abuse and neglect. That is not to imply that every parent *will* harm his or her child. The intent instead is to encourage the nurse to approach her practice prepared and able to assess the possibility of child abuse and neglect as she would nutritional status or immunization history or any other aspect of child health. As with many other socially unacceptable facts, no adult will acknowledge the maltreatment of a child unless he or she is given an open opportunity to discuss it. No professional nurse will give an adult the opportunity to ask for assistance in child-rearing if she does not suspect that every parent has the potential for problems. No child maltreatment will be found by the nurse who never suspects it.

ASSESSMENT

The nursing care begins with assessment. Before any action can be taken, data are collected systematically. Assessment for potential or actual child abuse requires the taking of a history and physical examination. The techniques of the two components of assessment can be approached using a variety of methods. It is not within the scope of this text to teach the beginning nurse basic questions to ask or how to palpate a lesion. Rather, this chapter, will attempt to identify areas of particular significance in the history and physical examination for child abuse and neglect. For ease of presentation, a particular history-taking and physical examination format will be followed; however, any thorough approach to assessment could be used.

History

Every nurse of necessity develops her own particular method and style of data collection. The location of nursing practice also requires the nurse to adapt the extent and method of assessment. The nurse in a well child clinic practices under different circumstances than the nurse in an emergency room. Each, however, is exposed to child maltreatment and should include assessment in this area routinely.

Gathering historical data about child

abuse and neglect can be stressful for both the nurse and the parent. Yet the nurse, by providing a conducive environment and using therapeutic communication techniques, can achieve maximum results.

It is essential that a nonjudgmental approach be maintained at all times. The role of the nurse does not require a judgment of the "rightness" or "wrongness" of certain client behaviors. Law enforcement and legal professionals accept responsibility for determining whether or not a crime has been committed. The nurse is also not in a position to punish or discipline parents who maltreat their children. If she expects to assist abusive and neglectful parents to "come to their senses" by expressing her own anger or threats to remove their child, she is actually only reinforcing to the parents that the use of aggression is appropriate to aid learning. The nurse is utilizing a subtle form of "beating some sense into them." Certainly aggression and, the less obvious, coercion are not the therapeutic approaches of choice to families who already experience an excess of violence in their homes. Eli H. Newberger and Richard Bourne identify that health professionals face multiple dilemmas in working with abusive parents. Social policies vary from those supportive of family autonomy to those recommending coercive intervention. Professional responses to child abuse are also dichotomized: compassion ("support") versus control ("punishment").[3] The various combinations of possible action responses are illustrated in Table 10-1.

Working with child abuse and neglect requires a skilled clinician who can establish a trusting, honest relationship with people who are most likely afraid to trust any professional. The nurse can provide the abusive and neglectful parent with an environment of support and concern. The nurse must approach the parent with compassion and by her questioning give the client the opportunity to voice his or her concerns and ask for help. The nurse's role is not to "cure" the child abuse and neglect. Rather, it is to assist the family to provide a safe and nurturant environment that promotes life, health, and well-being for all its members.

Table 10–1 *Dilemmas of Social Policy and Professional Response*

Response	Family Autonomy	Versus	Coercive Intervention
Compassion ("support")	1. Voluntary child development services 2. Guaranteed family supports, e.g., income, housing, health services		1. Case reporting of family crisis and mandated family intervention 2. Court-ordered delivery of services
Versus			
Control ("punishment")	1. "Laissez-faire." No assured services or supports 2. Retributive response to family crisis		1. Court action to separate child from family 2. Criminal prosecution of parents

Reprinted with permission from Eli H. Newberger and Richard Bourne, "The Medicalization and Legalization of Child Abuse," *American Journal of Orthopsychiatry*, 48, No. 4 (October, 1978): 593–607.

Nursing Care of Abused Children

From the moment of her first contact with the client and family, the nurse should present herself in a manner that is open and honest. The initial meeting begins with the nurse introducing herself and clearly stating her purpose. The setting for the interview with the abusive and neglectful parent should ideally be quiet and private. In those facilities where no quiet and private location exists, the nurse can work toward making the administration aware of the need. An example would be: "Hello, Ms. G. I'm J.H. I'm a pediatric clinical nurse specialist. What that means is that I'll be talking with you and asking you some questions about your daughter Sally's health, previous to today. I'll also be doing a physical examination of Sally." The specific description of the nurse's purpose helps to allay some of the parent's fears and also set the framework for the nurse-client encounter.

The nurse next seats herself so that her eyes are at the same level with those of the parent. She neither wishes to tower over the parent nor be dominated. The seating arrangement is such that no desk or other inhibitive object comes between the nurse and the client. The nonverbal message to the parent is "I'm interested in what you have to say and would like to help you to help yourself."

The nurse continues to be supportive and compassionate throughout her questioning. Detailed interviewing about sensitive subjects, potential or actual child abuse and neglect, can be very difficult for the parent. If the parent is too threatened by the approach of the nurse, he or she is unlikely to be completely open and honest. The nurse in turn, gives the parent every opportunity to share concerns or problems with childrearing while remaining cognizant of professional responsibilities.

The nurse begins the health history of a child who is known or suspected of being abused just like any other history-taking session. There are two reasons for this. First, the nurse can follow the sequence of questioning that she is familiar with and thereby increase her ability to attend to parent responses rather than a new or different format. Second, history taking *always* begin with parent concerns and progresses from the general family history (nonthreatening) to specific child history (more threatening). The nurse will be able to demonstrate her sincere concern for the parent before she asks about parent-child interactions and problems.

Eliciting parent concerns is a particularly important aspect of history taking. The parent's concerns are likely the reason the child was brought to the health facility to begin with. The nurse, by giving the parent's concerns or problems primary importance, is demonstrating that she is interested in and values the parent's opinion. The initial inquiry can be as simple as "Is there anything in particular that you are concerned about or that I should pay particular attention to?" If no area is identified, the nurse will want to follow up with "If you think of anything as we go along, please do not hesitate to bring it to my attention."

As the nurse and parent progress through the history, the nurse avoids being accusatory or confrontive. Clinical experience has revealed that giving parents an opportunity to voice areas of need or weakness can be far more productive than any accusation. The following excerpt from an actual interview demonstrates this point:

Nurse: Who helps you care for the children?

Client: Nobody.

Nurse: You mean you have to be the parent *all* the time?

Client: Yes.

Nurse: That's pretty hard work.

Client: It sure is. Sometimes I just can't stand it. And that B., he just really seems to know how to aggravate me.

Nurse: Tell me about that.

Other questions that help to illicit the information of concern are: "How do you discipline your children?" or "When was the last time you spanked him?"

The power of listening can never be underestimated. The nurse can make great progress in data gathering and establishing trust with the parent by just listening. Abusive and neglectful parents are often isolated physically and socially from other adults. The opportunity to voice their worries and fears to a compassionate listener can actually be therapeutic for the parent. Further, due to the complex nature of child maltreatment, long-term interventions are almost always necessary. A firmly established trusting relationship between nurse and parent is essential for achievement of client goals. Listening to the parent from the very first encounter is critical to the development of parent trust in the nurse.

It is also desirable to interview the parent with the child present at times and absent at others. The interaction between the parent and the child can be particularly informative. During an extensive history-taking session almost every child becomes wearied and bored. The parent's method of handling the child and the child's behavior can tell the nurse a great deal about factors that may be contributing to abuse and neglect in the home.

Further, interactions between parent, child, and nurse during a stressful situation can provide an excellent opportunity to assist parents in using alternative child-rearing behaviors. For example the nurse may wish to address uncontrolled behavior to the child: "I know it's scary to come to the clinic." Another approach directed toward the parent might be: "Many children feel nervous the first time they come here, because they don't know what's going to happen. You don't need to do that to him (hit him, yell at him, hold him down). Let's let him calm down with this book."

Table 10-2 provides a simple but thorough listing of historical findings that can indicate potential or actual child abuse and neglect. The table has been set up such that the "at-risk responses" listed in the right-hand column do not all necessarily mean that abuse or neglect of a child has taken place. The "at-risk responses" include obvious evidence of abuse and neglect (child in foster home or other institutional placement for abuse/neglect) and less obvious indicators of potential child abuse and neglect (poverty, single parent, chronically ill child). The "at-risk responses" are intended as clues that require interpretation and clinical judgment.

A brief clarification of terms is necessary at this time. The medical diagnosis "failure to thrive" is often automatically taken as a euphemism for child neglect. A child admitted to a hospital pediatric unit is often treated by health professionals as a "poor little victim" and the parent as "obviously unfit." The reality is that "failure to thrive" is very much like "fever of undetermined origin," a broad medical diagnosis that gets the child a hospital bed and

Nursing Care of Abused Children

Table 10-2 *Child History—Indicators of Potential or Actual Child Abuse and Neglect*

Area of Assessment	At-Risk Responses
I. Primary Concern/Reason for Visit	Historical data that do not fit with physical findings
	Vague complaints about child
	Inappropriate delay in bringing child to health facility
	Reluctance on the part of the parent to give information
	Inappropriate parental reaction to nurse's concern (overreacts or underreacts)
	Hyperactivity
II. Family Health History	
A. Parents	Grew up in a violent home (abused as child, observed mother or siblings abused)
	Low self-esteem
	Little knowledge of child development and care
	Substance abuse
	Adolescent at birth of child
B. Siblings	History of abuse and/or neglect of siblings
	Large family
	Several young, dependent children in family
C. Other Family Members	Other history of violence or violent death
D. Household	Violence and aggression used to resolve conflicts and solve problems
	Poverty
	Single parent
	No friends, neighbors, or other support systems available
	Problems between parents, especially sexual
	Other stressors
	a) unemployment
	b) death in the family
	History of child foster home or other institutional placement for abuse/neglect
III. Child Health History	
A. Prenatal	Unwanted pregnancy
	Difficult or complicated pregnancy
	Adolescent
	Wanted a baby so that "I would have someone to love."
	Little or no prenatal care

(continued)

Table 10-2 (Cont.)

Area of Assessment	At-Risk Responses
B. Birth	Caesarean section
	Prematurity
	Low birth weight
	Birth defect
	Immediate separation of parents and child
	Child not of preferred sex or appearance
C. Neonatal	Separation of parents and child
	Neonatal complications and serious illness
D. Nutrition (If necessary include 24-hour dietary recall)	History of feeding problems (frequent change of formula, colic, difficult to feed)
	Inappropriate food, drink, or drugs
	Dietary intake that does not fit with physical findings
	Inadequate food or fluid intake
E. Personal/Social	Child described as "bad," "different" or difficult to care for
	Parent has unrealistic expectations of child
	Multiple school absences
	Difficulty in school
	History of phobias, running away from home, or delinquent acts
	Poor peer relationships or no peer relations
	Sexual problems in child (excessive or public masturbation, age-inappropriate sexual play, promiscuity)
	Substance abuse
F. Discipline	Use of physical punishment especially in an infant or adolescent
	Use of an object to administer physical punishment
	Excessive, inappropriate, inconsistent physical punishment
	History of parent "losing control" and/or "hitting too hard"
G. Sleep	"Doesn't sleep," "Awake all night"
H. Elimination	Inappropriate, excessive home treatment of constipation
	Enuresis
	Violent toilet training
I. Growth and Development	History of excessive autostimulation
	"Hyperactivity"

Nursing Care of Abused Children

Table 10–2 (Cont.)

Area of Assessment	At-Risk Responses
	Developmental delays
	Excessive aggression or passivity
J. Illness	Chronic illness or handicap
	Disability requiring special treatment from parents
K. Operations/Hospitalizations	Operations or illness that required extended hospitalization
	Parent refusal to have child hospitalized
	History of suicide attempt
L. Diagnostic Tests	Evaluation for failure to thrive or other problem that would explain injuries and/or lack of weight gain
	Severe anemia
	Elevated lead level
	Parent refusal for further diagnostic studies
M. Accidents	Repeated
	History of preceding events does not support actual injuries
N. Safety	No age-appropriate safety precautions
O. Immunizations	None or only a few
P. Health Care Utilization	No consistent provider
	Parent "shops" for hospital care
Q. Review of Body Systems	Changes in previously reported data
	Pertinent data not previously reported

time to find out what is really wrong. Certainly there are neglected children who have at one time or another been labeled as "failure to thrive." For this reason the medical diagnosis has been included among the "at-risk responses" in Table 10–2. It is also true, however, that almost every chronic illness of childhood can present itself as a failure to thrive. Parents whose child is admitted to a hospital with the possibility of finding out their child has a chronic, possibly terminal, illness are in need of expert care, not merely tolerance. The medical diagnosis of "failure to thrive" therefore, requires the nurse to be most skillful in her use of the tools of assessment and evaluation to assure the exactly right plan of care.

It is particularly important to consider historical data in light of physical examination findings (see Table 10–3). The information acquired from the history may cause the nurse little or no alarm, and yet when contrasted with data from physical examination may reveal quite another picture. The parent may give a history of a restless, irritable, difficult to feed infant. Upon observing the parent feed the child, the nurse observes a crying infant who immediately quiets when fed, sucks hungrily

Table 10-3 *Physical Examination of the Child—Indicators of Potential or Actual Child Abuse and Neglect*

I.	General Appearance	Marked passivity or watchfulness
		Fearful, anxious, hyperactive
		Malnourished-looking
		Constant hunger in an infant
		Poor hygiene
		Inappropriate dress for weather conditions
		Excessive detachment by parent
		Physical handicap
II.	Vital Statistics	
	A. Height	Failure to gain height and/or weight as expected when compared to growth charts
	B. Weight	
	C. Head Circumference	Less than 3rd percentile rank
		Drop off in previously identified growth trends first in height, then weight, and finally head circumference
III.	Skin	Excessive or unexplainable bruises, welts, or scars, possibly in various stages of healing
		Cigarette or dip burns
		Wasting of subcutaneous tissue
		Infected or untreated wound
		(Skin lesion recording may most accurately be done on a diagram of the body)
IV.	Head	Bald patches on scalp
		Subdural hematoma
V.	Eyes	
VI.	Ears	
VII.	Nose	
VIII.	Mouth	Bruising, lacerations
		Gross dental caries
		Venereal infection
IX.	Neck	
X.	Chest	
XI.	Abdomen	Intraabdominal injuries
		Abdominal distention
		Pregnancy
XII.	Genital/Urinary	Urinary tract infection
		Vaginitis
		Venereal infection
		Bruising, bleeding
		Severe diaper rash
XIII.	Rectal	Poor sphincter muscle tone
		Bruising, bleeding
		Venereal infection

Table 10-3 (Cont.)

XIV. Peripheral Vascular	
XV. Musculoskeletal	Skull or facial fractures
	Fractured femur
	Green stick or spiral fractures
	Limited motion of an extremity
	Multiple fractures in various stages of healing
XVI. Neurological (Includes Denver Developmental Screening Test)	Developmental retardation
	Limited motion of an extremity

and quickly falls to sleep after feeding. Or, a parent may report that the child was left momentarily unattended in a bath tub while the parent answered the telephone. Upon returning the parent states, he found the child had accidentally turned on the hot water. Physical examination findings reveal second- and third-degree burns of the four distal extremities only. It is therefore not merely the history or physical findings in isolation that are important. It is the combination of the two sources of data and the *descrepancies* that exist between them.

The general appearance of a child is also important. The child's appearance includes not only the manner of dress, but also the behavior of the child during the assessment phase. The nurse who assesses the child can compare the affect, development, and growth of each individual against the generally accepted norms.

Every contact with parents and their children is an opportunity for the nurse to assess and intervene. The child abusing and neglecting parent may be particularly observant of the nurse's behavior as they are often anxious and desperate for help. The nurse in the manner of her interaction between both parent and child is demonstrating to each alternative behaviors. A physical examination need not be a socially acceptable means of frightening, controlling, and hurting children. Instead the nurse can establish trust, identify strengths, and still conduct a thorough assessment.

Nursing Diagnosis

The last step in the process of assessment is the development of appropriate nursing diagnoses. Potential or actual child abuse and neglect can result in a variety of nursing diagnoses. The needs of the individual child and family are used as a basis for nursing diagnosis development. Therefore, there is no one set nursing diagnosis for children who have the potential for or have actually experienced abuse or neglect. A sample nursing process (Table 10-4) with nursing diagnoses has been included in the chapter to aid the reader in understanding assessment.

PLANNING

The planning stage of professional nursing care requires the development of both goals and interventions. Goals in the case of child abuse and neglect are realistic, multidimensional, and both long-term and short-term. Nursing intervention with child abuse and neglect is based upon the three levels of prevention. The plan in the case of child abuse and neglect must of necessity be prioritized. The safety of the child must always be the first concern of the nurse. However, the development of interventions requires caution that responses to child abuse and neglect are not attempts to control.[4]

Goals

Goals are client oriented and whenever possible developed with the client. When mutually-agreed upon goals are developed, "noncompliance" becomes much less of a problem. Mutually-agreed upon goals can even be growth producing for the abusive and neglectful parent. By working with the parent to identify realistic goals in an area of mutual concern—child welfare—the nurse is actually helping the parent to improve his or her problem-solving capabilities. Further, the nurse is again demonstrating to the parent that his or her opinions and participation are important—that the parent has value. Attention to and reinforcement for parent strengths contributes to increasing the parent's self-esteem and self-care capabilities.

However, conflict can arise when the abusive and neglectful parent does not identify the same problems as the nurse. To the parent, strict corporal punishment may be absolutely essential to the development of a healthy child. The parent may not perceive violent childrearing practices as a problem that requires set goals aimed at their elimination. The nurse may be tempted to impose her own goals upon the parent. Certainly in those cases where the safety of the child is questioned, the parent's wishes cannot always be strictly adhered to. However, in the majority of abuse and neglect cases, the safety of the child can be assured and the parent's perception of problems generally followed. The nurse who sets her own goals exclusive of the parent will likely experience great frustration and disappointment when the goals are not achieved. This is not to say that problems identified by the nurse but not the parent should be forgotten. The nurse should, instead, realize that the problem now becomes helping the parent to identify the nurse's original area of concern. Until both parent and nurse identify the same problem areas, no goals can be developed or action taken to achieve them.

Child abuse and neglect is such a complex problem that all the appropriate goals would be impossible to list. Goals are identified in reference to the appropriate nursing diagnosis. For example, the nursing diagnosis "Alteration in parenting related to inappropriate discipline" might appropriately be associated with the goal "Parent will demonstrate age-appropriate discipline within one week." However, in another family the goal might instead be "Within one week the parent will verbalize the developmental characteristics of a 6-month-old child." The reader is again referred to the sample nursing process (Table 10-4) for additional examples.

NURSING INTERVENTION

Professional nursing interventions to child abuse and neglect cover a broad spectrum.

Nursing Care of Abused Children

The nurse is concerned about the hospitalized infant who is severely neglected. However, she would be remiss if she failed to be equally concerned about the societal problems that contributed to his or her condition. E. H. Schein states, "The new values call for the professional to be an advocate, to set out to improve society, not merely to service it, to become more socially conscious, to be more an initiator than a responder."[5] The nursing literature on child abuse and neglect tends to reflect nurses as "responders"; the majority of the publications describe nursing interventions in the case of overt abuse and/or neglect. Nurses work in the community, but with few exceptions have not written about their responsibility and activities in the wider advocacy against child maltreatment.[6] The following discussion attempts to highlight some of the societal problems contributing to child maltreatment that require professional nursing intervention.

Primary Prevention

Primary prevention of child abuse and neglect includes all interventions that prevent maltreatment of children. Also included under primary prevention are child health promotion activities with both well and "at-risk" populations. The type of professional nursing intervention at this level varies with the location and nature of practice.

Prenatal

The importance of prenatal obstetrical care has long been identified as essential to an enjoyable pregnancy, uncomplicated birth, and a healthy newborn. The prenatal period is also an excellent time to promote positive parent-child interactions and prevent child abuse and neglect.

Many pregnant women and their partners regularly attend prenatal classes that help them to understand the process of pregnancy and prepare them for the birth of their child. Future parents, in general, tend to be a very receptive audience. Their interest in the pregnancy, labor, birth, and the newborn makes them an ideal group for primary prevention of child abuse and neglect. In addition, prenatal classes are usually taught by nurses.

The teaching of prenatal classes provides anticipatory guidance to the expectant family. The nurse prepares the families for the expected changes associated with each phase of pregnancy, labor, and delivery. She assists the family in their gradual understanding, identification, and acceptance of their expected child. The nurse can do this by helping the family to develop a mental picture of their child. Preparing for the soon-to-arrive child by gathering supplies, acquiring a crib, and discussing possible names all help the family to accept and enjoy the changes associated with birth. The addition of a new member to any family is associated with stress. The nurse who prepares expectant parents by way of anticipatory guidance will greatly decrease the likelihood that stress associated with childbirth will later contribute to child maltreatment.

Parent classes also provide a regular meeting time for families who have at least one thing in common, pregnancy. The nurse teaching prenatal classes should allow some time at every class for general socializing. A fifteen-minute milk and juice break will give expectant parents an unstructured time to share experiences and possibly establish support systems. A scheduled reunion of the group one or two months postpartum can provide the parent group with another opportunity to socialize and "get out of the house."

Prenatal classes are ideally associated with child development or parenting classes for parents after the birth of the child. Preparation for parents to participate in group classes during early childhood begins early in the childbirth education course and is an ongoing primary prevention.

Prenatal classes, though largely focused at preparing the expectant couple for childbirth, do so within the larger group, the family. That is to say, the woman may give birth with the assistance of her male partner, but the impact of the newborn affects all the family members. The nurse teaching prenatal classes can prepare and remind the expectant parents that behavioral changes are likely to be noted in children already in the home. The addition of a new member to the family is stressful. An older sibling's behavior in response to the birth can further increase family stress. Primary prevention of child abuse and neglect is therefore aimed at both the newborn and older siblings.

Although the majority of the childbirth education class is spent discussing physiologic changes associated with pregnancy and preparation for labor and delivery, practical decisions such as diaper services versus disposable diapers or breast versus bottle feeding can be as important as any other aspect of prenatal education. A parent who has fewer worries about the cost of a new family member will have more energy to enjoy the newborn.

The prenatal period is also associated with frequent and regular visits to health care facilities. Such visits are often associated with waiting rooms occupied by several pregnant women and their partners. Nurses can utilize this time to offer education, conduct support groups, or a combination. The prenatal period provides the nurse with numerous opportunities to creatively promote health in the expectant family.

Hospital

An ideal place to intervene to prevent child abuse and neglect is the delivery room at the time of the birth of the child. Marshall H. Klaus and John H. Kennell report that "there is a sensitive period in the first minutes and hours of life during which it is necessary that the mother and father have close contact with their neonate for later development to be optimal."[7] The nurse who works on the obstetrical unit can support parents in their first few minutes and hours with their baby. This support can be provided by encouraging mother-infant contact as soon as the mother is ready. Usually the mother, after a quick look at her newborn child to assure its wellness, needs to "catch her breath." This occurs often as the placenta is delivered and any suturing completed. When the new mother is ready, she and the father should be given some private time to "take-in" their new infant. Klaus and Kennell recommend that the parents spend thirty to forty-five minutes with their nude newborn, the child's body temperature maintained by an overhead heating panel, with as few interruptions as possible. They further recommend that instillation of silver nitrate eyedrops be delayed until the parents have had the opportunity for extended contact with their newborn during the first hour of life.[8]

Mothers are encouraged to participate in the care of their children as soon as they are ready. Maintaining newborns in a nursery separate from postpartum mothers may inhibit the parents' ability to develop a healthy relationship with their children. The rooming-in of the newborn with its mother during hospitalization has been shown to correlate with fewer subsequent cases of parenting inadequacy and therefore is encouraged.[9] The nurse can further use the daily, extended contact between mother, father, and newborn to praise and reassure the parents. Criticism of parent behavior can be replaced with identification of strengths where they exist.

Along with the traditional class on bathing the baby, the nurse on a postpartum unit can prepare mothers and fathers for what they can expect when they go home. They should be reminded to expect the infant to cry, awake, and require feeding approximately every three hours throughout the day and night. They need to hear once again that being a parent is hard work. Parents can be encouraged to identify and call upon others who can help them adjust to the changes and stress they will experience. The nurse can assure them that the lack of sleep they will experience does not go on forever and that it is OK to ask for help.

Nursing intervention may be even more important in the case of the birth of a handicapped or a premature infant. These infants are frequently whisked away from parents in order to initiate life-sustaining measures. These parents are unable to experience the desired early contact with their children and are further grieving for the loss of their ideal imagined infants.[10] Nursing interventions include emotional support to the family of the infant, encouraging parents to have contact whenever possible with the child, and the education of parents in the care of their child. Parents are encouraged to be as involved as possible in the daily childcare. Many neonatal intensive care units now routinely encourage active parent participation. Nurses can advocate such policies in hospitals where they do not already exist.

The handicapped child or the child who is hospitalized for long periods, particularly during infancy, is a particular concern to the nurse who practices on a pediatric unit. Leo Stern in a study of fifty-one abused children observed that "one-third of these children had either been seriously ill in the newborn period or had a persistent congenital defect."[11] Again, the separation of the parent and child or the existence of some anomaly is associated with child maltreatment. It may be simplistic to think that prematurity or birth defect alone predisposes a child to abuse or neglect. Chronic health problems, particulary in offspring, are a source of stress. In addition, financial strain, the missing of work, the need to identify alternative sources of other childcare may occur. Primary prevention of child abuse and neglect in the case of the premature or handicapped child includes attention to more than just the child. The professional nurse includes among her interventions contact with community social agencies, childcare services, community health nurse visits, and parent groups, wherever appropriate.

Community

Nurses in the community are in a particularly good position for primary prevention. Community health nurses go into people's homes or see them elsewhere (clinic, school) during the course of their daily life.

Nurses who practice within the schools can intervene with the adolescent who is just entering the childbearing years. Nursing interventions include sex education programs that allow adolescents to be knowledgeable about sexuality and contraception. The decision of when and if to have children can be made more intelligently if the adolescent and young adult are well informed about the prevention of pregnancy. Child development courses that expose the adolescent to the realities of being a parent can also assist the potential parent's decision making. Should the adolescent become a parent, she or he is more likely to understand her own child's behavior for having been exposed to information about child growth and development.

The pregnant adolescent presents another opportunity for primary prevention of child abuse and neglect. Pregnant adolescents can be presented with the options available to them. Should the choice be made to keep and raise the child, the nurse can work closely with the mother-to-be.

It is important that the nurse approach the pregnant adolescent with the same respect she would give to any other client. The last thing that the pregnant adolescent needs are recriminations from the nurse. The nurse who seeks to punish or lecture the adolescent on past behaviors ceases to be therapeutic. Where the adolescent father is also involved in prenatal planning, the same nonjudgmental, supportive approach is appropriate.

Group programs for pregnant mothers that allow them to complete their education by assisting with childcare, parent education, and peer contacts are very useful. Adolescence can be stressful in and of itself. Programs that attempt to acknowledge these stresses and promote parenting skills take a realistic and beneficial approach to adolescent parenthood.

Nurses who provide care to children and their parents routinely include anticipatory guidance as part of their health promotion. Parents can be prepared for the various behaviors and changes in their children as they grow and develop. For example, the negativism of a two-year-old may not be as aggravating to parents if they have been forewarned to expect it and understand it is normal for that stage of development. Further, parents need to be prepared to be angry and to want to hit their child. The nurse can problem solve with the parents to identify alternative methods of dealing with their frustration and anger.

Nursing care also involves the nurse in assisting families to see their strengths and resources. Parents are routinely praised for evidence of good childcare. Even if there are ninety-nine problems with childcare identified by the nurse, the parent can be praised for the one aspect of positive parenting. The routine inclusion of praise to the parent as part of well childcare cannot be emphasized enough. Parents rarely hear what they did right from health care providers. It is important that evidence of skillful parenting be acknowledged and rewarded. Praise from the nurse can be easily included during the history or physical examination. For example, "You've really done an excellent job at seeing that your child has a nutritious diet." Or, "Her skin is so beautiful. I can see that she's really getting the kind of care she needs." Parents are usually pleased and surprised to have their hard work noticed. By her praise of good parenting, the nurse is increasing the likelihood of its continuing, helping the parent to see his or her strengths, and increasing parent self-esteem. Parents should also be encouraged to spend some time away from the children; they can be supported and reassured that time for themselves is not selfish. One approach acknowledges that "you can't be the parent all the time." An excellent way to give both parents and preschool children time apart is to enroll the child in Head Start or some other stimulating preschool program. Clinical experience has revealed that Head Start is a blessing to many parents and a delight to the children. Head Start has also been shown to assist children in their personal development, that is, increased self-esteem, advanced reading, arithmetic, and language achievement scores at all grade levels, even fifteen years after Head Start experience. In a long-term follow-up of individuals at nineteen to twenty-two years of age, those who had attended Head Start had a higher high school completion rate, a greater likelihood of attending college, less tendency to use welfare, a higher rate of employment, and lower arrest rates than those who attended no preschool.[12] Programs like Head Start were developed to help break the cycle of poverty. Considering the major contribution that poverty makes to family violence, the nurse who is truly a client advocate will work for the continuation of programs that intervene to assist the poor.

Many working mothers fear that because of their absence from their children much of the day, they must devote the remainder of the day to their son or daughter. The consequences of working at least eight hours per day at paid employment plus another eight hours devoted totally to the needs of a dependent child is a woman who is literally working two jobs, but being paid only for one. Working mothers can be encouraged to take time for themselves away from the responsibilities of childrearing. Parents living together also need time away to maintain the non-child related aspect of their relationship.

Social Interventions

David G. Gil in his article "Violence Against Children," clearly identifies several changes that must take place if maltreatment of children is to be eliminated in the United States.[13] Gil's suggestions are examples of the most basic and potentially the most pervasive form of primary prevention. The nurse who is more than just a "responder" can be actively intervening at the social policy level described by Gil.

Briefly, Gil recommends that efforts be made to change the cultural sanction for the use of physical force, in all areas, against children. He says that "changing this aspect of the prevailing child rearing philosophy, and developing clear-cut cultural prohibitions and legal sanctions against such use of physical force, are likely to produce over time the strongest possible reduction of the incidence and prevalence of physical abuse of children."[14] Gil does not suggest that children be treated with such permissiveness that they are never punished. He recommends that constructive, educational, nonviolent discipline be used. As he goes on to point out, "rarely, if ever, is corporal punishment administered for the benefit of an attacked child, for usually it serves the immediate needs of the attacking adult who is seeking relief from his uncontrollable anger and stress."[15]

The other major intervention suggested by Gil is the active pursuit of the elimination of poverty and racism. Social inequalities that prevent individuals of every race from experiencing the same opportunities result in the overrepresentation of minorities in the lowest socioeconomic strata. In addition, current social policies now allow for levels of poverty that were heretofore unacceptable. Racial discrimination and poverty contribute in a complex fashion to child maltreatment. The professional nurse cannot expect to eliminate the maltreatment of children by family education or support alone. The culture and social environment in which the harming of children occurs and is at times, condoned, requires nursing intervention.

Gil recommends that comprehensive programming be undertaken in every community to reduce abuse and neglect of children. Included in each community program should be:

a. Comprehensive family planning programs including repeal of all legislation concerning medical abortions...
b. Family life and education counseling programs for adolescents and adults in preparation for, and after marriage...
c. A comprehensive, high quality, neighborhood based, national health service, financed through general tax revenue, and geared not only to the treatment of acute and chronic illness, but also the promotion and maintenance of maximum feasible physical and mental health for everyone...
d. A range of high quality, neighborhood based social services geared to the reduction of environmental stresses on family life and especially on mothers who carry major responsibility for the childrearing function...
e. ...a system of social services and child care facilities geared to assisting families and children that cannot live together because of severe relationship and/or reality problems.[16]

Nurses can include Gil's or similar recommendations as part of primary prevention of child abuse and neglect at the community level. The framework for the existence of child abuse and neglect lies in the larger community sphere. Its impact is seen in the family.

Recently a breakthrough was achieved toward increasing funding available toward prevention of child abuse. Michigan's 1982 income tax forms had a new option for taxpayers: a box which permits persons receiving a refund to check off two dollars (or four dollars if joint return) for child abuse prevention. Funds collected from the check-off will be placed in a Children's Trust Fund within Michigan's Department of Treasury.

One-half of the money collected each year will be invested, and one-half will be spent for local child abuse prevention programs. Funds will be distributed by a citizen's board, appointed by the governor, for local child abuse councils and local prevention services through hospitals, churches, schools, and other community organizations.

Secondary Prevention

At the moment a child experiences harm at the hands of parents or some other responsible adult, professional nursing interventions are termed "secondary prevention." The goals of secondary prevention are early diagnosis and intervention to prevent recurrence. At the time of secondary prevention, injury has already been done to the maltreated child. Professional nurs-

Nursing Care of Abused Children

ing interventions are aimed at limiting the impact of child abuse and neglect.

Hospital

The most important type of secondary prevention of child abuse and neglect is the early identification of the maltreated child. In the case of the nurse who practices in an acute care setting, abused and neglected children may or may not be medically diagnosed at her first contact. Some forms of child abuse and neglect are not readily obvious. (See Tables 10-2 and 10-3 for a complete listing of pertinent assessment findings.) Some children will be admitted directly to pediatric or intensive care units with the diagnosis of child abuse and/or neglect. Other children with reported "accidental" injuries seen in emergency rooms will more correctly be identified as abused and neglected. Nursing interventions, although still secondary prevention, will be focused on limiting the consequences of the maltreatment and preventing recurrence.

The less obviously maltreated child is the one who is encountered by the nurse in the hospital and medically diagnosed as other than abused or neglected. The child with a fractured femur who "fell out of bed" certainly is in need of health care to aid in the healing process. However, reduction of the fracture alone is profoundly inadequate treatment.

The first step in early identification of child abuse and neglect is a thorough nursing assessment. Other professional nursing interventions may involve consultation with other health professionals. Diagnostic tests that would definitely determine child abuse and neglect usually require a physician's order. The nurse, with her extended, intensive contact with hospitalized children and their parents, coupled with thorough assessment and theoretically based knowledge, often has the greatest insight into family health needs. The nurse will want to accurately record her assessment and bring it to the attention of other professionals involved in the care of the child and family.

Child abuse and neglect should be dealt with in a collaborative fashion by a group of health professionals. Ideally, a child abuse and neglect team exists in every hospital. The team is composed of interested representatives from several different professions—nursing, social work, medicine, and so forth. The child abuse and neglect team meets on a regularly scheduled basis and as needed to review suspected cases, develop plans of care, and educate other members of the hospital community. Child abuse and neglect teams can be invaluable resources and aids to the early detection and treatment of child maltreatment. An important nursing intervention is to work to develop multidisciplinary child abuse and neglect teams in hospitals where they do not already exist.

Multidisciplinary efforts in the case of child abuse and neglect are extremely important. J. Michael Cupoli and Eli H. Newberger point out that neither health nor social interventions by themselves will allay the impact of child maltreatment.[17] However, interdisciplinary management of child abuse can be difficult. In an article from the physician's perspective on interdisciplinary management of child abuse, Newberger identifies several factors that prevent professionals from various disciplines from working most effectively. Professionals from one discipline are often ignorant of the conceptual basis for practice of another discipline. Thus, communication between members of different disciplines is often poor and compounded by institutional isolation. Sometimes confusion exists between professionals of various disciplines as to who should take what management responsibilities. Some professionals display a chauvinistic attitude toward other disciplines and/or generally distrust or lack confidence in colleagues in different fields. Newberger suggests that, in general, all professionals suffer from too much work, a sense of hopelessness, punitive attitudes and public policies, and cultural isolation from clients. The result is often multiple professionals functioning independently in a fashion that can hurt, not help, violent and neglectful families.[18] For the benefit of the family the nurse can therefore see that a coordinated approach to child abuse and neglect between professionals takes place. The nurse is actually in a prime position to coordinate such multidisciplinary functioning. At the very least the nurses can be systematic and thorough in their assessments and assertive in their interventions if the best interests of the maltreated child and his or her family are to be served.

Community

The professional nurse in the community at the level of secondary prevention of child abuse and neglect also actively pursues early case finding. Assessment of the family in the home is an excellent opportunity to observe interactions between parent and child.

Once child abuse and neglect have been identified, the professional nurse's next intervention is to report the fact to the appropriate child protective agency. Mandatory child abuse and neglect reporting laws exist in every state and hold the nurse legally responsible to report all cases (see Chapter 15 for detailed discussion). The reporting of actual or suspected child abuse and neglect immediately calls forth other helping professionals. The nurse, however, cannot automatically assume that "everything will be taken care of." Whenever possible the abusive and neglectful parent is advised of the nurse's concern over both the child and the parent. Many nurses assume that abusive and neglectful parents do not want help, that they are content in their maltreatment of their child. It is possible that some parents do not wish to change their behavior, yet clinical experience more often reveals anxious, frightened people who do not want to lose custody of their children, but fear what harm they may do in the future. Advising the parent of the nurse's concern for the well-being of the child may allow the parents to more easily utilize protective agency assistance. Parents often suffer under the misconception that the sole function of protective service agencies is to remove children from their families. Child protective agencies often offer a wide range of services from crisis telephone lines to emergency respite childcare services. In addition, some parents are better able to understand their having been reported to child protective services when it is explained that the nurse is required by law to make such a report.

Undoubtedly, some parents will react with anger and hostility to having been reported to protective services regardless of the nurse's tact. At other times, the nurse may not be able to tell the family of her plan to report them to protective services. Reporting parents as abusive and neglectful to child protective services is never easy. It is especially difficult to advise the abusive and neglectful parent that such a report is about to be made by the nurse. The nurse may fear that she is shattering trust and breaking a confidence. The parent's angry response to the nurse may initially give the impression that the relationship between client and nurse has been completely destroyed. However, by her honesty, the nurse is also demonstrating that she respects the parents enough to deal with them openly and directly, that she is consistent in doing what she says, and that she is dedicated in her concern about both parent and child. The initially difficult task of advising the parent of the impending report can pay off in the long run.

The focuses of secondary prevention following the reporting of child abuse and neglect are the elimination of recurrence and the limitation of the disability that already exists. Once the safety of the child has been assured, interventions to prevent recurrence of child abuse and neglect can be initiated. Interventions focus upon the family rather than the adult-perpetrator and child-victim alone.

In the few instances in which child abuse and neglect is committed by a mentally ill parent, intensive treatment by the appropriate professional should be aimed at alleviating the illness. Ninety-five percent of the adults who abuse and neglect children are not psychotic and therefore likely would not benefit from traditional psychiatric treatment.[19]

More commonly, abusive and neglectful parents are experiencing tremendous stress combined with inappropriate methods of childrearing. Quick action by the professional nurse to alleviate some of the family stress can work not only to prevent recurrence of child abuse and neglect, but also demonstrate to the family the nurse's commitment and ability to "deliver." The power of concrete interventions like emergency housing, supplemental food, and short-term childcare should *never* be underestimated. Bernard Horowitz and Wendy Wintermute describe an emergency fund set up in New Jersey precisely for the purpose of providing direct services to child abusive and neglectful families that were not covered by any other resource.[20] One of the results of the pilot study was the realization that small, immediate stress-reducing interventions could successfully eliminate the need for larger, later agency action.

More long-term stress-reducing interventions call for the nurse to involve the family in whatever social and economic assistance programs exist in the community. Even limited social and economic assistance may be enough to reduce the strain on the family and allow them to attend to alternative methods of coping and childrearing. Ideally, the level of poverty of families would not merely be decreased in the case of poor, abusive, and neglectful families, but the cause of their poverty would be addressed as well. For example, if a father is laid off from his job as a manual laborer, he would be provided with assistance in retraining, thereby increasing his ability to get a satisfactory job, raise his status of living, and allow his family to be self-sufficient. Although the financially independent, nonpoor family may still commit child abuse and neglect, the chances of it occurring are significantly less.[21]

Bryan D. Carter, Ruth Reed, and Ceil G. Reh report that both long-term (mean period of intervention was 5.44 months) and short-term (mean period of intervention was 1.55 months) multidisciplinary (nurse, paraprofessional, nutritionist, social worker) work with abusive and neglectful mothers was able to significantly impact upon all variables (home management, childcare, safety, communications, nutrition practices).[22] The majority of the responsibility for coordination of the various services rested with the nurse. Intervention techniques employed by the nurse included relationship building, modeling of appropriate methods of childcare, psychological support to the mother, collaboration with mother in planning health care, and coordination of other agency services.[23] Modeling and reinforcement of desirable behaviors was utilized.[24]

Kathleen Scharer describes a similar approach in professional nursing practice with abusive and neglectful families.[25] She describes the nurse's role in terms of six subroles: Mother Surrogate, Managerial, Technical, Teacher, Nurse-Psychotherapist, and Socializing Agent.[26] Essentially, nursing interventions are focused at gaining trust, role modeling, teaching problem solving and limit setting, attending to the parent, and facilitating the development of extrafamily resources. In both Carter's and Scharer's suggested interventions with abusive and neglectful families, nurses are called upon to use the full range of their skills. The reader is referred to Table 10-4 for an example of the varied and complex nursing interventions identified for three nursing diagnoses at the level of secondary prevention.

Kinds of nursing interventions and their necessary emphasis will vary from family to family. Unfortunately, nursing research that investigates the effectiveness of various nursing interventions is sadly lacking. The time has come to move beyond discussions of definitions and suggested interventions based upon one clinician's experience to a systematic investigation of nursing interventions in child abuse and neglect.

Social Interventions

The complex nature of child abuse and neglect and the need for multidisciplinary involvement has been presented. The nurse concerned about the status and treatment of children is likely alarmed at the dramatic cutbacks of social services to children and their families. The very nature of child abuse and neglect requires the involvement of many disciplines, and yet, the exact agencies that are needed the most by families with the fewest resources are the agencies that experience the most severe funding cuts. The individuals who preach the sanctity of the American family are often the advocates of the elimination of the few services that might help a family stay nonviolent and together. The American Bar Association's Juvenile Justice Standards Project has gone one step further by citing the low prevailing quality of protective child welfare services in the United States and therefore recommending a sharp *restriction* of access to those services.[27] A technique suggested for decreasing the number of referred cases of child abuse and neglect is the change of mandatory reporting to discretionary reporting.[28] Social policies and beliefs that promote such a backward movement of child welfare services are of great concern and a focus of intervention for nursing.

Over the past twenty years, the problem of child abuse and neglect has become more familiar to both the professional and general public. It is impressive to note that 40 percent of the cases of child abuse and neglect reported to child protective services in 1977 came from friends, relatives, and the general public.[29] Approximately forty-six percent of the reports were from professionals (education, health care, law enforcement, social agency).[30] Unfortunately as many cases and possibly even more went unreported. William N. Friedrich reports that after a two-week media campaign in Houston, Texas, aimed at educating the public and professionals about their role in child abuse, a significant increase in reported cases of child abuse occurred.[31] The greatest apparent effect of the campaign was on the professionals, and the increase in reports came under the category of the "less severe" type of abuse (soft tissue abuse, abuse with neglect). "Possibly the campaign had the effect of increasing potential reporters' awareness of the many types of abuse rather than just the severe types like burns, fractures, and gunshot."[32] As has been suggested in previous chapters (see Chapter 5), large numbers of incidences of child abuse and neglect go unreported. Nurses, then, have a responsibility to see that media campaigns like the one described by Friedrich take place in their community. Until these families are identified and given assistance, the child-victim will likely continue to suffer.

Tertiary Prevention

Child abuse and neglect ideally is never allowed to progress to this stage of intervention and yet as social resources are eliminated, more and more children are likely to be identified for the first time at this late stage. Tertiary prevention is the level of intervention that is required when the damage of child abuse and neglect is done and the disability is irreversible. The goal of tertiary prevention is rehabilitation to the maximum level of functioning possible within the limitations of the disability.

Tertiary prevention is further necessary when, after thorough assessment and interdisciplinary consultation, it becomes clear that the abusive and neglectful family cannot safely function. Of necessity the child is removed from the home either voluntarily or by the action of the court. At the time of the removal, the child is placed in an alternative living arrangement, usually a foster home. In certain areas where emergency custody programs exist through the courts, the nurse in such facilities will find herself in an excellent position to provide services from crisis intervention to health promotion.

Foster home placement for an abused and neglected child is often identified as a "temporary" action designed to provide care to the child when the family cannot. Andre P. Derdeyn reports, however, that in Massachusetts in a cross-sectional study, 60 percent of the children in foster care had been so for four to eight years.[33] Interestingly, one of the factors impeding return of children to their families, cited by the Columbia University longitudinal study of children in foster care in New York City, was the extreme poverty of the mothers.[34]

Derdeyn goes on to discuss that often foster home placement is not temporary, and also that many children live in multiple homes during their placement. Adoption is often an impossibility. Even if a family wished to adopt a child, the biological parents less often wish to give up custody. It appears that foster children, in the eyes of the court, have even fewer rights than children in general.[35] Derdeyn recommends permanent foster placement for children who cannot be returned home or placed up for adoption.[36]

Institutions as a whole, whether they be foster homes, group homes, or large child welfare institutions, are generally unacceptable and in no way beneficial to the abused and neglected children in them, according to Malcolm Bush.[37] The 370 children surveyed by Bush lived in a variety of settings at the time of the study. The majority of children living in institutions "felt less comfortable, loved, looked after, trusted, cared about, and wanted than children in any other form of surrogate care (foster home) or than children who had been returned to their original families."[38] In general, institutions were reported to be run on the basis that the children in them had "problems" and were in need of treatment.[39] Another frequent comment by the children interviewed by Bush was the environment and activities were organized primarily to facilitate the running of the institution.[40]

When the abused and neglected child is in poor physical condition as the result of parent maltreatment, the nurse can utilize interventions based upon healing and restorative principles. For example, the malnourished infant requires nursing interventions that alleviate the child's alteration in nutrition. The burned child experiences the same alterations in skin integrity as any other burn victim. In addition to physical needs, the abused and neglected child is likely to have difficulties relating to adults, be limited in communication, and otherwise developmentally delayed.

The appropriate nursing interventions directed at the psychological, social, and developmental needs of the abused and neglected child at the level of tertiary prevention are rehabilitative. The harm done to the abused and neglected child is irreversible, and nursing care must seek to limit the extent of the disability as much as possible.

As always, the nurse first addresses the safety of the child. As has already been discussed, often when the child's safety can be secured, the living environment is hardly desirable. The child experiences an unsafe, unhealthy childhood in the home of his biological parents only to be moved, "for his own good," to a safe but still questionably healthy alternative home. It is unlikely that an abused and neglected child would learn how to successfully be a parent in either setting.

The most important intervention for the abused and neglected child is the securing of a positive, loving home. If the home of the biological parents cannot be made safe, then the nurse should support the other professionals involved in the welfare of the child in foster home placement. Ideally, the biological parents' home should be made safe and the child returned as soon as possible.

The plan of care with the abusive and neglectful parents would include interventions that reduce stress on the parent, increase parent self-esteem, problem-solving skills, and knowledge of child development. Family counseling and therapy are most likely necessary to terminate the maladaptive family members' interactions. The reader is referred to Chapter 8 for a detailed discussion of overall family nursing care.

While in foster care the abused and neglected child is in need of ongoing nursing intervention. Indeed, it is possible that the nurse will be the only consistent person in the life of the child in the transition from abusive and neglectful home to foster home. The nurse seeks to assure that the foster home provides the child with an environment that is supportive, understanding, consistent, and nonviolent. Often the move to a foster home involves relocation to another part of town. Nursing intervention can see to it that schooling and health care services continue in the new location where past services left off. A child need not restart his or her immunizations just because no one kept track of the shot records.

Nursing intervention aimed at helping an abused and neglected child overcome past trauma may include psychological therapy and/or special education for the emotionally disturbed. The child who does not require special assistance in the school still needs to have the support of his or her school nurse who receives a referral on the child from his or her public health nurse.

The preschool child can also be involved in an educational program appropriate to his or her needs. Many abused and neglected children have received either no developmental stimulation, or the wrong kind. As soon as possible, they need to experience developmentally appropriate, positive stimulation.

Many severely abused and neglected children experience permanent physical disabilities as a result of their maltreatment. These children are entitled to many of the same state, federal, and charitable health and financial benefits available to other disabled children. The nurse can see that the abused and neglected child utilizes all available services as soon as possible in an effort to reduce the impact of physical disability.

It would seem that leaving an abused and neglected child in an unsafe home is unacceptable. However, placing a child in a foster home, group home, or state institution is also no solution. The energies of the nurse, in the case of child abuse and neglect, are best directed toward an earlier level of prevention, ideally primary. Social policies in the United States must become intolerable to the nurse until children are given the same rights and opportunities as granted by the Constitution as adults.

It should also be pointed out that all three levels of prevention of child abuse and neglect may be necessary in the nursing interventions with even one family. For example, the professional nurse may become familiar with a family as she intervenes to safely return an abused child to his or her home from foster care (tertiary prevention), while securing supplemental food program benefits for underfed siblings (secondary prevention) and providing health promotion to parents of a healthy newborn (primary prevention). The demands upon the nurse are great and require skillful, creative nursing care.

EVALUATION

The final step of the nursing process is evaluation. It is at this point that the professional nurse reviews what changes have occurred based upon the identified goals. Again, the nurse must be realistic in her evaluation of child abuse and neglect. She can also praise even small evidences of progress. Praise to a parent who is having difficulty in childrearing can be a new experience and a strong reinforcer.

SAMPLE NURSING PROCESS

A sample nursing process in a case of child abuse and neglect has been included in this chapter to demonstrate how each of the four steps can be applied to a hypothetical case. A brief description of the case has been recorded. An in-depth assessment composed of both historical and physical findings would naturally have preceded its development. The total assessment is not completely reported. In addition, each child and family are unique and require individualized plans of care. The sample nursing process (Table 10-4) is included as a starting point for professional nursing practice.

Summary

Nursing care of the abused and neglected child is approached from a family framework and based upon the limited available nursing research. The use of the nursing process in practice with abusive and neglectful families involves four steps—assessment, goals, planning, and evaluation. Assessment for child abuse and neglect can be included in the practice of every nurse who provides care to children and their families. Particular attention should be paid in assessment to certain warning signs that can indicate potential or actual abuse. Although three levels of prevention of child abuse and neglect are discussed, nursing practice should be directed toward primary prevention as no level of maltreatment of children can be acceptable to the nurse whose philosophy is to promote the life, health, and well-being of her clients.

Table 10-4 *Sample Nursing Process*

Brief Background

Kent is a 15-month-old white male who is admitted to the general pediatric unit of the hospital with a medical diagnosis of child abuse and neglect. Kent lives with his 22-year-old mother and 2 siblings. The family's sole source of income is Aid to Dependent Children. Kent's mother describes him as a "difficult" child who willfully disobeys her and refuses to be toilet trained. She reports that he holds his bowel movements "just to make me angry." In addition, Kent's mother reports that he "won't eat" and drinks only Kool-Aid in his bottle. Kent's mother is the primary caretaker who knows no one in the neighborhood and moved to the area to be with Kent's father who has since deserted the family.

The nurse's physical examination of Kent includes, but is not limited to the following:

General Appearance	Thin, 15-month-old white male who appears to watch all activities in the room, but remains quiet and passive through all procedures including subsequent blood drawing.
Vital Statistics	Height and weight below 3rd percentile.
Skin	Multiple discrete, circumscribed 1 cm. in diameter second-degree burns in various stages of resolution about the distal arms and legs. Scant purulent drainage noted at lesions.
	Generalized decreased subcutaneous tissue.
Neurological	Abnormal score on DDST (Failed language and personal/social).

Nursing Care of Abused Children

Table 10-4 (Cont.)

Three of the nursing diagnoses are identified in order of priority:

Family Nursing Diagnosis
I. Potential for subsequent violence (child) related to lack of parent support systems, inadequate financial resources, lack of knowledge (child development), and ineffective parent behavior

Client Goals	Nursing Intervention	Evaluation
I. Family will not experience additional violence as evidenced by: A. Short term (Prior to discharge) 1. No additional child injuries during hospitalization.	I. The nurse will: A.1.a. Provide continuous, but discrete supervision of mother-child interaction 1.b. Provide mother with age-appropriate to child safety precautions- for hospitalization.	As the nursing process is still in the development phase, no evaluation is possible. When appropriate, evaluation should be ongoing and based upon the achievement of identified family goals as evidenced by stated criteria.
2. Demonstration of nurturant behaviors by parent toward child	2.a. Role model nuturant childcare behaviors for mother, especially during bath, play, and feeding b. Encourage mother to actively participate in daily childcare c. Praise mother's attempts at nurturant behaviors expecting closer approximations of goal QD	
3. Mother's voicing of factors contributing to past episodes of violence toward child	3.a. Spend at least 20 minutes QD encouraging mother to talk about herself b. Use therapeutic communication techniques to elicit factors contributing to violence toward child	

(continued)

Table 10-4 (Cont.)

Client Goals	Nursing Intervention	Evaluation
	c. Use therapeutic communication to increase mother's awareness of factors contributing to violence against child	
4. Mother's identification of alternative methods of expressing anger	4.a. Use therapeutic communication and problem-solving techniques to assist mother in identification of nonviolent expressions of anger	
5. Mother's identification of key aspects of child behavior and development during the toddler stage.	5.a. Provide mother with information about child development b. Demonstrate to mother how information about child development can be used in daily life (discipline, play, feeding, toileting)	
6. Mother's agreement to participate with child protective and other agencies	6.a. Provide mother with information about child protective and other agencies b. Contact appropriate agencies and establish client contact prior to discharge c. Reassure mother that all agencies are concerned with child safety and helping her to care for her child	
B. Long term (6 months postdischarge) 1. No additional child injuries.	B.1.a. Referral to public health nursing for continued, intermittent monitoring of child, home, and family	Long-term evaluation will be carried out by the public health nurse following the family and

Nursing Care of Abused Children

Table 10–4 (Cont.)

Client Goals	Nursing Intervention	Evaluation
	b. Public health nurse will have contact with mother and child prior to discharge c. Public health nurse will secure and coordinate child protective and other agency services to family	will be ongoing, and based upon achievement of identified family goals as evidenced by stated criteria.
2. Improved DDST age-appropriate score	2.a. Public health nurse will enroll child in an educational pre-school program b. School will educate, encourage, and support mother in parenting skills c. Public health nurse or school will administer DDST 6 months post-discharge	
3. Demonstration of consistent nurturant parent behaviors	3.a. See I.B.1.a. b. Public health nurse will continue activities described in I.A.2.a. and c	
4. Documented demonstration of mother utilizing nonviolent methods of dealing with anger	4.a. See I.B.1.a. and c.	
5. Demonstration by mother of age-appropriate techniques of child discipline	5.a. See I.B.1.a b. See I.B.4.a c. Public health nurse will praise all attempts by mother to use nonviolent discipline.	
6. Documented active participation with other agencies.	6.a. See I.B.1.a and c	

(continued)

Table 10–4 (Cont.)

Client Goals	Nursing Intervention	Evaluation
7. Documented use (as appropriate) of alternative child-care services	7.a. See I.B.1.a., 2.b b. Public health nurse will provide information to mother regarding daycare centers and emergency child-care services c. Public health nurse will use problem-solving techniques to assist mother in identifying friends and/or relatives who might assist or exchange child-care	
8. Mother's participation in social or other organizations (church, school, etc.) that increase circle of acquaintances.	8.a. Public health nurse will assess mother for areas of social, educational, recreational, religious, or community interest b. Public health nurse will provide information about appropriate organizations in community and arrange for personal contact as desired c. Public health nurse will praise all evidence of mother decreasing her social isolation	

Child Nursing Diagnosis
II. Impairment of skin integrity related to second-degree burns and poor hygiene

Client Goals	Nursing Intervention	Evaluation
II. Client will experience improved skin integrity during hospitalization (2 weeks) as evidenced by: A. Healing of skin lesions	II. The nurse will: A.1. Note size, shape, location, and condition of lesions 2. Exact diagram of lesions	As the nursing process is still in the development phase, no evaluation is possible. When appropriate, evaluation should be ongoing and based upon the achievement of identified family goals as evidenced by stated criteria.

Nursing Care of Abused Children

Table 10–4 (Cont.)

Client Goals	Nursing Intervention	Evaluation
	will be recorded and included in initial nursing assessment	
	3. Skin lesions will be cleaned and gently debrided after 15 minutes of soaking during A.M. bath	
	4. Lesions will then be left open to air	
	5. Progress of lesions will be monitored	
	6. Provide adequate diet (see Nursing Diagnosis # 3)	
B. Decreased signs of infection (redness, tenderness, swelling)	B.1. Monitor vital signs	
	2. Monitor skin lesions for increased redness, tenderness, and swelling)	
	3. Monitor laboratory data, 1. CBC	
	4. Keep client's fingernails clean and short	
	5. Inform mother of all signs of improvement	
C. No new skin lesions	C.1. Monitor client's skin QD	
	2. Provide supervision of mother-child interaction	

Nursing Diagnosis
III. Alteration in nutrition (less than body requirements) related to lack of parent knowledge and inadequate financial resources

Client Goals	Nursing Intervention	Evaluation
III. Client will experience adequate nutrition during hospitalization (2 weeks) as evidenced by:	III. The nurse will:	As the nursing process is still in the development phase, no evaluation is possible. When appropriate, evalua-

(continued)

Table 10–4 (Cont.)

Client Goals	Nursing Intervention	Evaluation

A. No loss in weight, height, or head circumference.	A.1. Provide client with age-appropriate diet QD
	Protein 1.8 (gm/kg)
	Energy 100 (kcal/kg)
	Fat > 30%, < 50%
	Carbohydrate 50–100 gm
	2. Record all food and fluid intake
	3. Provide a varied selection of food (color, taste, texture)
	4. Prepare food so that it is mild and of comfortable temperature
	5. Provide 3 nutritious finger food snacks (10:00 A.M., 3:00 P.M., 7:30 P.M.)
	6. Provide a pleasant, quiet environment for eating
	7. Encourage mother's involvement in feeding
	  a. Serve as role model to mother
	  b. Provide information to mother
	  c. Praise mother's efforts to assist in attainment of goal and identify strengths
	8. Weigh QD
		tion should be ongoing and based upon the achievement of identified family goals as evidenced by stated criteria.

B. Good skin turgor and moist mucous membranes	B.1. Provide client with adequate fluid intake QD 120–125 ml/kg 2. Record all fluid intake 3. Offer 4 oz. of fluid (vary type) every waking hour 4. Encourage drinking from cup a. Assist as necessary	

Table 10–4 (Cont.)

Client Goals	Nursing Intervention	Evaluation
	b. Praise mother and child for efforts	
	5. Measure urine-specific gravity each shift	
C. Laboratory findings that show no worsening of physical condition	C.1. Monitor laboratory tests and alter diet as necessary	
D. Mother's identification of key aspects of child behavior and development during the toddler stage and appropriate available resources	D.1. Inform mother regarding available supplemental food programs 2. Recommend parent-child educational daycare center to mother 3. Contact social service agency to arrange for enrollment prior to discharge	

Chapter 10

1. Kathleen Scharer, "Nursing Therapy with Abusive and Neglectful Families," *Journal of Psychiatric Nursing and Mental Health Services* 17, no. 8 (September 1979): 15.

2. Kathleen Scharer, "Rescue Fantasies: Professional Impediments in Working with Abused Families," *American Journal of Nursing* 78, no. 9 (September 1978): 1483.

3. Eli H. Newberger and Richard Bourne, "The Medicalization and Legalization of Child Abuse," *American Journal of Orthopsychiatry* 48, no. 4 (October 1978): 596.

4. Ibid, p. 595.

5. E. H. Schein, *Professional Education: Some New Directions* (New York: McGraw-Hill, 1972), p. 3.

6. Norris L. Davis and Glenda H. Johnson, "A Way of Caring: Nurses Initiate Community Action to Prevent Child Abuse," *AORN Journal* 27, no. 4 (March 1978): 631–35.

7. Marshall H. Klaus and John H. Kennell, "Maternal-Infant Bonding," in *Maternal-Infant Bonding*, ed. Marshall H. Klaus and John H. Kennell (Saint Louis, Mo.: C. V. Mosby Co., 1976), p. 14.

8. Marshall H. Klaus and John H. Kennell, "Human Maternal and Paternal Behavior," in Klaus and Kennell, *Maternal-Infant Bonding*, pp. 88–89, 94–95.

9. Susan O'Connor et al., "Reduced Incidence of Parenting Inadequacy Following Rooming-in," *Pediatrics* 66 (August 1980), pp. 176–82.

10. John H. Kennell and Marshall H. Klaus, "Caring for Parents of a Premature or Sick Infant," p. 160; and Nancy A. Irvin, John H. Kennell, and Marshall H. Klaus, "Caring for Parents of an Infant with a Congenital Malformation," p. 169 both in Klaus and Kennell, *Maternal-Infant Bonding*.

11. Leo Stern, "Prematurity as a Factor in Child Abuse," *Hospital Practice* 8, no. 5 (May 1973): 119.

12. David P. Weikart, "Research Report" (Ypsilanti, Mich.: High/Scope Educational Research Foundation, 1980).

13. Gil, "Violence Against Children," *Journal of Marriage and the Family* (November 1971): 646-48.

14. Ibid., p. 646.

15. Ibid., p. 647.

16. Ibid.

17. J. Michael Cupoli and Eli H. Newberger, "Optimism or Pessimism for the Victim of Child Abuse?" *Pediatrics* 59, no. 2 (February 1977): 312.

18. Eli H. Newberger, "A Physician's Perspective on the Interdisciplinary Management of Child Abuse," *Psychiatric Opinion*, no. 2 (April 1976): 13-18.

19. Blair Justice and Rita Justice, *The Abusing Family* (New York: Human Sciences Press, 1976), p. 48.

20. Bernard Horowitz and Wendy Wintermute, "Use of an Emergency Fund in Protective Services Casework," *Child Welfare* 57, no. 7 (July/August 1978): 432-37.

21. Leroy H. Pelton, "Child Abuse and Neglect: The Myth of Classlessness," *American Journal of Orthopsychiatry* 48 (October 1978), pp. 608-17.

22. Bryan D. Carter, Ruth Reed, and Ceil J. Reh, "Mental Health Nursing Intervention with Child Abusing and Neglectful Mothers," *Journal of Psychiatric Nursing and Mental Health Services* 13, no. 5 (September/October 1975): 13.

23. Ibid., p. 12.

24. Ibid.

25. Scharer, "Nursing Therapy with Abusive and Neglectful Families," pp. 12-21.

26. Ibid., pp. 15-19.

27. Juvenile Justice Standards Project, *Standards Relating to Abuse and Neglect* (Cambridge: Harper & Row, Ballinger Publishing Co., 1977).

28. Ibid.

29. *National Analysis of Official Child Abuse and Neglect Reporting: 1977.* p. 31.

30. Ibid.

31. William N. Friedrich, "Evaluation of a Media Campaign's Effect on Reporting Patterns of Child Abuse," *Perceptual and Motor Skills* 45 (1977): 161-62.

32. Ibid.,

33. Andre P. Derdeyn, "A Case for Permanent Foster Placement of Dependent, Neglected, and Abused Children," *American Journal of Orthopsychiatry* 47, no. 4 (October 1977): 605.

34. S. Jenkins and M. Norman, *Beyond Placement: Mothers View Foster Care* (New York: Columbia University Press, 1975).

35. Derdeyn, "Case for Permanent Foster Placement," pp. 605-607.

36. Ibid., pp. 607-610.

37. Malcolm Bush, "Institutions for Dependent and Neglected Children: Therapeutic Option of Choice or Last Resort?" *American Journal of Orthopsychiatry* 50 (April 1980): 239-55.

38. Ibid., p. 244.

39. Ibid., p. 249.

40. Ibid., p. 251.

Nursing Care of Children of Violent Families

Bonnie Westra

"Shelter"

big old house
creaks and moans
til mothers come
and children's sounds
fill its empty rooms
little familys
with shattered dreams
and broken hearts
run from daddy's fist
to this
a shelter home
refuge from
sweet love
gone amiss

Susan Venters

Reprinted from *Every Twelve Seconds*, compiled by Susan Venters (Hillsboro, Oregon: Shelter, 1981) by permission of the author.

Physical abuse against children has been the focus of helping professionals for the past twenty years. More recently, abuse of women has become a concern to society. Children from violent families, who may not themselves be the actual victims of physical abuse, exhibit problems that should also be of concern to nurses. Children from violent families are at high risk for many problems because they must cope with and adapt to an environment that is disorganized. Some children adapt with minimal problems, while others suffer. Child abuse literature, including sexual abuse, has identified problems those children experience. Yet few problems have been documented systematically about children from families where women are abused, or siblings of abused children. Studies regarding families experiencing marital discord, separation, and divorce indicate children from these families to be at high risk for emotional, social, and physical problems. The purpose of this chapter is to describe the application of the nursing process to children of violent families.

INCIDENCE

One can only surmise the number of children from violent homes. Incidence statistics for both child and wife abuse vary widely and are potentially misleading. (see Chapters 4 and 5.) Estimates of abuse against children have ranged from 6,000[1] to over 1.17 million cases per year.[2] Abuse against women, based on a nationally representative sample of American families, was estimated at 1.8 million cases per year.[3] Based on the assumption of two children per family, the number of children from violent homes would range from 3.8 to 6.6 million per year. This is a conservative estimate of children in violent homes.

SOCIAL LEARNING THEORY

As described in Chapter 2, social learning theory can be useful as a background for providing care for children of violent families. It provides a framework for assessment of potential problems and intervention techniques for children from violent homes.

Children acquire attitudes, values, and behaviors through two kinds of learning: direct tuition and active imitation. Direct tuition is the intentional teaching of behaviors through using rewarding and punishing consequences. More complex patterns are learned through observation and active imitation of attitudes and behaviors. Through observation, children not only acquire behaviors, but also the emotional responses of the models and even the appropriate settings for emitting emotional and behavioral responses.

Through awareness, children learn to perceive the model's behavior and anticipate consequences. By memory of performance and its consequences, children can repeat behaviors even when the model is not present. However, motor responses must be developed to perform behaviors. A child must reach a point of maturity where he or she has the capability to perform an activity before the behavior, which may have been learned earlier, will be demonstrated. Motivation for performance is based on the consequences of behavior.

Learning may occur without immediate performance, if motivation to learn is sufficient. Immediate reinforcement for behavior motivates performance. Motivation to imitate a model is strengthened if the model is nurturing, receives positive reinforcement for a behavior, is similar to the observer, and/or has prestige or control over resources.[4]

Children copy other's behavior, in particular, those with whom they have the closest relationships. Children learn to imitate methods of coping with stress, particularly that of their parents. It is not uncommon to see children from violent families deal with their anxieties by becoming aggressive. Other reactions include withdrawal, such as that seen by the child abuse victim or woman who has been abused. Because violent families often isolate themselves from neighbors and community agencies, parents are the primary adult role models, even more so than in the nonviolent family. How parents treat each other models for the child how to interact with others. Parents demonstrate their own feelings of worth and acceptance. Studies of wife abuse and child abuse describe parents in these families as having a low self-concept. Parents teach children ways of behaving, both by what they do and what they say.

In violent families, inadequate stimulation may occur due to the disorganization and resulting consequences for all involved. Stimulation and a range of experiences are important for optimal intellectual development. Involvement and reinforcement from parents is necessary for development in children. Yet this may not occur when there is violence in the family.

CHILDREN OF BATTERED WOMEN

A study was conducted to assess development of children from homes where women were abused.[5] Based on theoretical indications and clinical experience, it was hypothesized that children in families where abuse against adult women occurred would have similar developmental problems to child abuse victims due to the impact of the violence in their home environment. There were indications that children from homes where the mother had been abused were at risk for being more aggressive; having poorer cognitive abilities; having poorer verbal abilities; and having poorer motor abilities than children whose families did not experience violence.

To test this hypothesis, a group of twenty children from wife abuse shelters, averaging five years of age, were tested on the McCarthy Scale, a Preschool Behavior Questionnaire. The tests encompassed physical measurements, a neurologic examination, an interview of the mother to gather health data, and a questionnaire developed by the researcher to measure the degree of violence experienced by the mother and nurturance of the child. Verbal, motor, and quantitative scale scores were all significantly lower when compared with scores of children from nonviolent homes. Children in the shelter with the abused mother demonstrated a lower cognitive ability and more aggressive behavior. However, heights, weights, head circumferences, and neurologic examinations were all normal, and both median and mean incomes of families were well above poverty levels. Children from wife abuse homes therefore displayed similar developmental delays to abused children in this study.

IDENTIFICATION OF CHILDREN OF VIOLENT FAMILIES

Nurses are in a position of identifying and intervening with children from violent families. They work in multiple settings where they have contact with childrearing families: emergency room and ambulatory care settings, pediatric units in hospitals, psychiatric and chemical dependency units, as well as schools and community settings. Nurses also work in less traditional settings, such as shelters for battered women, churches, and children's groups like the Brownies. The multitude of settings provide wide access to children who may be from violent families.

Further, nursing education, including extensive developmental theory and health promotion concepts, provides excellent preparation for working with children from violent homes. The process of interviewing, observing each child's behaviors, and comparing them with norms, are essential skills. With a bio-psycho-social background, nurses can assess and intervene on varying parameters. The skills nurses possess make them ideal to work with children from violent homes.

HIGH-RISK CHARACTERISTICS

Nurses rarely have children present or be referred with a diagnosis of "child from violent family." Violence in the family is seldom talked about, even when a good relationship has been established. The nurse must be sensitive to selective clues within the family that are high-risk characteristics. These may be problems regarding the children, the parents, or the interaction between the two. When high-risk characteristics are present, a more in-depth assessment for family violence becomes necessary.

Chapters 8, 9, and 10 have described the indications of risk for child abuse and wife abuse. Families exhibiting these characteristics need careful assessment for violence. In addition, whenever specific developmental delays are the reason a child is referred, an assessment of why these delays exist should include family stress, family ability and manner of coping with stress, and in particular, indications of violence.

Individual children from violent families may display the effects of the violence in a variety of ways. Ann Haas states, "The way in which the child learns to adapt or cope with the family violence is unique." They frequently have poor social adjustment, a low self-esteem, and difficulty with learning. Children have a tremendous amount of guilt, feeling that somehow they are responsible for the discord in their family. The only consistent factor in these situations is that these children have a high risk of problems.[6]

The author's own clinical experience with children who live with violence in their lives has revealed some additional behavior patterns. The children may become withdrawn. Change is difficult. Some act afraid. They may be afraid of adults, generalizing the violence seen at home to other adults. They are afraid of the victim at home, as well as the offender, feeling that the victim may turn against them. They may even be afraid of other children.

Role reversal between parent and child has been noted in child abuse families. Observations in shelters for battered women support this phenomena also occurring when the woman has been abused. Adults in violent families often have unmet needs. Their ability to meet the needs of children, at times, may be limited. As a means of gaining acceptance and love, children may take on the role of caring for the adult or parenting younger children. For instance, one seven-year-old, when asked where her mother was when the baby was crying, stated, "She's had a busy day and is resting. I'll take care of the baby." When children take on the "caretaker role" then time and energy is preempted from getting their own needs met through the usual activities for their stage of development.

Aggression in children from violent famlies is not uncommon. It has been observed in shelters for battered women that children may use hitting and kicking to get the mother's attention. Children have learned that violence is one way to get their way when playing with other children. Some children turn the violence on themselves. Others may just display very active behavior, throwing things or destroying property for no obvious reason.

Physical symptoms, either real or imagined, are not uncommon. Some children develop nervous habits such as nail biting, or hair pulling. Regressive behavior, such as bed-wetting has been frequently reported by wife abuse shelter staff. A child may turn from being a relatively tidy child to developing sloppy habits, either in eating or dress.

Children assume different adaptive behaviors. Some try to appease the offender and in some cases offer themselves as the victim. Others may try to protect the victim or to "make it up" to the victim. Often the story is heard in a shelter from an abused woman that she could live with the abuse, but when her child tried to intervene in the violence, she felt the need to leave. Some children try to remove themselves from the situation by either going to their room, going outside, or running away. Violence at home is a common precipitator for runaway adolescents.[7]

It is important to not only identify characteristics of children from violent families, but also characteristics of the families. Many times the nurse may be seeing a family for various reasons and observe characteristics of families that may be experiencing violence. (See Tables 8-1, 9-1, and 10-2.) Through identification of these families, the nurse, then, can focus on the children to see if they are having difficulty, or she can attempt to prevent potential problems.

To further delineate possible pertinent influences on children of violent families, a framework of selected characteristics of child abusing parents and battered women and their spouses has been used. These characteristics are presented in Tables 11-1 and 11-2.

The adults partially described in Tables 11-1 and 11-2 are the major role models

Table 11-1 Selected Characteristics of Abusive Parents (Martin)[1]

Immature and dependent. The dependence may be on the child, on a treatment setting, or on the therapist
Social isolation
Poor self-esteem
Difficulty seeking or obtaining pleasure
Distorted perceptions of the child
Fear of spoiling the child
Belief in the value of punishment
Impaired ability to empathize with the child's needs and to respond appropriately

[1] From Harold Martin, ed., *A Multidisciplinary Approach to Developmental Issues and Treatment* (Cambridge, Mass.: Ballinger, 1976), pp. 13–14.

for children of violent families. The modeling of behavior and interaction with these adults strongly influences the learning that takes place in the children and may result in problems for them. Based on the characteristics of role models in child abuse and wife abuse families, the following interactions in violent families between significant adults and children can be anticipated in many cases.

1. Limited interaction between parents and children. If parents who abuse a child have a high degree of unmet needs, their ability to fulfill the needs of children is limited. Women who are abused often view their role as the primary caretaker of the children, yet they frequently display a high degree of physical complaints as well as helplessness, limiting their energy to interact with the children. Their spouses tend to have traditional values, not taking responsibility for childrearing.

2. Inadequate role modeling of appropriate behaviors to facilitate development in children. Since violence is being used as a means of dealing with stress, children may be learning ways to avoid stress (e.g., withdrawal) which may in turn prevent them from performing behaviors necessary for healthy development. Children are also learning that violence is a way of obtaining things,

Table 11-2 Selected Characteristics of the Battered Woman and the Batterer (Westra)[2]

Battered Woman	Batterer
Low self-esteem	Low self-esteem
Traditional values (i.e., responsibility for chilren and home, submissive toward male partner, etc.)	Traditional values (i.e., breadwinner in family, decision maker for family)
Guilt	Blames other for his actions
Severe stress reactions and psychophysical complaints	Pathologically jealous
Helplessness (including symptoms associated with depression)	Dual personality (i.e., violent or hostile at home but pleasant in front of outsiders)
	Severe stress reactions
	Uses sex as act of aggression

[2] From Bonita Westra, "Battered Women and Child Development" (Master's thesis, University of Colorado, 1979), p. 11.

and controlling the environment. Violence precludes a nurturing environment, at least some of the time.

3. Role reversal between parent and children. Adults in violent situations have many unmet needs. Children may be viewed as someone to take care of them. Children may stay home from school to care for a sick parent, avoid playing with peers to perform household tasks the parent is unable to perform, or take over parenting younger children. "Covering up" for parents who are unable to perform their usual tasks is not unusual.

In describing behaviors of children, of parents, and interactions that may exist in violent homes, it is important to realize that not all situations are alike. Not all children have obvious problems. Violence does not exist all the time. There may very well be many positive factors occurring in the lives of children from violent homes. Some battered women have stated that they stayed in an abusive situation because their spouse was a good father. Children also are exposed to other role models and interactions than those with the parents. Because they are exposed to violent models and a potentially nonnurturing environment, these children can be considered at risk for problems, but cannot be assumed to have them. It is the process of assessment that would determine the need for intervention, if any, and what type would be the most appropriate.

ASSESSMENT TECHNIQUES

Nursing care of children of violent families requires an understanding of family dynamics. Assessing this provides information about the child's ability to get along with others as well as who are the important persons in the child's life. The extent and nature of contact with extended family members should be assessed, and also other relationships should be noted. It is important to determine if the child attends a daycare center, school, and so forth. When a child has problems getting along with others, it is helpful to know if this exists only at home, in relation to authority figures, or just with peers. Careful attention to family and interaction dynamics while conducting the history and physical exam will ensure a more complete assessment.

History

The history serves an important interpersonal function as well as a means of gathering data. During the interview, a relationship is established between parent(s), child, and nurse. Those relationships affect the accuracy of information gathered and therefore the outcome of intervention. It must be a sensitive interchange, a process of interplay of people, their thoughts and feelings.

The process of interviewing children generally includes an adult, most often the mother. Most information is gathered from the parent; however, it is important to include the child in the interview, asking the child questions. Observations of the child during the interview provide a rich source of data; that is, does the child sit quietly, look around inquisitively, or run around uncontrolled? It must be remembered in addressing the child, to take into consideration his or her developmental stage.

The developmental stage determines the types of questions children are able to answer, as well as the phrasing of questions.

To begin the interview, an initial greeting and introduction to the child and parent are extremely important. The nurse should see that all persons are introduced and the family member's relationship stated. An explanation of the nurse's role should be given. This helps the family know what to expect.

Interviews involving children require special considerations. Talking on eye level with the child will decrease the sense of "that big person," and establish rapport faster. Nurses will have a much better communication and will encourage more productive exchanges of information if they take time initially to make the parent and child comfortable. Small talk provides time for all to get a feel for each other. One way of doing this is asking children about favorite TV characters, their best friends, or pets. Children from violent families may not be responsive initially to the nurse, displaying withdrawal, or they may be difficult to contain. Flexibility in conversing with the child is important.

An agenda for the visit should also be explained before proceeding. It is helpful to give the parent and child an opportunity to ask any questions they may have before proceeding with the interview. Once the opportunity to state their concerns takes place, they may feel more at ease and open while the rest of the assessment process is accomplished. It is important to answer any questions the child has promptly and directly, to alleviate any fears she or he may have. If questions are complex or emotionally laden, it may be best to explain that these will be answered after more information is known, while assuring the parent the issue is not being avoided and their concern is respected.

At times, competition between parents and child for attention from the nurse may occur. Unless the nurse is sensitive to this occurring, the interview may suddenly deteriorate. Two methods of coping with this problem can be helpful. First, reemphasize to the parents that information will be requested from the parent and some from the child. Second, provide the child with an activity, such as drawing, while attention is focused on the parent. At a later point, spend a moment commenting on the drawing. These actions reclarify how the interview will progress and provides the child with a distraction that is fun and interesting.

The purpose of information gathered must be explained. In hospital situations, the purpose may seem more clear, but in situations in which the role of the nurse may be less understood, concern may exist about why the nurse is asking certain questions. It is important to explain this, and stress to the parent that information given is confidential. The exception is if the child is potentially in danger of being harmed, in which case suspected abuse must be reported and appropriate action taken to protect the child.

The personalities of all involved will affect the outcome of the interview. For example, adolescent parents have needs unique to their stage of development. Often adolescents have not completed their task of deciding who and what they want to be. Superimposed on this task is that of parenting plus a disorganized, violent home. The total effect of these is often withdrawn or aggressive behavior. The nurse needs to become aware of the parent's feelings and relate them to the behaviors and reasons for the behaviors. It may take a considerable time to establish trust in the interview process. Avoiding a judgmental attitude, or one that appears as if the nurse is parenting the adolescent, is important. Encouraging talk about positive parenting skills or personal accomplishments and showing support for these whenever possible helps the adolescent to feel competent. Nurses need to be aware of their own personality characteristics to direct their behavior in interaction with those they are interviewing.

Factors affecting the nature of the interview include length of time for interview, number and variety of issues to be discussed, attitude and feelings of parent and child. Flexibility and sensitivity of the interviewer are the key to a successful interview. The interviewer must be able to change the structure of the interview to meet the needs of the parent and child.

The goal of a successful interview is to obtain complete information efficiently, while maintaining flexibility. Therapeutic techniques of interviewing are used, including open-ended questions as much as possible. Structuring the questions so that they do not hint at the right answer provides unbiased information. Thus, "tell me about John's behavior" is preferable to asking "does John act aggressively?" It should be mentioned early in the interview that some questions may be difficult to answer and if that happens, the nurse should be asked to explain more clearly what she means.

Interviewing children to obtain a health history provides limited information until the child is above elementary school age. Children may be able to recall if they have seriously hurt themselves, been really sick, or ever gone to the hospital or emergency room. Specific information such as diseases, extent of injury, immunization status, allergies, and so forth, are difficult for them to recall. Family history, other than recent events in the immediate family, is also difficult to obtain from children. At the same time, the child's perceptions of events are important; therefore, both parent and child should be interviewed, either together or separately.

The child's personality influences the way in which he or she reacts to the environment. Many children from violent homes may show signs of developmental or emotional problems. However, it has been shown that not all children develop problems. Children with particular temperaments are at higher risk for difficulties.

Children differ in their temperamental attributes from the time of birth. Infants have been shown to vary in energy output or level of activity; regularity of their biological cycles; adaptability; and intensity of emotional responses.[8] These temperamental attributes later in life have been associated with ability to cope and adjust to life or tendency to develop emotional or behavioral problems. Studies have supported that children characterized as difficult to care for and nonadaptive have had a higher incidence of behavioral difficulties than those who are easily adaptive.[9] Thus, the history needs to include questions about early behavioral characteristics to indicate children particularly at risk in violent families.

The specific format used for the nursing history of a child will be determined by the practitioner's education and clinical setting. An indication of other areas particularly important to include for children from violent families is available in Table 10-2.

Physical Assessment

The physical exam is an integral part of the assessment of children of violent families (see Chapter 8). Another extremely important part of the physical assessment is a development assessment. Children from violent families are at risk for developmental problems, necessitating a detailed developmental assessment. Formalized developmental screening instruments, such as the Denver Prescreening Developmental Questionnaire, the Denver Developmental Screening Test, the Dial, or the Vineland Maturity Scale provide specific information on developmental progress.

Interpretation of developmental assessments requires more skill than actually doing the assessment process. It is not easy to interpret information obtained from a one-time setting to be a complete picture of the child's performance. Indeed, that is exactly what the assessment signifies, how the child is doing that day. To have a more accurate picture of the child's overall performance, an ongoing assessment is needed. Other observations, such as the child in different settings, interactions with other people, and so forth, help provide a more comprehensive picture.

The number of times a child will be seen influences the style in which an assessment can be done. In the case of an ongoing relationship with the child and his or her family, brief updates of the developmental history and appropriate observations of the child will suffice to add to the original thorough developmental assessment. However, periodically, a more formal evaluation should be undertaken, or less obvious problems may be overlooked.

The relationship of the nurse and family also influences the type of information that can be obtained, as well as the manner in which it is obtained. Some parents may have difficulty in communicating, either because of their own limited communication skills or their unwillingness to share information. This is especially true when the family and nurse have not known each other very long. Violent families tend to be isolated and not very trusting of community agencies. The nurse may, therefore, pose a threat to these families. Thus, it is important for the nurse to use observations of developmental activities and screening instruments as well as the information obtained from the history to assess development.

Social learning theory states that learning is a product of personality interacting with the environment. The developmental assessment measures the environment or interaction with the environment, not what is possible for the child to accomplish. Measuring achievements by developmental screening provides an indicator of problems or delays in development. Developmental screening tests do not indicate why, but rather what exists.

Other tests used in the usual assessment process are screening tests for behavioral and psychological problems, such as the Behar Preschool Screening Test, which measures disturbed behavior. Screening tests indicate a need for further information and should not be interpreted as absolute data. They serve a useful purpose only if they are used in conjunction with other sources of data.

Self-concept is a particularly important area in assessment of children of violent families. Ways of measuring self-concept include observing the child, having the child draw human figures, talking with parents or teachers, or having the child complete a written test. One method of observation is using play, which is discussed later. Use of figure drawings of self and family provide information on how children perceive themselves and their relationship in their families. A type of written test is the Coopersmith Self-Esteem Inventory, which can be used with children ages nine through adolescence.[10] There are fifty-eight items on a self-report scale. The scale not only measures total self-esteem, but also includes measures about home/family, peer/social, and academic achievement.

Assessment Through Play

Play is the work of children. Through play, children develop skills, learn appropriate interaction, and develop a positive self-concept. Much can be learned regarding a child's development by asking about and observing a child's play. Play is influenced by the toys and opportunities available to the child. Parents should be asked about the use of toys, that is, does a child understand what to do with them; the patterns of play, that is, does the child repeatedly play the same way or try new ideas; approach to play, such as curious and exploratory; and age-appropriate play, that is, plays side by side or collaboratively with other children.

Play changes depending on the developmental stage of the child. During infancy, play is centered on pleasurable sensation. It consists of repetitive exploration using the body, primarily sucking. Toddlers and the preschool child use dramatic or perceptive play, which is a reenactment of everyday life situations. Dramatic play continues into school age, when imitation of significant adults and interpersonal relationships occur. Playing house or school are typical examples of this type of play. Preadolescents and adolescents employ games with rules. A competitive nature exists in adolescents; sports provide a means of dealing with this as well as developing coordination. Using the mode of play suitable to the stage of the child enhances the nurses understanding of the child.

Speech Delays

How children play reflects their understanding, which is especially important in assessing speech delays. Children should be given toys, such as combs, telephones, or trucks to see if they use the toys in the appropriate manner. Assessing a child's ability to imitate reality can demonstrate whether speech delays are expressive (talking) or receptive (understanding), therefore determining the type of intervention needed.

Feelings

Play is also a good source of information about children's feelings, thoughts, and social relationships. Using toys such as dolls, puppets, clay, or paints allow children to express feelings and concerns. Children use fantasy play to enact their concerns. It is important for the nurse to realize that the content of play should not be taken literally, but rather the feelings expressed should be noted.

One method of assessing children's feelings is through the use of puppets. Children enjoy making up stories and using puppets to enact them. Initially, the nurse may have to demonstrate how to use the puppets by acting out a story. Gradually, the child, with encouragement, will join in or do a show by him or herself. Some children are shy and will require considerable prompting. A theme about an animal or friend could be suggested. It would be advisable not to start off with an emotionally laden topic, such as the family, unless the child demonstrates readiness to do a show about something from his or her family. The nurse observes the general theme and feelings elicited and at times asks questions about how the puppet is feeling. This not only provides an assessment, but also initiates a therapeutic process as the child begins to become aware of feelings.

Social Development

Social development can be ascertained by the degree to which children interact with others in a cooperative manner. Therefore, observing children playing in a group situation is useful. One method of doing this is described in the following example:

> While living at a shelter for battered women, children were taken to the playground. They could use any of the equipment if they did so safely. It was observed that eleven-year-old Sandra constantly cared for her four-year-old sister, Suzie. Suzie was demanding attention, wanting Sandra to push her on the swing, catch her on the slide, and so forth. If Sandra tired of this and wanted to climb on the monkey bars, Suzie would fall, pretending to hurt herself. Sandra would spend the next ten minutes trying to comfort her. On the way back from the playground, Suzie demanded Sandra carry her. When the nurse attempted to intervene, stating she would carry Suzie, or walk with her, Sandra insisted on carrying Suzie. Suzie did not interact with any of the other children her age, even when they asked her to join in with them.

This brief observation serves as the basis to begin gathering data about a potential problem area. One concern is that Sandra strongly plays the mother role. One might question if this is her usual role in the family. Is she doing this to the point where she is not meeting her own needs of developing peer relationships? At age four, Suzie should begin playing with other children. She demonstrated a high degree of dependence. It would be important to know if this also occurred in other settings. Observations of children at play provide the opportunity to assess children's social development, which is incorporated with other information.

Self Concept

Observing children in a group, working on a cooperative project, provides observations for the nurse to assess the child's self-concept. The feelings of competence, adequacy, and worth compared with cultural norms provide the basis for the self-evaluation in forming the self-concept. Children compare themselves with their peers, and receive feedback about their acceptability in the group. The following is one method of using the peer group to measure self-concept.

The nurse can form a group of children from the same developmental level to work on a project, such as putting on a play. The children should determine the content of the play. If they are not able to, the nurse can provide a theme for them or remind them of a story with which they are familiar. If possible, a box of various clothes and props for them to use should be available. A set time to practice before giving the play to the nurse should be established. During the time they practice, the nurse can make notes about their behavior, or the behavior of the specific child with whom the nurse is working.

The types of observations that are helpful include the role the child assumes, that is, leader, follower, noninvolvement with the group; the child's ability to carry out the designated role in the play; the child's feedback from peers as well as type of feedback given to peers; and, the child's feelings of accomplishment from completing the performance.

In working with children through play or any other mode, it is important to work with them where they are and not push them into trying to relate to the nurse's concerns. It takes time for children to trust the nurse (this may not happen at all). Some children have a very strong denial system which has survival purposes for them. They may choose to deny any problems or unhappiness, and this is their right. The nurse's role may be one of providing distraction for a short time, which in itself can be enjoyable and therapeutic for the child. At the same time, the nurse is demonstrating a positive image of an adult figure.

Behavioral Observations

Observation of behaviors provides another means of assessing children from violent homes, who display behaviors that are of concern to parents, teachers, or childcare workers in shelters for abused women. Regardless of the setting in which the problems are identified, a systematic assessment should be done. Behavior problems need to be clearly described, such as, "Suzie demands that Sandra take care of her constantly." Next, the nurse needs to know when the behavior occurs. Does this only happen when Sandra is alone with Suzie, or does it occur all the time? Is there any time that Sandra is around Suzie that Suzie is able to do things for herself? Does Suzie do things for herself when Sandra is not around? What reinforcers continue the behavior? For instance, does the mother demand that Sandra keep Suzie content? Does Mom baby Suzie every time she whines? Is Suzie's behavior a problem? If the nurse is the only one perceiving Suzie's behavior as a problem, any attempt at intervening will fail. Questions such as these will identify antecedent events, problem behaviors, and reinforcers of behavior.

Nursing Diagnosis

During the assessment process, much information about the child, environment, and interactions within that environment has been gained. Many potential problems could be identified, based on the assessment information. It is also important to identify behaviors that are positive as well as ones that are problems. Using the assessment data, groupings of information should be made that support possible explanations for the identified problems. For instance, if the child has a delay in speech, what are the possible causes? Is it an articulation problem? How much reinforcement does the child receive to talk? Does the child understand what is being asked? Is the child attentive during the assessment process? Does the child have a hearing problem? The assessment data should provide clues for the observed behavioral problem. This information can then be added to the nursing diagnosis in the related section. Intervention strategies can thus be aimed at the reasons for the behavior.

PLANNING

The first part of planning is of course the formation of goals with the parents and child. The behaviors being dealt with are often complicated, and therefore, it is important that small-step, short-term goals be formulated so that they can be reinforced until the long-term, eventual goal is reached.

Although the focus of this chapter is specifically on nursing care of children from violent homes, it is imperative that plans be developed to concurrently work with the family. Unless factors in the family are changed that precipitate and continually reinforce difficulties these children are experiencing, little will be gained.

It is also useful to identify support persons other than the parents in developing the plan. In complicated behaviors, or ones that are difficult to extinguish, positive reinforcement from all support persons enhances the likelihood that the behavior will change. Part of the planning process will be to inform these people and enlist their help in identifying useful, reinforcing interventions in their area of interaction with the child.

NURSING INTERVENTION

Intervention strategies employed in working with children from violent families focus on modeling behavior, reinforcing desired behaviors, or extinguishing negative ones. These can focus on either the child, parent, or interaction between the two. There is not a single type of intervention that is *the* correct one. If one approach does not work, then another must be tried, or several in conjunction. Often working with children requires this combination of approaches. The main focus of interventions to be discussed in this chapter is the nurse working individually with the child using self as the model of behavior or reinforcing behavior in the child. This does not decrease the need to work with the parents. Children are dependent on their families, and changing the home environment would provide a broader and more lasting behavior change. These approaches have been addressed in Chapter 8. There are several different classifications of individual interventions which will be described: developmental stimulation, play-oriented therapies, group therapy, and behavior modification.

Developmental Stimulation

Developmental stimulation is the process of providing experiences and reinforcing activities for children to help them achieve their optimal potential. It requires the provision of necessary toys or equipment and interaction with the child to reinforce desired behaviors. Children from families with a history of abuse showed delays in speech and gross motor skills as well as overall intellectual development.

Stimulation of Speech

After careful assessment and subsequent identification of speech delays and determination of possible cause, a stimulation program should be planned. For instance, suppose a three-year-old has a delay in speech which is due to lack of understanding. The nurse might plan to see the child for thirty minutes one to three times a week for six to eight weeks, before reevaluating the child. During each session, everyday objects or toys representing them could be used. The nurse would show the child how to use the object, talking about its use. Then the child should be encouraged to use the object. The nurse should reinforce the appropriate use of the object. Other activities would include using simple storybooks with pictures. The nurse would read the story to the child, pointing out in the picture what is being read. The nurse then should ask the child to point out objects in the picture. Simple questions to be asked of the child might be, "Is the ball round?" to begin to introduce abstract concepts as the child progresses. Through constant interaction with the child and reinforcement for behaviors, the nurse can improve developmental lags.

Stimulation of Other Developmental Tasks

There are many types of activities that provide stimulation for children. Activities should be selected based on the child's stage of development. Table 11-3 provides an example of such activities. In working with children, the nurse will also want to consider involving parents or others who have frequent contact with the child. In this manner, the nurse is also changing the modeling of behaviors the child is observing in the parents and providing a positive model of how to interact with the child.

Play-Oriented Therapies

Therapeutic play is the opportunity provided to children to express their feelings in a semistructured play experience. It can range from structured activities like drawing or use of dolls to observation of children at play. In considering the use of play therapy, the nurse should be cognizant of the usual style of play appropriate for the child's developmental stage. Charles Schaefer's book *The Therapeutic Use of Child's Play* discusses types of play, including styles, theory and techniques.[11]

Table 11-3 *Developmental Stimulation*

Age	Activities
0–4 months	Mobile on crib
	Talking to and touching baby
4–8 months	Squeeze toys
	Hard toys to chew on
	Patty-cake and peek-a-boo
8–12 months	Pull toys
	Music and dancing
	Put objects in container and pour out
1–2 years	Push toys
	Walking and climbing with help
	Toys to manipulate: cubes, cup, lids
2–3 years	Reading out loud
	Excursions: zoo, walks
	Clay play
3–4 years	Pasting and painting
	Swinging and climbing
	Simple puzzles
	Blocks
4–6 years	Chores in house
	Cooking and water play
	Coloring, painting, and pasting
	Doll or puppets music and games to synchronize hand and foot

Source: Adapted from Stanley Coopersmith, *Washington Guide to Promoting Development in the Young Child* (Seattle: University of Washington School of Nursing).

Play therapy can be conducted either individually with the child or in a group. It can be used both as an assessment process and as therapy. It provides a view of the child's world. Three suggestions for consideration before beginning are: use appropriate techniques to gather intended data, review family data to focus on specific concerns, and keep in mind questions that guide the interaction with the child.

The nurse can use the same form of play for both assessment and intervention. The previously mentioned group of children putting on a play is one example. During the rehearsal, the nurse might be required to intervene by setting limits on aggressive behavior or destruction of property. If a child dominates the group to the point where it might become nonfunctional, the nurse might suggest an alternative to the conflict. If a child refuses to participate and is dominating the group's attention through this means, the nurse might suggest that the group go on without that person, ignoring the behavior. For the most part, the nurse should play the role of the observer and intervene only when necessary. The effect of these interventions, if necessary, provides the nurse the opportunity to role model appropriate ways of handling conflict and extinguishing unacceptable behaviors.

Another method of using play therapeutically involves the use of a play kit with a variety of toys to choose from, that is, dolls, cars, dishes, and other objects to imitate reality. The nurse should introduce the experience to the child by stating that there are some toys that can be played with and the child can stop playing any time he or she becomes tired and wants to quit. During the play time, the nurse should ask questions about what is going on, to clarify the child's feelings and experiences.

Through playing with toys, children decrease their anxiety and fear. If the feeling gets too high, the child will quit and should not be urged to continue. When the child demonstrates inadequate methods of problem solving, the nurse can suggest alternative strategies, depending on the focus of the session. If the focus is strictly to deal with feelings, this would not be appropriate.

Older children do not appreciate using toys. Instead, asking them to draw pictures, prepare a television script, or write a story is helpful. If children use drawings, ask them to tell a story about the drawing. The general mood can easily be assessed. J. H. D. Leo's *Children's Drawings as Diagnostic Aids* is a good reference for further assessment and interpretation of drawings.[12]

One technique that elicits feelings of children in a nonthreatening manner is drawing to music. The nurse selects a variety of records representing different moods. Paper and colors are provided. Children are informed that different songs will be played during which time they can draw a picture for each song. The picture can be any color. It can be a specific picture of an object or just any design. Before starting each drawing, children should try to look inside themselves and see how the music makes them feel, then draw a picture.

After the drawings have been completed, the nurse should review the drawings with the child (this can be done with a group). The nurse would ask about each picture and how the music made the child feel. Sometimes, the nurse may have to put the record on for just a moment to remind the child of the song. The emphasis at the end of the session is that some songs make us feel happy and some make us feel other emotions. Some situations in our life make us feel that way, too. Children can choose to listen to certain types of music that make them feel good when they may not be feeling that way. This type of group not only helps children to identify their feelings and one way in which they are elicited, but also to learn that they can elicit those feelings in different situations.

Storybooks and coloring books have been designed to help children deal with their feelings. One is *This is a Coloring Book for Kids Whose Moms Get Hit*.[13] Child advocates in shelters for battered women have had children color pictures and talk about the pictures while coloring. This provides an opportunity for children to talk about how it feels when mommy gets hit. *Red Flag, Green Flag People* is a coloring book used to help children problem solve situations and alternatives to prevent sexual abuse.[14] Other storybooks, to be read with children, focus on feelings about divorce, being alone, getting mad, and friendship. The nurse can use activities such as coloring and storytelling to help children process their feelings.

Play Therapy with Parent and Child

One method of therapeutic play emphasizes developing a positive relationship between parent and child. The role of the nurse is that of teacher. She teaches the parent how to use play to help the child become aware of his or her feelings, build a child's trust and confidence in the parent, and build a child's confidence in him or herself. It is important for the parent to be open to the child and accepting of the feelings expressed.

Setting up the Play Session

First, a time must be set aside. Initially, it should be half an hour, once a week. That time should not be interrupted. Individualized full attention breeds confidence and trust between parent and child. A room for play where things cannot be spoiled or broken allows for freedom in play. A variety of unbreakable toys reserved just for play sessions should be available. These toys are selected to be used by the child to enact feelings. Usually little explanation to the child is necessary. The parent explaining they want to spend time alone with the child is sufficient.

Role of the Parent

Establishing an atmosphere of acceptance for the child is the role of the parent. The child takes the lead in the type of play. (The right not to participate must also be respected.) Full attention should be paid to the child's actions, feelings, and what he or she says. Parents can help the child become aware of feelings by reflecting these back, out loud to the child. For example, "that makes you mad." Parents show acceptance of the child's action by stating such things as "you're really hitting your doll hard." No judgment is made of the child's behavior in this manner. Through this type of involvement, parents can try to understand their children's feelings.

Setting Limits

Some restrictions may need to be made and rigidly adhered to. A warning should be given if the child exceeds the restrictions and the play session ended if the child is unable to stop the behavior. Limits include no hitting, hurting, or endangering the parent in any way; if the child leaves the play session, he or she may not return; and a sharp implement may not be used to poke any toys.

The value of teaching parents how to use this method of therapeutic play are several. Parents learn how to use time with their children in a positive manner. They demonstrate an acceptance to the child. An opportunity is provided to the parent to gain a better understanding of the child's feelings, especially toward family members and him or herself. Parents may even learn more about their own feelings toward the child. Parents in violent homes often feel the need to control the actions of children and have unrealistic expectations of their performance. By having the child "take the lead," parents may realize the benefit of children's play and the level of their performance. Many women who are abused deny their children's awareness of the abuse. In fact, this type of play with the parent and child involved can provide the child with a way to express fears and concerns, since there often is awareness of the tension and physical abuse.

Group Therapy

There are many alternative ways to be therapeutic while working with children. By the age of five or six, children are beginning to move away from parents and interact and play in groups. This is a natural association in which to relate fears, decrease anxiety, and bolster their self-concept. Depending on the stage of the child, composition of the group, setting and purpose, different types of groups for children may be helpful. It is advisable to focus more on behaviors and feelings that are readily identifiable in the group. In-depth analysis may be used with groups, but does require specific training.

Developmental Stage

The developmental stage of a child influences ability to communicate, as well as content. During the preschool stage and early schoolage stages, there is limited ability to perform certain cognitive functions, that is, relate cause-effect, reason, and so forth. Therefore, talking out problems and solutions will not be an effective way to work with the child. At later stages, children are able to perform these functions. Younger children have limited verbal capacity and awareness of feelings. A type of group that utilizes play, therefore, will be most helpful in younger children, whereas, in late childhood activities may be useful, but discussion or group therapy utilized with adults may also be used.

Setting

Setting, which includes location and time, affects the type of group activity to be used. It is important, as with other therapeutic measures, that a quiet, comfortable and nondistracting location be used. In one situation, the school library proved to be unsuitable for a group. This was an inappropriate setting, since the children were constantly looking at books, asking if they had read this book or that one. This disturbed the group process.

Identifying the time when children are most comfortable is important, that is, not before meals or bedtime. Physical needs have priority over any imposed activities. Furthermore, time should be kept to a half hour with young children and not more than forty-five to sixty minutes with older children. Attention spans do not go beyond these limits.

Composition of Groups

Some groups encompass several developmental stages, but as a general rule, children from just one developmental stage should be included. As mentioned earlier, children from different developmental stages have varying abilities and interests. The exception to this rule would be when the purpose of the group is to role model behavior for younger children or to use older children to reinforce behavior in younger children.

Personality characteristics should be considered in the composition of the group. A child who is not able to contain his or her behavior will only become disruptive in a group. But variety in personalities may complement each other, helping to reinforce the "OKness" of unique characteristics of the individuals.

No more than six to eight persons should be in a group, with six being the ideal. Too many make it difficult to give attention to all members.

Purpose

Groups can be used to accomplish several purposes, such as encourage positive interaction between peers, enhance self-esteem, share experiences, or deal with feelings. Often groups accomplish more than one purpose. In determining the composition of the group or the activities to be used, the purpose must always be kept foremost in mind. For instance, having children draw to music may help them identify feelings and decrease anxiety, but it does not improve interactions among peers, unless discussion about the pictures is also included. On the other hand, observing children in natural play, such as at a playground, provides opportunity for the nurse, as well as peers, to give feedback on behavior. At the same time, there is a potential opportunity to process feelings. Keeping the purpose of the group in mind guides the style in which the group is conducted.

One group technique that focuses on improved peer interactions was used with a group of five children, ages eleven and twelve. One girl was referred to the school nurse for poor grooming and inability to get along with classmates. Another girl did well with school work, but was quiet and withdrawn. The remaining three children in the group were selected for their ability to get along with their peers.

The five children met with the school nurse for five weeks, forty-five minutes each time at 1:00 p.m. on Thursdays. The library was used due to lack of a more appropriate setting. Initially, an explanation for meeting was given and the purpose of the group was explained, that is, spending time together getting to know each other and getting along. Meeting time, place, length, and limits (the children were expected to stay, pay attention, make no derogatory remarks) were established. The variety of activities that would occur were discussed.

An example of one session included reaffirming the purpose of the group, limits, and explanation of activities. Each group started by having members state one thing they liked about another member. Initially, this was difficult. The nurse role modeled a variety of compliments, such as you do well in spelling, I like that you listen well to others, and I like your green shoes. The nurse also role modeled how to receive compliments. One activity was having each member tell one thing they did well or enjoyed outside of school.

Using a group that requires verbal interaction with boys and girls ages eleven and twelve was beneficial. Preadolescence is a stage in which peer relationships are becoming more important, adding value to the group experience. Girls and boys are discovering they are different, but distinct sexual identities do not interfere with interaction. Children this age were able to learn to give and receive compliments. They also got to know each other for positive qualities not displayed in the classroom, such as water skiing and building a go-cart. A common bond was made within the group over five weeks.

Another group technique utilizing children from various developmental stages could include children in a shelter for battered women. The ideal time would be after a meal, when children are not tired. A room with limited distractions should be used. The purpose of the "get-together" should be stated as "this is the time for us to talk about when Mommy gets hit. We're going to talk about how you feel when this happens and what you can and cannot do about it." The nurse should encourage children to talk about how scary it feels. Other feelings that might exist should be encouraged. Children have a tremendous amount of guilt, feeling in some way they are responsible for the violence. By encouraging children to identify this feeling and by reassuring them that they did not do anything to make the fighting happen, the nurse can allay that sense of guilt. Children need to be made aware that they should not get in the middle of the physical violence. They need to establish a plan not to be hurt. When the children brainstorm ways to keep safe the nurse can support acceptable plans and explain why some plans may not be the best. Through this type of group, children from wife abuse families can process their feelings and plan for their safety.

Behavior Modification

Through a systematic program, behavior modification can become an effective tool. Nurses need to assess what factors precede an undesired behavior and what factors reinforce that behavior. Nurses can use behavior modification in three ways to change behavior: teach a new behavior, reinforce existing desirable behaviors, and eliminate problem behaviors.

Children from violent families may exhibit a number of problem behaviors, which are attributed partially to learning that occurs in the home environment, that is, aggressive behavior. Aggressive behavior has been shown to achieve results, such as obtaining desired objects or control over others. The nurse can teach a child an alternative method of obtaining desired results and then use reinforcement to establish the behavior. One alternative is teaching the child how to ask another child for an object instead of using physical force. The nurse then should work with the adult involved in the situation, that is, parent, teacher, and so forth, to reinforce each time this behavior occurs, immediately at the time it occurs. After continual reinforcement, the desired behavior will occur with more frequency, replacing the aggressive behavior. Eventually, when the behavior of asking for an object occurs on a regular basis, reinforcement should be cut back to an intermittent basis. The child's ability to obtain what he or she wants in a friendly manner will also result in improved relationships with others, which in itself becomes a reinforcer.

Behavior modification can be used not only to teach and establish new behaviors, but also to reinforce existing desirable behaviors. When a problem occurs, an existing positive behavior should be reinforced that may interfere with the undesired behavior. For instance, John, who is ten years old, insisted on writing all over Jimmie's paper when they sat at the same table. John was careful never to destroy his own paper and in fact was very neat. The nurse might suggest that John and Jimmie do their work jointly on the same paper for a week. Praise should be given for neatness when they work together. After a week, intermittently, John and Jimmie should use separate pieces of paper and praise should continue for neatness on both pieces of paper. Eventually John and Jimmie would return to using separate pieces of paper all the time with only intermittent praise to both for neatness.

Another alternative for dealing with this problem may be to use aversive stimuli. John enjoys his work being neat and tidy. Every time he scribbles on Jimmie's paper, Jimmie's paper would be given to John to recopy. The increase in work for John eventually would decrease his behavior, especially if done at recess. Punishment or aversive stimuli needs to occur immediately, contingent with the undesired behavior, and should be done consistently to be effective.

In using behavior modification, complex behavior problems can be changed. More complex patterns require the process of shaping, that is, reinforcing parts or subgoals of the final goal. More complex patterns usually also require the use of positive reinforcement for new behaviors, existing behaviors, and extinction of undesirable behaviors. Change does not occur overnight. The more complex and long term the behavior, the longer it will take to change it.

Table 11-4 is sample nursing process intended to illustrate some of the issues involved with nursing care of children of violent families. A brief description of the situation is presented, and is intended only as a starting point.

EVALUATION

Evaluation of nursing care of children from violent families is based on established goals. It must be an ongoing process. Furthermore, subgoals should be the focus for evaluation, as well as the eventual overall goal.

Children from violent families present with a variety of problems, ranging from speech and motor delays to behavioral disturbances. A variety of goals may be established, based on identification of problems. Goals, stemming from social learning theory will focus on the environment that precipitates or supports problems, characteristics of the child, or the interaction between the two. Intervention strategies employed attempt to model desired behaviors, reinforce new or existing positive behaviors, or extinguish negative behaviors.

Problems experienced by children in violent homes are thought to be a result of learning over a period of time. Long-term behaviors require a lengthy intervention to achieve the final goal of optimizing the child's potential. Short-term goals need to be established and provide the basis for evaluation. For example, in working with a child who has low self-esteem, one related factor might be ability to interact with other children. This, in turn, might be influenced by poor grooming. Small goals, such as not having excessive body odor, keeping hair neat, or wearing clothes that are clean, would be short-term goals. These goals are steps in the eventual process of improving self-esteem.

Nurses may have limited interaction with children. Goals established must be realistic if the nurse and child are to experience a feeling of accomplishment in evaluation of the goal. For instance, a child may be seen in the emergency room for a minor laceration after falling while trying to hide in the dark during a violent episode between the parents. The nurse can establish a trusting relationship with the child, demonstrating to the parents how to explain a procedure that may be painful. The nurse can also demonstrate providing support to the child by stating that it is OK to cry if it hurts. The method of evaluation would be observation of the parents' ability to do the same. Referral of the family would be indicated if the emergency room nurse can take no further action personally.

Nurses may have the opportunity to work with children over an extended period of time. When this occurs, more extensive goals may be evaluated such as the ability to express feelings by having the puppet talk about a situation, or building a clay object and then smashing it. Other goals that can be evaluated include improved interaction with peers as evidenced by ability to play together for thirty minutes without conflict, or sharing toys while playing together.

Some goals, such as eliminating developmental delays, can be measured by an improvement of a score on a developmental screening test. The use of formalized tests provide objective data to measure changes. If the nurse did not see an improvement in performance, a reassessment of the cause of the problem or associated factors should be made. The intervention used may need to be changed.

Evaluation is not the final step in the process of working with children from violent families. Evaluation is an ongoing process. Working with children requires flexibility. The nurse must continually be sensitive to the interactions and readjust as necessary.

Summary

Children of violent families, whether siblings of abused children or offspring of battered women, are at risk for developmental and emotional difficulties. These children are at present only haphazardly identified and critically underserved. Nursing needs to be aware of the research just beginning to demonstrate the possible needs of these children, as members of families experiencing violence, and to be alert for them in a variety of clinical settings. Social learning theory is suggested as a viable basis for assessment and nursing interventions. Such interventions include play-oriented therapy, developmental stimulation, group therapy, and reinforcement techniques. Additional theory-based research into the effects of violence on

Nursing Care of Children of Violent Families

all family members and the outcomes of nursing interventions remains to be done. The potential for nursing involvement in theory development and research in the area is essentially untapped.

Table 11-4 Sample Nursing Process

Brief Background

Susan, age 10, was referred to the school nurse for poor grooming. Susan seldom washed her hair, and it was frequently disarrayed. She wore the same clothes to school for almost a week at a time, even when they had become soiled. Peers teased her about smelling bad. The teacher reported no one wanted to sit next to her or work with her. Susan came from a middle-class family where both her parents worked. The school nurse called Susan's mother and found out that she was concerned about Susan's appearance. Susan had a variety of clothes which were clean. Susan's mother said they had an ongoing battle to get her to take a bath and shampoo. The nurse noted from the school record that there was a history of alcohol abuse and violence in the family. Susan's sloppiness was especially evident after weekends and days off.

Nursing diagnosis: Self-care deficit (dressing/grooming) related to low self-concept

Client Goals	Intervention
A. *Short Term:* Susan will identify extent of problem at end of one week	A.1. Nurse to give mother flow sheet for daily documentation of Susan's grooming, problems at home, and reactions to grooming
	2. Nurse to call mother on Monday and Thursday to assess frequency of bath, shampoo, brushing teeth, changing clothes, problems at home, reactions of family to grooming
	3. Nurse to review with teacher and Susan sheet of Susan's daily grooming (hair, body odor, dress, problems at school, peer/teacher reaction) to establish a baseline
B. *Short Term:* Susan will help formulate behavior modification plan at end of two weeks	B.1. Nurse to meet with mother to discuss if any identified problems preceding sloppy appearance
	2. Nurse to discuss with teacher plan to change behavior
	3. Nurse to meet with Susan to discuss concerns and plan

(continued)

Table 11-4 (Cont.)

Client Goals	Intervention
C. *Short Term:* Factors precipitating Susan's poor grooming will be discussed by mother and Susan as evidenced by: 1. Susan discusses occurrences (positive as well as negative) over weekend at home 2. Mother discusses occurrences at home preceding Susan's poor grooming 3. Mother will relate home factors to Susan's feelings about herself and her manner of grooming	C.1. Nurse to discuss with mother and Susan that individual meetings be held biweekly to identify precipitating factors to Susan's poor grooming 2. Nurse to encourage Susan to discuss both positive and negative occurrences at home over weekends and days off 3. Nurse to encourage mother to identify home factors preceding Susan's poor grooming 4. Nurse to discuss with mother Susan's grooming as a way of showing her feelings in relation to other events
D. *Long Term:* Susan will demonstrably improve appearance at end of six weeks as evidenced by: 1. Reports of improved appearance by teacher and mother 2. Flow sheets indicating improved grooming patterns	D.1. Nurse to encourage mother to praise Susan when appearance neat and ignore sloppy appearance 2. Teacher to praise neat appearance, especially with peers present and ignore sloppy dress 3. Teacher to send Susan to wash herself and comb hair during recess when dirty 4. Nurse, with mother's approval and financing, to take Susan for hairstyling 5. Susan to spend 30 minutes in office with nurse weekly helping with small pleasant tasks, if appearance reported good that week 6. Nurse to discuss with Susan positive outcomes of improved appearance and increase Susan's awareness of resulting changes

Evaluation of nursing interventions are based on achievement of goals as perceived by client and as indicated by criteria met.

Chapter 11

1. Harold Martin, ed., *A Multidisciplinary Approach to Developmental Issues and Treatment* (Cambridge: Ballinger Publishing Co., 1976), p. 2.
2. Murray Straus, "Family Patterns and Child Abuse in a Nationally Representative American Sample," in Helfer and Kempe, *Child Abuse and Neglect*, vol. 3 (London: Pergamon Press Ltd., 1979): pp. 213-25.

3. Ibid.

4. Albert Bandura, *Aggression: A Social Learning Analysis* (Englewood Cliffs, N.J.: Prentice-Hall, 1973).

5. Bonnie Westra and Harold Martin, "Children of Battered Women," *Maternal-Child Nursing Journal* 10 (Spring 1981): 41-54.

6. Ann Hass, personal correspondence, 1982.

7. Ellen Dunwoody, "Sexual Abuse of Children," *Response* 5, no. 4 (July/August 1982).

8. Bonita Westra, *Battered Women and Child Development* (master's thesis, University of Colorado, 1979), p.11.

9. Michael Rutter, *Helping Troubled Children* (New York: Plenum, 1975), p. 110.

10. Stanley Coopersmith, *Coopersmith Self-Esteem Inventory* (San Francisco: W. H. Freeman & Co., 1967).

11. Charles Schaefer, ed., *The Therapeutic Use of Child's Play* (New York: Arnson, 1979), pp. 219-26.

12. J. H. D. Leo, *Children's Drawings as Diagnostic Aids* (New York: Burner/Mazel Publishers, 1973).

13. J. H. D. Leo, *This is a Coloring Book for Kids Whose Moms Get Hit* (St. Paul, Minn.: Region XII Battered Women's Consortium, 1980).

14. Joy Williams, *Red Flag, Green Flag People* (Fargo, N.D.: Rape and Abuse Crisis Center, 1980).

The Nurse and the Police: Dealing with Abused Women

James Bannon

12

INTRODUCTION

One of, if not the most, frustrating and intransigent problems confronting the working police officer is wife abuse, or as it is known in law enforcement, domestic violence. The officer feels poorly equipped to deal with these calls for service in any meaningful way. His or her training is inadequate or nonexistent. Agency policy is unclear, nonexistent, or contrary to general policy.

As a result, the officer detests, resents, or avoids to the greatest extent possible any involvement in domestic violence cases, or alternatively, gives them short shrift. This chapter will attempt to examine some of the issues that have caused police officers to adopt "hands-off" attitudes toward domestic violence. This is the first of four chapters addressing the interface of law enforcement and the legal system with the profession of nursing in the area of family violence.

SCOPE OF THE PROBLEM

Historically, no data have been collected on domestic violence separate from assaults generally. With rare exceptions in the past, no effort has been made to research the issue in such a way that reliable estimates can be made of the number of such assaults that occur. Thus, "guesstimates" range from 50 percent to one-third of all married dyads are commonly thought to have some violent encounters.

In attempting to achieve some notion of the size of the problem, this author, along with Marie Wilt, a criminologist, undertook a study in Detroit, Michigan, in 1972.[1] The findings of that study, published by the Police Foundation, indicated clearly that at least 50 percent of all domestic assaults are never reported. Additionally, it became clear that even fewer assaults are reported by the victim herself. Frequently, children, other family members, or residents in the household will notify the police. Neighbors, themselves disturbed, will often call as well.

Although it has proven difficult, if not impossible, to find hard data for the simple reason no such data are collected, it is widely believed that in many jurisdictions fully one-third of all calls for service are domestic violence calls. Of course, in larger jurisdictions with multiple crime problems, the ratio of such calls drops off dramatically. It should be understood that the reason for this decrease has nothing whatever to do with the actual incidence of abuse. On the contrary, it is related to the work load of the agency and the policies of that agency designed to manage its work load.

In Detroit, Michigan, in the years 1980, 1981, and 1982, the average monthly calls for police response to domestic violence cases for the city were about 3,900 to 4,000. These numbers are for all types of calls related to domestic violence. For many reasons, which we will discuss, it is believed that this represents only a fraction of the total number of actual incidents.

One of the most notable facets of law enforcement attitudes toward domestic violence is the seeming indifference of police administration to the physical safety of its officers in responding to domestic violence calls. Federal Bureau of Investigation reports consistently indicate that about one-third of all police fatalities occur when responding to social conflict calls. It is further believed that most of these are domestic violence calls although it is impossible to state with precision. Similarly, a large proportion of disabling injuries, that is, those requiring either hospitalization or release from work due to injury, are the result of attempted interventions in domestic disputes. For the above reasons, it would seem that the competent police administrator would have wanted to develop strategies for successfully dealing with these cases. Unfortunately, this has not been the case.

While the author will and does indict the police for failure to adequately address the issue of abused women, in fairness, it should be pointed out that many police attitudes flow directly from the society of which they are a part.

It is much too complex an issue to explore in this chapter, but the reader by now is aware that historically wifebeating has been regarded in most societies as legitimate male behavior (see Chapter 4). It has been sanctioned by the courts, by the clergy, and by public opinion. There has and remains a very strong belief that the male assumes the responsibility for regulating the behavior of all in his household. Therefore, it is expected that at times he may be required, in fulfilling his role, to mete out physical discipline.

It is true that in some socioeconomic groups in our society these expectations are carried out with greater public notice than in others. However, there is no reason to believe that there are substantial differences in attitudes about the appropriateness of the behavior. There are, of course, differences in reporting, in interventions, even in the location on the body of assaults by members of the upper socioeconomic strata. These differences have to do with such diverse matters as living arrangements of the poor, lack of privacy, lack of alternatives for the victim and the abuser, differential concerns over public image of the affluent, and, not to be forgotten—the most important consideration of the affluent—the risk of monetary and status loss in the event of dissolution of the marriage.

Please note that the author is not unaware of the increasingly popular "less than married" relationships. When the term "married" is used, it should be taken to mean any cohabitation which features consensual sexual access and economic interdependence. This definition *would not* exclude homosexual relationships. It *would* exclude casual sexual liaisons. The author believes that the battering syndrome necessarily contains within it a requirement of dependency—social, economic, legal and emotional—which inhibits or overcomes the natural instinct to flee or vitiate the assault on one's person.

Traditional socialization of male/female children carries within it all the ingredients necessary to cast the male in the dominant role, the female in the passive. However, dominance and passivity as conditioned responses would not be adequate to explain violence in the relationship.

There is a need to look to other socialization issues as they pertain to female/male differences. Most notable are the male required strengths of body and spirit. Men don't cry; they are physically strong, brave. They fight their own battles. They will not be cowed by another, nor will they suffer any interference with their affairs. Meanwhile, the female child is taught not only is it okay to cry, to be sensitive, frightened, and dependent, but that it is also the most feminine thing to do. Moreover, the more feminine she is, the more she will attract her polar opposite, that is, the masculine, physical male.

Since Americans are socialized to believe that the male is acting appropriately and the female has the burden to recognize and surrender to this, it is also expected that all accommodation will be made by her. It is her responsibility to satisfy, pacify, give in to the demands of the male. She fails as a wife if she does not. She fails as a woman if she fails as a wife. Most often, it is her sense of failure that inhibits her from telling others of the abuse she is absorbing.

There is an additional cultural impediment to effective police intervention in the black community which maintains a basic distrust of the historically predominantly white criminal justice system. For reasons we have discussed, the police lack policy, training, or mandate develop unorthodox remedies to problems. In the black community, this sometimes led to the abuser himself being beaten by the police. Two things happened. First, the victim was reluctant to call the police for fear they would deal too harshly with the abuser. Second, the abuser would in turn retaliate against the police by reabusing the original victim.

Much more definitive information on the role of the female/male socialization in the issue of spouse abuse is presented in Chapter 4. It is entirely too complex and lengthy an issue to be more than mentioned here. What is important to keep in mind is that all of us have been exposed to the same conditioning. While we may not all be violent nor all be victims of violence, our thoughts on these matters are directly related to our common socialization. Thus, police officers have been conditioned to believe in and to aspire to the "macho" man image. In fact, many have been attracted to law enforcement because of its seeming comportment with the masculine role model. Later we will discuss the effects this could and often does have on their behavior.

HISTORICAL BACKGROUND

Traditional Police Response

While minor differences existed in police response to domestic violence calls in different parts of the country, the net result was virtually the same no matter where the assault occurred. Changes began to occur in the late 1960s and continue today. The changes have been slow, sporadic, and reluctant. An attempt to give some of the reasons is presented here.

First, it must be remembered that the police not only are a part of their own society, sharing in its beliefs and values, but also only one component of the criminal justice system. The other components are the prosecutorial, the courts, and corrections. Not only do these other components share social values with their society, they also have different interests and concerns than do the police on any given issue.

The police officer might desire to make

an arrest and lay a charge against a man who has beaten his spouse, even if only because he is tired of going back to the same household repeatedly. The prosecutor, on the other hand, may not want to proceed due to his belief that the victim will not follow through, or more importantly that it will affect his conviction rate. The court may also be reluctant because of concerns with an overloaded docket or the alternatives available if the spouse is convicted.

It then becomes clear to the police officer that the other components of the system simply do not want to see these cases. The officer also sees that his own agency does not value domestic violence arrests. Sometimes this realization is direct. The universal statement in police manuals that reads: "You should remember that domestic assaults are civil in nature and arrest should be avoided if at all possible," is the classic example.

In the first place, although the statement is universally used in police procedural manuals, it is untrue. Domestic assaults are legally no different than stranger-to-stranger assaults. For whatever reasons, police administrators over the years have adopted an assumption of noncriminal behavior for the act of a man beating his wife. There is nothing in the law that permits the police executive to do this, yet, the premise went unchallenged until 1975, when lawsuits were lodged in Oakland, California, and in New York City.

These class action suits, settled out of court, sought simply to have the police treat domestic violence as a crime just like any other crime, which they legally are. Police procedures have been changed to eliminate this language in most but not all parts of the United States.

Even more pervasive and influential to an officer's judgment on such arrests, however, was the silent message that was given. There simply was no recognition by the officer's superiors of the value of superior service to domestic violence victims nor of arrests for domestic assault. The latter was a function of only being allowed to actively pursue court arrests that went on to prosecution. Since so few of these cases did, no credit accrued to the officers. Add to these direct messages the fact already discussed, that these cases often end in an assault, sometimes fatal, of the officer, and it is not difficult to imagine the police officer wanting to avoid all involvement.

However, the dilemma is obvious. The police officer is required by his dispatcher to respond to a domestic violence call, yet the agency is ambivalent at best, if not actually hostile, to such calls. The officer has a policy that tells him to avoid arrest if possible. The prosecutor does not want these cases, nor does the court. The police officer has no training in how to handle these matters and he may well believe that physical resolution of conflict is the appropriate solution. His superiors will not recognize superior performance. And lastly, while the officer is spending an inordinate amount of time attempting to do what the officer knows that he is not competent to do, the other work is backlogging. Or worse yet, from the officer's perspective, he is losing the opportunity to do "real" police work that is not only personally satisfying, but also obtains both public and agency acclaim. This is "the stuff that promotions are made of."

The author has often noted that in thirty-three years of experience, he has never seen an award for excellence given to an officer for successful resolution of a domestic violence case. Except posthumously that is!

It is obvious that the officer has to employ some strategy to get away from the scene. Since he has not been given the tools to function in these cases, he is compelled to develop personal, informal, often unorthodox, remedies. Over time, the solutions may progress from the simplest admonitions of future arrest to both parties, to highly complex sociopsychological strategies far beyond his academic capacity.

An example of the latter occurred a few years ago in a large metropolitan area. At the time, a certain police precinct was largely an all-black ghetto. This police officer, though white, had migrated from the deep South. Although he had only an eighth grade education, he seemed to have the country philosopher wisdom often remarked by some authors.

In those days, most family assaults seemed to occur on weekends—the time of greatest drinking and social interaction. The man would come home "under the influence" and assault the woman, and the police would be called to the scene. Our hero would have both parties brought to him at the station. He would declare their differences irreconcilable and divorce them on the spot complete with pseudolegalistic jargon. He would order them to come back on Sunday night or early Monday morning at which time he would talk to them for a while, get agreement that their differences were at least temporarily reconciled. At that time he would pull out an old dog-eared Bible, Gideon, I believe, place their hands on it, and remarry them. Interestingly enough, since at the time this state was a common-law state, this was the closest many of his clients had ever come to a formal ceremony.

Unfortunately, this methodology, while seemingly effective for this officer and his clients, only came to light because of a trial board hearing in which he was fired. It seems he had been charging a fee for the service. This officer had bragged that during all the years he had performed this service, he had never lost a client to domestic homicide.

Despite his limited formal education, the cracker-barrel philosopher had discovered that he could temporarily defuse some of the abuser's anger, protect the victim from further immediate harm, and keep the relationship intact. These were desirable goals in most people's view at that point in time. Such short-range goals are no longer considered appropriate for the victim, the abuser, or the agency.

Unfortunately, this relatively benign, if not beneficial, strategem was the exception rather than the rule. Most police officers confronted with the frustration of having to do something but lacking the training, the support, and the mandate, would frequently fall back on their masculine role images. They would simply "beat the hell" out of the abuser, or at least make that threat to. Knowing the effects of pain or the threat of pain on inhibiting certain behavior, many claim this was *not* an ineffective device.

Unfortunately, the message it delivers is that physical violence is in fact under some circumstances an appropriate vehicle for invoking authority. We need to remember that the abusive male sees himself as the authority figure. The lesson he learns is not that violence is wrong but that he needs to be more circumspect so that other authority figures who also use violence are not called.

Between the two extremes just described are countless other variations of police behavior. Some officers without formal training would attempt to counsel the parties, perhaps doing far more harm in the long run than if they had actually beaten someone. Others, and this is by far the most common approach, would slough off the complaint by telling the victim to see the detectives Monday through Friday between the hours of 9 A.M. and 5 P.M. They would not take a report even though it was clear a crime had been committed. The officer knew full well that those detectives themselves had a full range of strategies to discourage the complainant's pursuit of a legal, criminal remedy.

The detective would try to dissuade the victim from prosecution, pointing out that she and the children would suffer adverse economic effects if she put her spouse in jail. It was likely, however, that in the detective's entire career, he had never known of an abuser going to jail.

The detective would explain the difficulty to be encountered in sustaining the prosecution, the inconvenience of multiple court appearances, the embarrassment of public disclosure, and so forth. Should the victim persist, the detective might well advise her to go home and think it over, to bring back medical proof of injury, to bring her assailant in the next time she comes back.

If in fact she persevered, the detective may ultimately have been compelled to submit a write-up to the prosecuting attorney, who would begin the process designed to discourage prosecution all over again. The attorney's tactics might include counseling (equally untrained), intimidation, insistence on medical proof, pictures of the injury, threats of a cross-complaint, and demands for an assurance bond (a cash bond posted to guarantee prosecution). As a last resort, the attorney may have offered her a so-called peace bond, a completely worthless document made out in appropriate legalese which was tantamount to being a promissory note to prosecute the abuser if he assaulted the victim within the time frame stipulated on the document. Since such a subsequent assault would have constituted another crime, no such commitment was necessary.

It was widely believed (and appeared to have been supported by the clients themselves) that in certain legally unsophisticated communities, the "peace bond" in fact did inhibit assaults. Unfortunately, what is not addressed is the notion that the violent behavior was only controlled during the time limits on the document. This implies that at all other times, the violence is appropriate.

One device, while illegal, at least had the dubious virtue of candor. This was the so-called call screening employed in Detroit, Michigan, from about 1965 through 1973 or 1974. Call screening was said to have become necessary because calls for service exceeded the department's capacity to respond to all calls. To reduce the work load, it was decided to interview the caller sufficiently enough to determine the exact nature of the complaint and make a conscious decision not to send a response unit in certain cases.

In Detroit, the domestic dispute was selected as the first type of call to be screened out. The rationale for this decision was once again the refusal of women to follow up on prosecution. No consideration was ever given to an attempt to enhance their willingness or capacity to prosecute, nor was any consideration given to the obvious history of the criminal justice system in discouraging prosecution.

It happened that later explanations pointed out that the policy had an escape clause for the victim that if a weapon was involved, the police would be sent. The victims, on becoming aware of this override, invariably alleged a weapon. Thus, the policy, it was said, was effectively vitiated.

Dr. Marie Wilt and this author took is-

The Nurse and the Police: Dealing with Abused Women

sue with this claim by raising the substantial objection that a police officer responding to an alleged assault with a weapon would react in an entirely negative fashion if there was no weapon. Often times he would even threaten to arrest the caller for having made a false felony report. To this day, it is impossible to estimate the residual effects of such a policy on a community long conditioned to rebuff when calling in a domestic violence complaint. It is certain that several generations will come and go before these effects disappear.

While it is not possible to quantify the effects previously mentioned, it is possible to look to one statistic which the authors of the study cited believe directly reflected the abandonment of the victim, that is domestic homicide. The investigators believe and continue to believe that the rate of such homicides rose dramatically as a direct result of the call screening policy.

Other researchers disagree with this interpretation, pointing out that all homicides had increased during the same period. However, domestic homicide was frequently not properly categorized as such because relationships did not and do not reflect a broad enough definition of domestic. The one used by this author—cohabitation with consensual sexual access and economic interdependency—is more functional.

Contemporary Developments

Although not proving the relationship between call screening and other policies designed to separate out wife abuse complaints from other crimes, the recent rash of widely publicized trials of women accused of murdering their husbands merit attention. Such trials are not new, but the defense being offered is. Women in effect are asking for an expansion of the self-defense doctrine based not on traditional legal issues, but rather on the failure of society and its legal system to protect them. Two notable Michigan cases come to mind. The first, involving Francine Hughes, was widely publicized. In the end, the legal position was not self-defense, but diminished capacity, that is, not guilty by reason of insanity. However, the facts adduced at trial clearly showed a victim forced by neighbors, family, friends, and the criminal justice system to rely on her own resources to escape the unending cycle of violence. She waited until her husband was asleep, soaked him in gasoline, and lit his bed. He burned to death.[2]

The second case, that of Janet Smith, is directly on point because it not only showed the same indifference of society and its system, but also led to an acquittal of Mrs. Smith on the grounds of self-defense. This defense prevailed despite the fact that the threat to her, thus the danger, was not contemporaneous with her killing of her husband. It was the accumulated experience of assault and inability to rely on the system for protection or redress. The reader is referred to *People v. Janet Smith*, Otsego County Circuit Court, 1978, for details of this case.[3]

In the early 1970s, several concurrent developments occurred which began to raise domestic violence from the position of a private problem to that of a public issue. First, the feminist movement, often embodied in the National Organization for Women, recognized the plight of the battered wife as an issue of national and immediate concern. The organization adopted this issue as a primary focus for consciousness raising and action programs.

At about the same time in Michigan,

two female law school students began to take an interest in the issue, desiring to focus the attention of fledgling lawyers on the matter. Their work, "Catch 22," became one of the first expositions available in writing.[4] The authors, Pat Micklow and Sue Eisenberg, are widely credited with disseminating information both to feminist organizations and professionals in related fields. Micklow and Eisenberg, in attempting to obtain hard data for their project, came into contact with Marie Wilt and this author who were engaged in the homicide/assault study already mentioned. The four of us began to share data and ideas.

Throughout the country, although not uniformly so, consciousness was raised and the media began to address the issue. There was confrontation between the criminal justice system and concerned women's groups. Some of this confrontation created far more heat than light, but in the end it began to stimulate an interest on the part of public officials in examining their own practices and procedures. At first, this self-examination was purely defensive. Later, some of the more sensitive administrators, prosecutors, and judges recognized and admitted the system's failures.

To their credit, police agencies were generally far more willing to critique and change than were the other components of the criminal justice system. However, there have been some false starts and unfortunate, unnecessary battles over detail that have been costly in terms of cooperation, and it may be well to look at some of them. First, there was a great deal of denial on the part of the police. This was countered by allegations that the police were frequently involved in their own violent personal relationships. Both sides were right to a certain extent, but both lost sight of the central fact that the police have both a private and a public face. It often happens that the police officer can and does function effectively in his public role, although privately he may engage in the same behavior he is required to police in his public role. Gambling, drinking, and traffic violations come readily to mind.

What got lost in this debate was the obvious fact that agencies control police behavior through policy. No policy existed, or if it did, it was contrary to the law. It was not necessary to enter the debate about private police behavior at all. Only if the policy was published and violated without sanction would one need to look at the issue of private behavior.

Another damaging and unnecessary debate was engaged in (and still is to some extent) over the assertions of criminal justice practitioners that their "hands-off" policy toward domestic violence was due to the failure of women to follow through on prosecution. Feminists responded strongly to this claim, taking the position that it was an outright lie. Some members of the feminist movement reacted vehemently because they simply could not understand how a woman could be abused and not want to pursue all available avenues of redress.

While criminal justice personnel insisted that it was true and relied on such myths as "She must have caused it, she likes it, she loves the guy," and so forth, feminists insisted it just was not true. In fact, it is true that there is a great deal of attrition in these complaints. Part may be due to the battered women's own socialization to expect and accept male dominance and physical punishment. Part may be due to her emotional and economic dependency or her legal confusion over her rights.

The point is missed that there is attrition in prosecution in all kinds of criminal prosecutions. The reasons are numerous, ranging from fear of retaliation to simple disgust over the awkwardness of the system. Yet only in the case of domestic violence victims is the failure to pursue the matter held against the victim in future complaints. Significantly, it is only in these cases that a pattern of attrition by some complainants is used to disenfranchise all such victims. This approach is the reason for the author having described the criminal justice system's response to domestic violence victims as a systematic pattern of discrimination every bit as pervasive as that practiced in race discrimination cases.

The question becomes, how is the class of victim fixed? It is clear that female victims of stranger-to-stranger violence do not experience this discrimination. Nor is the boundary fixed by the state of marriage or cohabitation since women who have long since terminated their relationships continue to be disenfranchised.

The author came to believe that the only common denominator among these victims was prior sexual access. Since there is nothing in the act of coitus itself to imply a surrender of autonomy on the part of the female, further reflection was needed.

The author concluded that consensual sexual access is widey interpreted in our society as denoting a proprietary right of the male over the female. While she may and is empowered to deny the conferring of property status through access to her body, once given, she no longer exercises control over its continuation. This property notion serves to explain abuser attitudes and behaviors. "I have a right and duty to discipline her." Since it appears to be a widely, if not universally shared notion, it also explains in what fashion the criminal justice system determines her to be less worthy of the rights extended to female victims of crime generally. It appears that once conferred, the property right can only be renounced by the man himself. He will not accept even legal dissolution orders. Many cases are on record of men periodically seeking out former wives and asaulting them, some after more than twenty-five years. Amazingly, these cases are usually treated by the criminal justice system as though the parties still cohabited.

Despite the skirmishes and occasional battles, there did arise a willingness on the part of many police executives to address the problem of their agency's neglect or outright hostility to the abused wife. It would be reassuring to report that once they had been made aware of their own culpability in contributing to the problems of conjugal violence, police executives immediately set out to correct the problem in the same way they would address a traditional crime control problem, that is, to look at and change policy, procedures, and philosphy where necessary, and to monitor compliance and address continued malfunctions in the organization. Such was not to be the case.

Basically, no policy or operational changes were made. The problem was thrown to behavioral scientists for recommendations as to how best to respond. These people in turn did not see spouse abuse as a crime in its ordinary sense, but instead saw it as an issue calling for an extraordinary approach.

What in fact ended up being proposed as the only workable solutions called for the police to see their role in interventionist terms. This intervention was not in the classic and legal form, through arrest and charge, but some other form of intervention requiring skills not presently available to most officers as counselors, mediators, conciliators. It was precisely what some of them had been doing for generations without the specialized training to perform that role. The concept then saw specialized teams of highly motivated, specially trained, and selected officers who would respond to the scene and attempt to reconcile any dispute. Experiments with such a schema were carried out and reported as highly successful. The result was replication in twenty-three cities in the United States at a cost of 8 million dollars.[5]

It only occurred to critics later that the "success" of police as counselors had been predicated on the criteria of "lack of callback" (the absence of additional calls to the police). Some suggest that success may not be the only reason for lack of callback. The parties may have moved, or they may have separated, or one could be dead. It occurs to this writer that a more likely scenario finds the victim unwilling during any future such conflicts to call for the team which, in her view, did not perform the functions she expected or felt were necessary.

In our society, police officers perform, for the most part, many different functions and duties, but central to our conceptualization of them when we are victims of crime is that they will arrest and charge the accused. What would be our reaction if we were victimized by a burglar, and the responding officer spent his time attempting to establish the culprits underlying desire or need to steal? Clearly the officer would not be performing the role we have come to expect of him. Should we be victimized in the future, such officers would not be called, and if they responded, they would not be welcome.

In short, a police officer therapist is a contradicition in terms. This is not to maintain that officers do not, in their daily routines, often and in many different contexts, function as advisors, counselors, and confidants. Yet there is a substantial difference in performing these functions on an ad hoc basis and in structuring them to routinely perform those functions.

In the first place, there is no legal basis for them to carry out these functions. Even the naive, poorly educated abuser knows the officer's right to intervene is based solely on his right to arrest. While such a person may not (but sometimes does) physically resist an extralegal intrusion into his home to deliver therapy, he does recognize his right to refuse to accept such an offer. This knowledge in fact allows him to maintain an element of power and control which he would not have in an arrest situation.

Unfortunately—at least to this author—such specialized therapist concepts persist in various parts of the country. In evaluating them, the reader is asked to remember that intellectually they are no different than the strategies employed for generations. The officers may be better trained, but no more empowered than they were formerly.

A somewhat different and slightly better approach has been attempted with improved results in certain large cities. This approach allows the officer to call for the professional assistance to counsel the parties. To the extent that this method is used only when arrest and charge are not possible or desired by the victim, it seems to offer a preferable option in that it does not alter substantially the traditional and expected role of the officer. Such an approach further does not violate the legal requirements of officer interventions because the parties agree beforehand to the arrangement.

In Detroit, the program has been operated by Family Service of Detroit and

Wayne County and places the trained professionals in the police precinct where they become an immediately available resource for the officer. The usual officer resistance to such programs, often predicated on the lack of immediate access to the social worker therapist, was thus negated. Moreover, this program gives the officer feedback so that he can appreciate his role in the process. In published reports, the project has been reported as resulting in 60 percent better follow-up rates by clients than standard referral methods.

Unfortunatey, the reports also reflect that if the programs were offered on a citywide basis, the Family Service case load would increase by about 800 percent. Since operational funds are limited, the potential for major expansion of this highly successful program is dim indeed.

In 1976, the Detroit Police Department adopted new policies and procedures for its response to domestic violence calls. First was the unequivocal policy declaration that interspousal assault was no different at law or in department practice than the same acts committed by strangers. Second, if the elements of a crime could be established, an arrest should be made if legally permissible. Third, a report of the crime was absolutely required. This report must be assigned to an investigator for follow-up and prosecution. In addition, medical documentation, pictorial evidence, and third-party witnesses were not required unless they were required in all other similar cases.

Because compliance with such major policy changes is often not complete or willing, a special computer program was established to permit administrators to monitor compliance. All domestic violence calls were coded in a thirty-nine hundred series. Whether these were injunction violations or homicides, they were so coded. Supervisors were required to test police performance in line with the new policies and procedures. They were to censure noncompliance and were to acknowledge superior performance.

All public-generated complaints of poor performance were followed up with complete investigations and punishment or corrective action taken when appropriate. Soon voluntary compliance became the norm, and only rarely are complaints received.

Recognizing that mere policy change unaccompanied by special training designed to overcome the myths surrounding domestic violence would not meet with success, Detroit determined to develop a training package. It was felt that two types of training were essential. First, a training model for the recruit would be more extensive than for an experienced officer. Because it would not primarily be geared to overcoming established preconceptions and experience, it would be substantially different as well as longer in duration.

Training of the tenured officer would be briefer, but would also attempt to change a set of attitudes and beliefs the officer had built up over a long period of time. It could also be expected that because these attitudes had been shaped by the officer's experience, his peers and agency, they would be extremely difficult to change. In fact, it was recognized that attitudinal change may not be possible. In such an event, only behaviors were thought to be susceptible to meaningful change.

Difficulty in developing the two required modules was encountered because staff could not identify any extant programs that sought to accomplish this agency's goals. Virtually every module reviewed was designed by behaviorists whose goal was clearly to train the officer as mediator, counselor, or therapist. Because it already had been decided that this was not the model Detroit desired, they were rejected. Finally, Detroit's own model was created.

Although this training curriculum is too long and complex to set forth here, some of the principles governing its design may be worthy of discussion. First, the decision was made not to confront the officer with his presumed lack of sensitivity, concern for the victim, or discriminatory behavior. It was assumed that none of these things were the officer's fault, but rather that of the system of which he was a part. Furthermore, the officer was not going to be regaled with horror stories of victims, after all, he had seen this firsthand. Perhaps he had seen incidents even more atrocious than the trainer. The woman's failure to follow through with prosecution, her tendency to return to the abusive male or to sometimes turn on the officer and assist in his assault would all be acknowledged as true, thus removing his source of denial or excuse.

The entire training module focused on the procedural and legal aspects of his involvement in the domestic call. The police officer would be instructed on the very real dangers inherent in these cases and how best to cope with them: what to be alert to and safeguard against; how to approach the scene, the situation; what to say to the parties; how to elicit information sufficient to arrest or make a report. The officer would be encouraged to do these things in sequence and to depart after having achieved the various levels. Only after it became clear that an arrest was not possible or desirable would the officer be given information which would allow him to offer further assistance through referral.

Officers were given complete and comprehensive information on other services available, which ones would be appropriate, and how the client could begin to use these services. They were equipped with referral forms that were also sent to the referred to agency, which was encouraged to feed back to the officer information on clients so referred. In every case possible, all private and public agencies offering services to abused women were asked to participate either directly or as resource persons during the actual training.

Although lectures, review of the law, department policy, and orders remained an integral part of the training, role playing was used extensively. At first, professional actors played the roles. Later the officers themselves did so. The skits were designed to examine some of the more prevailing myths as well as the dynamics of spouse abuse itself. The officer was assisted in formulating his own understanding of each of these situations.

The training was neither preachy nor righteous, but sought to direct the officer to the inevitable conclusion that here was a victim, in every sense of the word, who required his professional police attention. Should she not avail herself of his help or that to which she was referred, she was no less worthy than would be any other citizen victimized by a stranger.

Although it was not a part of the program, officers often came to the conclusion that not only was this victim equally entitled to police protection, but due to the extraordinary circumstance of living with the abuser, she might, in fact, have an even greater need to be protected. It became clearer to the officer why the abuser was in need of a strong, direct, and clear message that his behavior was wrong.

An unanticipated but nonetheless welcome side effect of this officer training was the relatively large number of police officers who recognized in themselves the propensity to use violence in their own relationships. Many of these sought professional help. As a result, the already existent Personal Affairs Section, heretofore specializing in alcohol and substance abuse, found itself offering counseling services for officers and their spouses.

Unfortunately, Detroit's deteriorating fiscal situation forced the postponement of this training before it was completed for the entire department. In addition, because only recruit and front-line officers were initially trained and these were laid off in fiscal cutbacks to be replaced by older but untrained officers, much of the anticipated benefit remains unrealized. As the city's fiscal situation improves, we hope we will be able to complete this program.

Although not directly a Detroit Police Department function, a series of events in 1977-78 are important to the police role in domestic violence.

The process of reviewing spouse abuse laws began with the formation of the Social Conflict Task Force. As the result of the work of the task force, a set of proposed legislation was introduced in Michigan's House of Representatives by the Honorable Connie Binsfield, of Traverse City. The proposed legislation which many, including this author, had recommended, sought to strengthen the hand of law enforcement and also provide for protective services for the abused spouse.

A joint legislative task force was formed which recommended legislation designed to achieve these goals. In 1978, the Michigan legislature passed these bills, and they were signed into law by Governor William Milliken. There are two distinct pieces of legislation, but since they thoroughly complement each other, they are always considered together.

The police-related issues of these laws will be discussed first. First, police officers are empowered to make arrests for misdemeanors not committed in their presence in spouse abuse cases. Previously, the officer would often be required to leave the victim in a continuing dangerous situation, lacking the power to arrest or the ability to defuse the situation. Second, a spouse abuse protective order for the first time made it a criminal offense to disobey the terms of the injunction. Heretofore, such violation was only civil contempt, and the officer could not arrest without a warrant for such violation. This law was amended in 1979 to permit extension of its protection to unmarried cohabitants, and even those married women not filing for divorce. Third, the law required all police agencies to report spouse abuse to the Michigan State Police so that a data base could be begun.

On the nonpolice side, the legislation created a Domestic Violence Prevention and Treatment Board. This board was empowered to expend state funds to establish and continue operating domestic violence shelters to house such victims. In addition, the board was charged with the responsibility for public awareness and education programs, as well as programs designed for the prevention and treatment of domestic violence.

The board now funds, in whole or in part, thirty-one shelter programs, four assailant counseling programs, a statewide toll-free number for referral and information, as well as a resource library and a media campaign. The latter features television and radio spots and a documentary film called "Appearances." In addition, the board conducts seminars and training programs for shelter personnel and assists in such programs for a wide range of professional groups, such as law enforcement, legal officers, courts, and medical personnel.

The author has been pleased to serve as chairperson since the inception of the Domestic Violence Prevention and Treatment Board. Unfortunately, the needs of battered women for shelters have severely hampered efforts in the public education, prevention, and treatment responsibilities of the board; these latter have suffered the inevitable setting of priorities inherent in the need to provide immediate protection and assistance to women most in need. These shelter programs offer an invaluable resource to police officers and professionals who generally encounter cases of domestic violence.

INTERFACE WITH NURSING

It is commonly thought that the first person to come into direct contact with the victim of domestic violence is the police officer. In fact, this is only partially true. The Wilt and Bannon study documented that at least 50 percent of all known domestic violence cases required medical treatment of some nature. It should also be recalled that only about 50 percent of all domestic violence cases are reported to the police. It is unknown what proportion of these respective ratios overlap, how many of the 50 percent reported to the police are the same as those seen by health care personnel.

It can be said with some confidence, so far there has been no significant effort to attempt to correlate the activities and knowledge of the two disciplines. The author believes, in fact, that medical administrators have openly opposed or resisted medical personnel playing an active role with the police in identifying these cases, cooperating in the obtaining of evidence and preserving it for subsequent presentation in court. It is suspected that potential legal liability for misassessment is not the whole story. Doctor-patient privilege is certainly an issue; there remains a substantial concern for privacy issues. One may be forgiven for also suspecting that it is more a concern with the potential loss of services of staff due to documentation and evidential needs that influences these judgments. A standard emergency room walk-in patient, bearing signs of blunt force trauma or perhaps stab/cutting wounds is a good example here. The patient is often accompanied by a man either actually or presumed to be the spouse. The health care professional seeing this patient is told that the injury occurred in a certain manner. The explanation is often improbable, if not impossible, yet, it is recorded and no further information is sought. In fact, the interview usually continues in the presence and obviously under the influence of the person suspected of causing the injury.

Despite state statutes either requiring or permitting medical personnel to notify local law enforcement agencies of the injury, no such notification, in fact, occurs for the most part. In those cases in which the authorities are notified, the file is so incomplete as to be virtually useless for evidential purposes. It is often impossible to even determine who made the notations on the file. Moreover, when the essential information is on the official medical record, law enforcement personnel will have extreme difficulty in obtaining this evidence without a court order.

Emergency room personnel should be

sensitive to and trained in the dynamics of domestic violence. They should be aware of its symptoms as well as the inherent need for the client to deny its occurrence, because of embarrassment, fear, confusion, or self-doubt. There should be a firm institutional policy of notification of authorities, along with a fixing of responsibilities for such notification. There should be a protocol established which would enable nursing personnel to elicit information regarding the nature of the injury and the patient's description of how the injury occurred. These documents should be separate from the medical records and should be of sufficient number to provide one copy to the law enforcement agency, the institution, and the person reporting.

Clearly from what has been said about staff responsibility, it is obvious that the hospital must take a leading role in establishing the policies empowering and supporting staff to carry out these functions. In addition, hospitals should assure that their assigned social worker staff be thoroughly familiar with spouse abuse. Such staff should be directed to follow up with patients who nursing personnel suspect are victims of domestic violence, but who may deny the cause of their injury initially.

A recent case came to this author's attention which dramatically illustrates the value of high levels of awareness, commitment to serve, and intelligent observation of nursing personnel. A patient was admitted suffering from what was diagnosed as peritonitis due to a ruptured colon. She casually related to one of her nurses that her husband routinely abused her by rendering severe blows to the stomach, sometimes with his feet. She denied, when questioned further by the nurse, that such an assault had preceded this particular admission. However, she did admit continuing distress since the last assault some weeks previously.

The nurse recorded this information and reported it to her supervisors who in turn notified the Michigan State Police. Officers interviewed the patient who denied that she had been beaten or that she had even told the nurse that such was the case.

A short time later, the patient died. The police agency reopened its case and was able to locate additional witnesses who could attest to the patient's having complained to them of the assaults. In fact, other corroborating evidence was obtained. The husband was indicted and awaits trial for second-degree murder. None of this would have been possible had the nurse ignored the patient's claim of prior abuse, failed to record it, or had not made the proper notifications to her supervisors or the police agency.

The most interesting aspect of this case is that the nurse involved and the state police detective who took a personal interest in following up the case, despite the patient's having recanted her story, had both participated in a community seminar on spouse abuse conducted by a local shelter program. Thus, both had had their own consciousnesses raised to the issue as well as their commitment increased to bring that heightened awareness to their respective professional lives.

Like police officers, nursing personnel wear at least two hats—their professional serving, caring hat as a health care professional, and their citizen, member-of-the-community hat as well. It is in this community context that nurses can provide almost as vital a service as in the professional milieu. They are uniquely qualified as sensitive caring professionals to convey to the community at large their knowledge of the magnitude and seriousness of the issue of domestic violence.

It is also true that by training and temperament, most nurses are superbly qualified to serve as volunteer staff in programs offering direct victim services. Yet, the capacity to serve is not limited to health care delivery. As a rule, nurses are excellent role models for women who lack the confidence in themselves necessary to break the vicious circle of dependency, low self-esteem, and feelings of entrapment. Often times, it is in association with such role models that the process of empowerment begins. Nurses generally bring to their professional lives a sense of caring and concern without the need to overpower the patient or to think for her. In other words, they enable the client to do for herself, rather than attempt to do for her.

Nursing personnel can make substantial contributions when they encounter, either professionally or personally, battered women. Some of the items they can address themselves to are briefly outlined here.

First, they should prepare themselves by learning as much as possible about the issue of domestic violence. They then are in a position to understand the concerns of the victim, and what the requirements for successful prosecution may be. Above all, they should be thoroughly aware of all the resources available in the community to the battered woman. In addition, the nurse should be familiar with her legal rights and responsibilities in relation to domestic violence. The nurse has some protection with respect to maintaining confidentiality (see Chapter 14). However, the nurse also has an obligation to report any weapon-related injury or suspicious trauma to the police.

Second, nurses should be aware that prosecution is not always possible. They should know something about the legal requirements and limitations on the prosecutorial possibilities. Nothing confuses the victim more than the well-intentioned but erroneous representation that arrest and prosecution are always possible. Well-intentioned insistence that the victim must prosecute is often counterproductive in that the victim who does not may feel some self-recrimination or even disloyalty if she fails to do so.

Nursing personnel should advise the battered woman that prosecution is probably available and should be pursued if the case meets the legal requirements for an indictment. Such personnel should also become familiar with those procedures in the local jurisdiction for appealing lower-level decisions which adversely affect the client's rights. Often times, such redress is available within the police organization itself. If not, many groups are often available in the community which are designed to act as advocates for the victim. These are legal aid groups, women's justice groups, and so on. Advice on the existence of such groups is always available through shelter programs, legal aid societies, and feminists groups.

Finally, nursing personnel should be familiar with the rudiments of evidence that may be required for presentation in court. As with rape victims, domestic violence victims often have a revulsion to articles associated with the crime itself. They may burn or discard bloody clothing, weapons, or other instruments used in various ways in the assault. It is not uncommon for the woman to shower, and change clothes prior to seeking medical or other professional help. It has even been recorded that the victim will call the police and then clean up, almost thoroughly obliterating all evidence of the assault, prior to opening the door for the responding officers. This behavior is difficult to understand if we do not or cannot appreciate the level of embarrassment the victim feels because she is a victim.

As a general rule, all physical and trace evidence should be preserved. Further, a record of witnesses should be obtained. It is important to specify to the client that a witness need not have actually seen the assault. They may have heard something or witnessed some part of the transaction not directly involved in the assault itself. These witnesses must be identified to the responding officers so their report will reflect this information. All physical evidence including medical diagnosis, X-ray, pictorial representation, and notes of medical observations must also be preserved and reported. Lastly and often most difficult, nursing personnel must make a commitment to testify in court as to their actions and observations. In many cases, this may well entail personal sacrifices in both time and perhaps wages.

Summary

To summarize this chapter briefly, the author would restate the obvious conclusion that domestic violence is a serious national problem. Its costs in emotional and physical pain are astronomical. Costs in real dollars through medical payments, lost wages, and other related costs are incalculable.

The problem is not, as it has been known in the past, a personal problem of the victim. The impact of domestic violence on society at large is so great that it becomes a clear public issue. As a public issue, it demands the efforts of all members of society to ameliorate its effects and attempt to interdict its tragic consequences.

Nursing professionals, in equal measure to the police, share in the responsibility to perform their duties in such a way that the domestic violence victim is not further brutalized by the system designed to protect and serve her. Clearly neither discipline has performed its duties as well as they might have. A major premise of this chapter is to specify nursing and law enforcement obligations, but more importantly to urge a joint, cooperative effort to do all in our power to redress not only past neglect but also future discrimination. Increased contact and exchange between the disciplines of law enforcement and nursing serve as avenues for mutually beneficial collaboration.

The real issue is violence generically. Violence is learned behavior, and it is learned in the home. However, it is differentially learned. That is, violence is appropriate male behavior, but inappropriate female behavior. Thus, one-half of our society is identified at conception as potential, if not probable, victims; the other half is identified as potential, if not probable, assailants—all without regard to who or what they are or to what they achieve or fail to achieve. Such genetic determinism should be repugnant to all of us—male and female alike.

Only through a conscious and combined effort will we ever be able to interdict the intergenerational transmission of violence by men against women.

Author's Note: Throughout this chapter, I have used the masculine "he" when referring to police officers. This was not just a sexist convention or a design to economize on energy and space. It was done self-consciously to point out to the reader that until the last four or five years, policing was almost solely a male-dominated discipline. The few "policewomen" there were did not work in patrol, thus did not respond to domestic violence calls.

It is far too soon to tell but who knows, perhaps neither this chapter or this text would have been necessary if in fact women had not been systematically excluded from patrolling our nation's cities in the past.

Chapter 12

1. James Bannon and Marie Wilt, *Domestic Violence and the Police: Studies in Detroit and Kansas City* (unpublished report for the Police Foundation, 1977).

2. Faith McNulty, *The Burning Bed* (Harcourt Brace & Jovanovich, 1980).

3. The citation is for the original trial as the case was not appealed.

4. Sue E. Eisenberg and Patricia Micklow, *The Assaulted Wife: "Catch 22" Revisited* (Ann Arbor: University of Michigan Law School, 1974).

5. *The Function of the Police in Crises Intervention and Conflict Management, A Training Guide* (Washington, D.C., National Criminal Justice Association, 1974).

The Nurse and the Police: Dealing with Abused Children

Isaiah McKinnon

Police are on the side of the victim perhaps more than any other professional group. They are the one solid group of professionals who see case after case of what happens to victims as they go through the legal process.[1]

The role of law enforcement in cases of child abuse and neglect begins with a report or suspicion of child maltreatment and ends with the securing of safety for the child. During the course of any case of child abuse and/or neglect, the police officer may be called upon to investigate suspected child injury, support other professionals as they investigate child welfare, or facilitate the attainment of health care for the maltreated child. The goal of preventing child abuse and/or neglect at every level is common to both law enforcement and nursing. The purpose of this chapter is to describe the role and responsibilities of law enforcement in cases of suspected or actual child maltreatment. In addition, the interface with nursing will be discussed so as to increase the sensitivity of both disciplines, law enforcement and nursing, to each other and facilitate a cooperative effort in the prevention of child maltreatment.

OVERVIEW

Generally, society believes that law enforcement officers' emotional responses to crimes become hardened due to the nature of their work. However, a problem such as child abuse and neglect raises the wrath of private citizens and the police alike when unfortunate defenseless children are subject to vicious beatings and cruel treatment. Child abuse is not exclusive to any particular geographic area, but is prevalent in many cities throughout the country. As evidenced in the national media, every ethnic, professional, and social group in the United States has been affected in some way by this crime.

There is no denying that young children of all ages are abused daily by parents or other family members. The child's body may be a montage of bruises and his or her buttocks may be permanently scarred as the result of numerous cigarette burns because the child wet his or her pants or could not stop crying, and yet it is possible that the child still loves the abusers.

The actual incidence of child abuse and neglect is difficult to ascertain as discussed in previous chapters (see Chapter 5). In Detroit, Michigan, the Detroit Police Department and the Detroit Department of Social Services keep various records of the cases of child abuse and neglect within the city. The total number of cases acted upon in an official capacity by the Detroit Police Department from 1979 through 1981 were as follows:

1979	647	Assault
	705	Neglect
1980	656	Assault
	587	Neglect

1981   573   Assault
        465   Neglect

The total number of children who die as a result of abuse or neglect in Detroit is not known. Procedures to increase the statistics collected and available on abused and neglected children in Detroit are currently being implemented.

DEFINITION OF CHILD ABUSE AND NEGLECT

To assist in identifying the instances of child abuse and neglect, law enforcement uses the following statutory definitions:[2]

Child: Means a person under eighteen years of age.

Child Abuse: Means harm or threatened harm to a child's health or welfare by a person responsible for the child's health or welfare which occurs through non-accidental physical or mental injury, sexual abuse, or maltreatment.

Child neglect: Means harm to a child's health or welfare which occurs through negligent treatment, including the failure to provide adequate food, clothing, shelter, or medical care.

VARIATIONS OF DEFINITIONS

According to the National Center on Child Abuse and Neglect's manual titled *The Role of Law Enforcement in the Prevention and Treatment of Child Abuse and Neglect* (1979),[3]

States and communities have a variety of definitions of child abuse and neglect; some are found in laws, some are found in procedures, and some are found in the informal practices of those agencies assigned to implement laws concerning child abuse and neglect.

It is important that nurses become familiar with the various formal definitions used by law enforcement officers in their community, which can be found in:[4]

Criminal Law Definition: Those forms of child abuse and neglect which are criminally punishable.

Juvenile Court Act: Those forms of child abuse and neglect defined in legislation which authorizes the court to require child protective services and, when necessary, remove children from their parents.

Reporting Law Definition: Those forms of known or suspected child abuse and neglect which require reporting by some persons and permit reporting by others. These reports activate the child protective process which can result in either juvenile court or criminal court action.

REPORTING CHILD ABUSE AND NEGLECT

It is a mandate in all states that professionals who are in contact with child abuse and neglect must report such crimes. Included in this mandate are law enforcement officers, educators, social workers, and health care personnel. It is important to note that in the reporting of "suspected" child abuse, no state requires the person reporting the alleged abuses to have absolute proof. The reporting person need not be certain, but should have "reasonable cause to believe."[5]

PROTECTIVE SERVICES

The Child Protection Law of Michigan Act No. 238, Public Acts No. 238, Public Acts of 1975,[6] defines child abuse and neglect as follows: Child abuse means harm or threatened harm to a child's health or welfare by a person responsible for the child's health or welfare which occurs through non-accidental physical or mental injury, sexual abuse, or maltreatment. Child neglect means harm to a child's welfare by a person responsible for the child's health or welfare which occurs through negligent treatment, including the failure to provide adequate food, clothing, shelter, or medical care. Protective services are social agencies designed to assure that children are protected from physical or emotional harm due to parental abuse, neglect, or exploitation, and to assist parents or guardians to function appropriately in providing the necessary care for their children.[7]

According to the Michigan Department of Social Services, protective services are necessary because children have a basic right to care, guidance, protection, and love required for normal health, growth, and development, and there is a need to protect these rights. Parents, when able, have a basic responsibility to provide their children with love, care, guidance, and protection—either through their own efforts or through the use of available community resources.

In Michigan, as in many states, the Department of Social Services is authorized by law to study and act upon reports of abuse, neglect, or exploitation of children. On the basis of their analysis, appropriate social services are provided to children, parents, or guardians to assure that any behavior or situation contributing to child maltreatment is corrected and/or that the child is otherwise protected.[8] Law enforcement officers, like other professionals who have as their concern the welfare of children, work closely with protective services.

LAW ENFORCEMENT INVOLVEMENT

There are many reasons for the involvement of police personnel in the treatment and prevention of child abuse and neglect. Most obvious is the fact that the police officers are most accessible to the community as a result of their twenty-four-hour, seven-day-a-week responsibilities. Second, there are the aforementioned legal and professional mandates that require law enforcement involvement.

Nationally, police have the initial responsibility for the investigation of circumstances involving the violation of law, prevention of crime, and preservation of peace. In addition, as will be explained in detail later, in many states, law enforcement personnel may also take into custody any child the officer feels is in need of assistance.

According to Sergeant David Mays, commanding officer of the Detroit Police Child Abuse Unit, the police officer has three basic responsibilities when handling child abuse and neglect cases:

1. A duty to report all suspected cases.

2. A duty to investigate all suspected cases.

3. A duty to provide emergency services to protect the child.[9]

If there is any suspicious conduct on the part of the parents or guardians or evidence of noticeable injuries, or scars (old or new) on the body of the child, the officer would have reasonable cause to enter the premises, forcibly if necessary, to protect the life and/or welfare of the child.

THE PATROL OFFICER

Traditionally the patrol force has been the backbone of the police department. The patrol officer is the first line of defense in the overwhelming majority of criminal acts, and this cannot be overemphasized in the protection of battered, defenseless children. Most importantly, in most states police officers are the only persons who can remove children from a location and place them in protective custody without a court order. In Michigan the statutory authority to remove a child from the home is as follows:

> Any municipal police officer, sheriff or deputy sheriff or state police officer, county agent or probation officer of any court of record may, without the order of the court, immediately take into custody any child who is found violating any law or ordinance or whose surroundings are such as to endanger his health, morals or welfare. Whenever any such officer or county agent takes a child coming within the provisions of this chapter into custody, he shall forthwith notify the parents or parent, guardian or custodian, if they can be found within the county. While awaiting the arrival of the parent or parents, guardian or custodian, no child under the age of 17 years taken into custody under the provisions of this chapter shall be held in any detention facility unless such child be completely isolated so as to prevent any *verbal, visual,* or *physical contact with any adult* prisoner. Unless the child requires immediate detention as hereinafter provided, the arresting officer shall accept the written promise of said parent or parents, guardian or custodian to bring the child to the court at a time fixed therein. Thereupon such child shall be released to the custody of said parent or parents, guardian or custodian.[10]

Under normal circumstances, before entering the domicile of any citizen the police must ask permission or possess a warrant or probable cause to arrest or believe that a crime is in the process or has been committed. More importantly, officers can usually enter a home if an emergency situation arises such as cries for help or if there is imminent danger to a citizen, other officers, or themselves. Traditionally, in Michigan, when dealing with family dispute calls the police officer does not have the right to enter a home without consent, a warrant, or probable cause to arrest.[11] However, if given the knowledge through informed sources that there exists the possibility of some kind of child abuse at a given address, the officer has a duty to conduct a preliminary investigation. This is not to imply that an officer has the right to enter a premises on "mere suspicion,"[12] which in fact is to say he cannot forcibly enter any premises to investigate legally without consent. In reality, the officer usually would conduct a superficial investigation, asking questions and attempting to see the child to determine the parent's and child's reactions and conditions.

INVESTIGATION

The primary concern of the investigating officer is the protection of the child. In doing so the investigator must determine whether:

1. The child is or has been abused;
2. The child is in danger at home;
3. Or if the officer must take immediate action to ensure the safety of the child.

Upon completion of these immediate concerns, the investigator must determine whether further police action is necessary and whether there is need for removal of the child from the home or involvement by protective services.

The traditional police role in child abuse cases involves the receipt of a report, an investigation, possible detainment, and prosecution. The involvement by police or child welfare personnel or the laying of charges typically requires the kind of justification observed in blatant and readily identifiable physical abuse cases.

In recent years, however, law enforcement agencies have been reexamining their responsibilities in the area of child protection. Police officers are becoming more sensitized to the problem. First, in child abuse situations most local police departments have improved their services in child advocacy, and in cases of child sexual abuse, the enlightened department will have a special team or unit of officers trained to make contact with the victim and family.

In Detroit, reports to the police department of child abuse and/or neglect are initially investigated by the uniformed officer who patrols the area. Investigative techniques vary with individual officers; however, once the officer is inside the house, he will usually quickly isolate the child and question him or her as to the nature and origin of the bruises or injuries. Second, the officer will do a thorough visual inspection of the child for injuries, including possible broken bones. Often it is extremely difficult for officers or other laypersons to detect nonvisible injuries because abuse may or may not be readily identifiable.

In those cases in which the patrol officer identifies or suspects non-sexual child maltreatment both the Detroit Police Child Abuse Unit and Detroit Child Protective Services are contacted. Sexual abuse is handled somewhat differently in Detroit and will be discussed in a separate section. The uniformed officer then either remains with the child until members of the Detroit Child Abuse Unit arrive or takes the child to a location, often an emergency room, designated by Child Protective Services.

The Detroit Police Child Abuse Unit is composed of a group of seven specially trained, sworn police personnel who handle only child abuse and neglect cases. These officers, as with the initially investigating patrol officer, work very closely with Detroit Child Protective Service workers in the investigation of each case of child abuse and neglect.

In most instances, the investigation into child abuse cases is difficult. A parent, or partner will often consciously refuse to provide corroborating information for the investigation in an effort to protect the abusive adult. Often, however, the parents' account of the child's injury will conflict not only with the nature of the child's injury, but also with the other partner's story.

Detroit police officers are instructed, as are most officers investigating child abuse cases, to take careful notice of the home and surrounding area. This may include pictures of the bruises sustained by the child, pictures of the child's living area, and pictures of other items of possible evidence. In addition, officers routinely will canvass the neighborhood for possible witnesses who had been strongly silent before, but will usually come forward once some official action is initiated.

The guidelines suggested in the *Role of Law Enforcement in the Prevention and Treatment of Child Abuse and Neglect* are useful in understanding the responsibilities and approach to child abuse and neglect of the specially trained police officer.[13]

> At the very beginning of the interview, the interviewer must try to determine the emotional state of the child. Is fear, hatred, defiance, shock, confusion, love, jealousy, or anger apparent? Is the child ready to tell the truth, lie, or exaggerate?
>
> The interviewers should attempt to gain the child's confidence. The interview should be conducted on a friend-to-friend basis rather than as police officer to child.
>
> The investigator should not appear to take sides against the parents. Under no circumstances should the interviewer indicate horror, disgust, anger, or disapproval of parents, child, or the situation. Children will often become defensive if they feel outsiders are critical of their parents, even if they feel the same way.
>
> The interview should be conducted in language the child clearly understands. Particularly in cases of sexual abuse, the officer should accept and use whatever terms of genitals and sexual acts the child uses while also asking for clarification and eliciting specific information regarding what has occurred.
>
> Children should be permitted to tell about incidents in their own way. They should not be pressed for details they may be unwilling or unable to give. The officer should limit questions to necessary information and should use open-ended questions whenever possible. Younger children may be more at ease if the situation is discussed in terms of fantasy.
>
> The interview should include a discussion of what will happen next and how the officer will use the information the child has given.
>
> If the child is an adolescent and the officer feels a "person in need of supervision" petition or a similar order will be necessary, the officer should so inform the child. The officer should also inform adolescents of their Miranda Rights.

SEXUAL ABUSE

At the time of the initial investigation by a patrol officer, if it is suspected or determined that sexual abuse has taken place, in Detroit, the Sex Crimes Unit and Child Protective Services are contacted. The Sex Crimes Unit in Detroit is composed of thirty-five to forty sworn officers who handle only sex crime cases. A review of research conducted by this author in the area of special police department sexual-assault units presents both current practices in Detroit and other large cities across the country.

In 1981 this author conducted a study to evaluate police training structures and procedures in the investigation of sexual-assault cases in U.S. cities with populations of 500,000 or more. Of the police departments in the twenty-seven most populous U.S. cities, twenty responded by completing a forty-seven-item questionnaire developed for the study. The results revealed the inconsistent, weak, and poor status of sexual-assault investigation, staff training, and record keeping in the police departments in the major cities of the United States.[14]

The majority of cities (nineteen) reported that their police departments had a unit or section that specialized in sexual-assault investigations. These units are largely composed of white males (65 percent) of the rank of police officer (63 percent). Of the twelve who responded to the question, ten departments reported that their special unit personnel receive some type of training in child sexual abuse. The number of hours of training in sexual assault varied from 4 hours in Baltimore, Maryland, to 480 hours in Kansas City, Missouri. The type of training also varied greatly. Only nine departments reported including training in crisis intervention, investigative techniques, victimology, and psychology of the victim.

The Detroit Police Department Sex Crimes Unit is composed of approximately equal numbers of male and female officers who usually work in two-person teams along with an evidence technician. The specialized unit is in operation twenty-four hours per day. Upon arrival at the home, or at police headquarters, the Sex Crimes Unit officers interview both the involved child and the adult. On some occasions the child is taken directly to a hospital emergency room and interviewed at that time. Extensive evidence is gathered at the home and emergency room.

INTERFACE WITH NURSING

The most likely time of collaboration between nursing and law enforcement professionals is when the child arrives at the hospital emergency room. The special unit or patrol officer usually brings the child into the health care facility as directed by child protective services. The investigating officers will have recorded the parents' story as to how the child received the injuries and relay it to the examining health care provider who may conclude that the injuries did in fact occur in the manner as stated.

It is also possible that physical examination will corroborate the law enforcement officers' suspicions that child abuse and neglect did occur. Under Section 6 of the Michigan Child Protection Law which is similar to that in many states, physicians are required to take certain actions.

> If a child suspected of being abused or neglected is admitted to a hospital or brought to a hospital for out-patient services and the attending physician determines that the release of the child would endanger the child's health or welfare, the attending physician shall notify the person in charge of the department. The person in charge may detain the child in temporary custody until the next regular business day of the probate court, at which time the probate court shall order the child detained in the hospital or in some other suitable place pending preliminary hearing. . . . [15]

The nurse can at all times be the advocate of a child. Where physician consent for admission to the hospital is necessary, the nurse can provide invaluable information and assistance if she is knowledgeable about the law and has already collaborated with the accompanying officer. The nurse's knowledge of child abuse and neglect, and ability to relate the gathered evidence to the larger issue of general child welfare, can increase the ease with which a child may appropriately be admitted to the hospital pending hearing.

At the time of contact at the hospital emergency room, the officer and nurse are in a sense exchanging responsibilities. The job of law enforcement personnel is to respond to reports of child abuse and neglect, investigate, and provide emergency services to protect the child. It is not the responsibility of the involved officer to stay with the child once emergency services have been secured. Instead, the officer must return to his or her duties in the community. Yet, the officer may feel very protective of the mistreated child and at the same time have the job of leaving the child with strangers, the health care professionals.

The nurse is also concerned about the welfare of the child. It is a great source of relief to the involved officer to see that the maltreated child is receiving immediate care and comfort. The nurse can be of greatest assistance by first quickly obtaining the pertinent information gathered by the officer accompanying the child. Then the nurse will ease the process of the officer leaving the child if she in some way lets the officer know that she is equally interested in the child and will secure the best possible care. The nurse can do this by stating to the officer that she understands the nature of his or her concern and briefly outlining what will happen to the child in the hospital. The officer can then be assured that the responsibility for the child has been transferred, and concerned care will be provided. The officer is then free to return to other duties in the community for which he or she is best trained.

The nurse in the community may also have reason to call upon assistance from law enforcement. The nurse, as any person, may call law enforcement if she suspects child abuse and/or neglect. For example, the nurse who suspects child maltreatment and needs assistance in a home visit may call upon law enforcement officers to accompany her. Child protective services frequently work with law enforcement in this fashion.

Upon completion of the initial investigation, removal of the child from the home, and verification that child abuse did in fact occur, the officer will, as appropriate, deliver the child to the department of social services which will file a petition to declare the child a ward of the juvenile court.

THE DETECTION OF CHILD ABUSE

With special training, police officers are able to identify a particular type of child abuse or neglect by recognizing physical and behavioral indicators in the child, and attitudinal indicators by the parents.

Trained officers are aware that the child abuse happens everywhere, in poor, middle-class, as well as well-to-do homes. It occurs in rural areas, suburbs, and in cities, and can involve one or both parents.

The law enforcement officer's initial response to child abuse and neglect cases is critical. The officer is called upon to make favorable impressions on all parties involved and evaluate the situation objectively.

GATHERING EVIDENCE

All aspects of the evidence-gathering procedures are important. They include physical, verbal, and photographic evidence as well as the officer's own observations. Additionally, this is one of the few instances in which hearsay "evidence," which can be submitted to the protective services agency, can be of major value in the decision of child placement, or subsequent court actions.[16]

In each area of evidence gathering, the nurse can assist the law enforcement officers as the situation allows. The interview of parents and child can be facilitated through the nurse's knowledge of growth, development, and crisis intervention. In the situation in which the law enforcement officer is gathering specific details of evidence, the nurse can serve as both a collaborator and as support to the family members.

Physical

Physical evidence includes the collection of all objective evidence involving any aspect of the suspected child abuse and neglect. This is done immediately and includes inspection of the child for signs particularly suggestive of child abuse and neglect (see Chapter 10). Specially trained officers know the conditions and jurisdictions requiring search warrants prior to any action.

Verbal

Verbal evidence include all utterances or statements made to or in the presence of the investigating officers. Hearsay evidence would be very prevalent in this area (see Chapter 15).

Photographic

Photographic evidence is perhaps the best means of presenting the severity of the abuse and neglect problem to the courts. These photographs are taken as soon as possible and should be in color to present the true life image.

Officer's Observations

Officer's evidence include the general condition of the home, physical condition of the child, parent's behavior, and reaction to the officer.

ARREST

The position of most progressive police departments is that arrest and prosecution for child abuse and neglect are not the best means of dealing with the abusive parent. These departments are of the opinion that the desired result is to protect the child from further harm and assist the adults in becoming better parents rather than punish a parent or separate a family. Assistance in this area can take several forms, such as improved services for families, homemaking services, employment counseling, and an attempt by all agencies involved to have a positive influence on the family. Nursing has always played a valuable role in the process of intervention with violent families. The methods of nursing intervention are discussed in detail in Chapter 10.

Summary

There is a need for early recognition of the abused or neglected child for the purpose of reducing or stopping the frequency of the acts. To date the focus has dealt with instances of child abuse and neglect after the fact. The goal of both law enforcement and nursing is to prevent abuse and neglect from happening. Recognition and identification of family problems as potential indicators of abuse and the alleviation of these problems aid in the prevention of these acts.

It is important for law enforcement agencies to be strong advocates for the prevention of abuse and neglect. This advocacy should be expressed through education not only of the respective officers, but the community as well. Additionally, departments should survey their departments for needed improvements in the areas of response, planning, and services to community agencies. Lastly, police departments must continue to work collaboratively with other professionals and participate in community awareness programs, explaining their programs and being receptive to newer ideas.

Chapter 13

1. Ann W. Burgess and Lynda L. Holmstrom, *Rape: Crisis and Recovery* (Bowie, Md.: 1979, Robert J. Brady Co., 1979), p. 92.
2. Detroit Police Training and Information Bulletin, Publication no. 78-5 (6 January 1978).
3. National Center on Child Abuse and Neglect, *The Role of Law Enforcement in the Prevention and Treatment of Child Abuse and Neglect* (Denver, Co.: 1979), p. 3.
4. Ibid.
5. Search and Seizure Information obtained in U. S. Supreme Court Case, Spinelli vs. U.S. 393 U.S. 410.89, Supreme Court 583.216. Ed. 2d 637.
6. Act #238, Public Acts of 1975, Section 722.621..722.636, Michigan Compiled Laws.
7. State of Michigan, Department of Social Services, Informational Pamphlet, Publication no. 105.
8. Ibid.
9. Personal interview, Sergeant David Mays, Commanding Officer, Detroit Police Child Abuse Unit, 21 September 1982.
10. Michigan Compiled Laws Ann. 712A.14.
11. See note 5 above.
12. Ibid.
13. *Role of Law Enforcement in the Prevention and Treatment of Child Abuse and Neglect.*
14. Isaiah McKinnon, "An Evaluation of Police Training Structures and Procedures in the Investigation of Sexual-Assault Cases in United States Cities with Populations of 500,000 or More" (unpublished dissertation, Michigan State University, 1981).
15. See note 10 above.
16. Role of Law Enforcement in the Prevention and Treatment of Child Abuse and Neglect.

The Nurse
and the Legal System:
Dealing with Abused Women

William O. Humphreys

14

THE LEGAL CONCEPT OF WIFE ABUSE

The concept of abuse of married women,[1] and the equitable handling of such cases, has been hampered by the convoluted thinking that appears to have prevailed in American legal thinking since its conception. This thinking has been based on the false premise that women are inherently unequal, and, as a result, must be placed under the authority of the men they marry—much as a child is under the authority of a parent. Indeed, as to her personal and property rights, the very legal existence of the wife was regarded as suspended for the duration of the marriage and merged into that of the husband.[2]

Because of this so-called merging of the husband and wife, the right of the husband to discipline his wife with physical force was tacitly accepted by society:

> For as he is to answer for her misbehavior, the law thought it reasonable to intrust him with this power of restraining her, by domestic chastisement, in the same moderation that a man is allowed to correct his apprentices or children; for whom the master or parent is also liable in some cases to answer. But this power of correction was confined within reasonable bounds, and the husband was prohibited from using any violence to his wife. . . .[3]

Despite this concept of the husband as a benevolent despot, the early English and American courts were filled with cases of husbands assaulting their wives,[4] and it was not until the late nineteenth century that the courts began to expressly repudiate the concept of the merging of interests.[5]

Legislatures began passing what came to be known as Married Womens Acts, or Emancipation Acts, about 1844. These acts were designed to secure to a married woman a separate legal identity, and a separate legal estate in her own property.[6] Because these acts pertained to property, however, many courts refused, and still refuse, to allow a spouse to maintain a civil action against the other for a personal injury.[7]

Thus an unsatisfactory situation presents itself to the legal community. Although a definition of assault and identification of the factors which determine the degree of the crime, have been a relatively easy legislative task,[8] no jurisdiction has promulgated a statutory defense based on the fact that the victim was only a spouse. Yet the legal profession, reflecting the views of society, has established a privileged status for domestic attackers which has been informally accepted by police, prosecutors, and judges in civil as well as criminal matters.[9]

The purpose of this chapter is to shed light on these legal aspects of the abuse of female partners. The civil and criminal avenues of the law are examined. Further, the actual recourses available to battered women are described. Finally, the interface of nursing and the legal system are addressed, with special attention to nurses' responsibilities to the victims and in the courtroom.

THE LAWS AND THE ABUSED WOMAN

A major complication in the effective disposition of wife abuse offenses is that these cases may arise under either the criminal or civil statutes, or both. The intentional infliction of physical injuries is generally considered a crime against society.[10] However, wife assault offenses are overwhelmingly disposed of in civil courts, primarily in divorce proceedings.[11] The reasoning for this is manyfold, but it would appear that the beliefs of domestic chastisement and the fiction of a woman's place are now cloaked in legal theories such as a constitutional right of privacy and claims of victim consent or noble, but misguided, attempts of preserving the family unit. Indeed, it would appear that courts go to great lengths to avoid legal intervention and at the same time do not condone the violence.

Civil Proceedings

In civil proceedings, a prime example of these legal acrobatics, and one which bears directly on the problem of wife abuse, is what is known as the interspousal immunity doctrine.[12] This doctrine set forth the proposition that a willful or negligent tort committed by one spouse against the other does *not* give rise to a cause of action in favor of the injured spouse.[13] Although the interspousal immunity doctrine gives the illusion of equal application, the respective roles of husband and wife have made the wife a far more likely victim of abuse than the husband (see Chapter 4).

It is therefore a sad commentary that so far as torts against the person (for example, assault, battery, and false imprisonment) are concerned, approximately one-half of the jurisdictions which have considered this question still refuse to permit any action between the spouses.[14] This is true even though the tort was committed and the action was begun before the marriage of the parties, or even when the action is brought after the marriage relation has been terminated.[15]

The main reasoning behind these opinions is the mistaken belief that each spouse has sufficient recourse through the criminal or divorce laws. This belief is simply untrue; it neither compensates for the damage done, nor covers all the torts which may be committed.[16]

Criminal Law

The theory of a constitutional right of privacy was first put forth in the criminal law by a North Carolina court in the case of *State v. Rhoades*[17] stating:

> However great are the evils of ill temper, quarrels and even personal conflicts inflicting only temporary pain, they are not comparable with the evils which would result from raising the curtain, and exposing to the public curiosity and criticism. . . . the bed chamber.

With these statements, the court invoked a right of privacy for the battering spouse which precluded the victim's use of the assault laws. This reasoning presents the unacceptable proposition of a "criminal assault" being viewed as a social problem or a domestic matter between the husband and wife.[18]

Yet no jurisdiction has chosen to exempt domestic assaults from the scrutiny of the criminal law.[19] An assault is not a mere "family quarrel." The incidents of domestic violence commonly result in serious physical injury or death for the woman,[20] and statistics indicate that 40 percent of all homicides involved interspousal killing.[21] Further weaknesses in this argument are pointed out by more recent court holdings that the right of privacy shields acts between two individuals only when both consent,[22] and when such acts do not impair any other person's safety and health.[23] For example, a husband may not prevent his wife from obtaining a legal abortion. A vision of a husband kicking or beating his wife with his fist certainly does not appear to be consistent with these holdings.

Thus, it is clear that although the right to a private family life may be a fundamental right, the courts have made it clear that it does not extend to the point of allowing one family member the authority of an overseer as to the others.[24]

In keeping with these, now somewhat archaic, legal views of the inviolate "family unit," and the wife as property, is the belief that a husband is incapable of raping his wife. This so-called spousal exemption is the result of some rather obscure reasoning by the courts.

It is believed that by consenting to marriage, a woman forges a *contract* which makes her body available to her husband at any time.[25] Therefore, in many states all the husband must do to legitimize his assault is to combine it with rape.

Further reasoning puts forth the belief that the possibility of false charges (in order to exact revenge or gain an advantage in property settlements) are more likely when the victim is the wife. Finally, the standard "family unit" argument is presented in the strange context of "jeopardizing" a marriage by thrusting the prospect of criminal sanctions into the ongoing process of adjustment in the marital relationship.[26]

These arguments require a certain myopia about the facts. There is some question about the validity of a contract which may be enforced by whatever means one party chooses, including violence. False charges may be filed in connection with any crime, and the judicial system deals with it daily. The difference is simply that it is a wife bringing the charges. The final argument presumes that the forcible rape of a wife is a matter which the wife can adjust to, and that such a relationship is capable of being saved at all.[27]

This type of reasoning, unfortunately, is seen throughout the judicial system as criminal charges against the husband are dropped under the pretext that the family would be denied the services of its main support.

This belief came about with the rise of mercantilism and the industrial revolution. This "revolution" signaled the demarcation of the economic and domestic spheres of life, in which domestic work, and therefore the domestic worker, were devalued.[28] This separation resulted not only in the extreme isolation and segregation of women, but also in their growing economic dependency on their mates.

This argument ignores the point that the criminal law is not so inflexible as to make its only remedy a jail sentence. As will be discussed later, an array of possible alternatives are available, ranging from peace bonds to treatment agencies. The critical point here, however, is that by the time law enforcement agencies are notified, the wife who seeks their protection has opted for health and safety regardless of the economic and societal risks.

THE ABUSED WIFE IN THE LEGAL SYSTEM

Aside from the many substantive law hurdles encountered by the abused wife, there may be a seemingly endless array of procedural obstacles to prevent a successful prosecution of the husband. Statistics indicate that only 2.7 percent of the women seeking to file complaints against their husbands actually succeed.[29] What are the reasons for this seemingly incredible attrition rate?

Prosecutors often view the problem of wife abuse as primarily a civil and personal matter, and therefore, out of their jurisdiction.[30] The prosecutor should view a case in terms of its legal viability and be concerned with the availability of the complainant, other witnesses, or tangible evidence of the crime.[31] However, in wife abuse cases, the focus is on whether the victimized wife is perceived as a "worthy victim" deserving of both the prosecutor's and the court's efforts.

It is fairly common knowledge that a prosecutor has considerable leverage in deciding whether or not to exercise his or her authority in any given case. Thus, a "worthy victim" must demonstrate that she did not deserve to be attacked and that in the face of her economic and physical difficulties, she will pursue the complaint against the husband.[32] To impress upon the prosecutor her seriousness to follow through on prosecution, an assaulted wife must often meet a so-called divorce test.[33] This test demonstrates her willingness to institute divorce proceedings against her husband.

It is this willingness to follow through that is the prosecutor's main concern, for the biggest problem reported in such cases is that victims of abuse who initially express interest in filing charges change their minds by the time of the arraignment or preliminary hearing.[34]

Assaulted wives drop charges or fail to show up in court for numerous reasons, most relating to prosecutorial attitudes. Many drop charges because they do not understand the criminal justice system and receive little or no information from the prosecutor about the steps in the process, or the likely consequences.[35]

The abused wife will also discover that filing charges and pursuing a complaint proves to be a tedious and time-consuming proposition. The woman finds that much work time will be lost, and that childcare would have to be arranged for a sometimes seemingly endless number of court appearances.

The simple fact is that family violence cases are difficult to prosecute:

> Often there are no witnesses to battering incidents except perhaps the children of the parties. There may be little or no evidence of the crime charged, because the victim did not get immediate medical attention and because bruises may have disappeared by the time the victim goes to court. Police reports are often inadequate or nonexistent.[36]

These reasons, as well as a lack of prestige in prosecuting these types of cases, and a desire to keep the overwhelming case load of most offices down, encourage a program that is geared toward discouraging the battered woman from pursuing her complaint. The prosecutor's attitude of "get rid of the complaint" may be based not on the seriousness of the injury inflicted or the possibility of recurrence, but on the likelihood of conviction and the benefit to the prosecutor's career.[37]

NEW BELIEFS, BETTER UNDERSTANDINGS

The legal system of the United States is based upon the simple premise that for every legal wrong there is a corresponding legal remedy. As has been pointed out, however, this has not always been true when the legal wrong is committed against one's own spouse.

In the last decade, as public awareness of the violence within the family has grown, legal remedies for abused wives have been studied, and new strategies for effective law-related prevention have been developed and implemented.

New laws, whether legislatively or judicially enacted, cannot by themselves change attitudes about the problem of domestic violence. What they do is provide the tools that battered women, and their advocates, can use to promote more effective court response and better services for violent families.[38]

Less than a decade ago, what was known as a peace bond was the most common sanction used in cases of wife abuse. A peace bond is a hybrid of the civil and criminal laws in that it is primarily a civil action which may carry the threat of a penal or financial penalty.[39] Although there is no statutory basis for the peace bond—reflecting the judicial belief that wife abuse is a civil or domestic matter—it gained acceptance as the remedy most appropriate for such "domestic affairs." Basically, the peace bond amounts to a judicial threat which may be exercised to control the future behavior of the assailant husband.[40]

There is some disagreement among legal observers as to the effectiveness of the peace bond, but many believe the device to be unenforceable and "a complete sham . . . (in which) the complainant and assailant are deceived into thinking it is enforceable."[41]

In response to these beliefs, the last five years have seen the passage of extensive legislation aimed directly at domestic violence. These laws have created specific remedies for domestic abuse and impose duties on courts that handle family violence cases.[42]

Civil

Possibly the most successful of these is the Protection Order Laws.[43] These orders differ from peace bonds in that they allow the court great flexibility, and the time required for enactment is much less. The laws vary widely from state to state; however, most allow the court to order an abuser to move out of a residence shared with a victim. This is arguably the most important form of relief available; it gives the abused woman an enforceable right to be safe in the home and establishes that the abuser rather than the victim should bear the burden of finding another residence.[44]

The court may order the husband to refrain from abuse of or contact with the victim, to pay support, restitution, or attorney's fees, and may restrict the use or disposition of personal property. The best of these laws and those operable in at least thirty-four states allow for a temporary protection order to be issued *ex parte*. That is, they may be issued almost immediately without the presence of the abusing party. Of course, a full hearing with both parties present is required before this order becomes permanent, but this legislation gives the battered woman the immediate protection which is so necessary.

Criminal Law

As has been stated previously, wife abuse was not traditionally treated as a crime. Thus, although every state has laws imposing criminal penalties for assault, battery, rape, burglary, and kidnapping, these laws often go unenforced if the suspect is a spouse and the damage inflicted is not too severe.[45]

> The benevolent non-arrest policy might be satisfactory in some instances if the husband/assailant responded to leniency and kindness by resolving never to resort to violence again. Unfortunately, the man is more apt to see this lenience as reinforcement for his abusive behavior. He quickly learns that lesser injuries, like a broken nose, are tolerated by the system and the probability of his being taken into custody is remote.[46]

This belief by the assailant is related to the fact that a police officer can make an arrest for felonies committed out of his or her presence, but must witness a misdemeanor being committed to make the arrest. The nature of most wife abuse cases would lead an officer to approach them from a misdeameanor perspective and avoid an arrest. However, many jurisdictions have now made spouse abuse a separate *felony* giving the officer greater flexibility in his or her response. The California Supreme Court has stated that

> (most interspousal attacks) are usually accomplished with fists and kicking. . . .The severity of the injuries are therefore not always capable of instant diagnosis. . . . An officer responding to a wifebeating case would ordinarily, in the exercise of caution and to avoid a charge of false arrest, only arrest the husband under the provisions of. . . . (the assault law) in extreme cases. Even the infliction upon a wife of considerably traumatic injury would tend to be treated by the arresting officer as a misdemeanor which would produce the consequences of the wife's being left in the home to face possible further aggression. But an officer given the alternative of arresting for a felony under the. . . (spouse abuse law) may do so. . . .[47]

This rethinking and revising of the statutes has removed many inequities. For example, the spousal exemption to rape laws have been removed in ten states. New Jersey's statute now reads, "No actor shall be presumed to be incapable of committing a crime under this chapter because of age or impotency or *marriage to the victim*" (emphasis added).[48] However, there are forty states where this legislative change is still needed.

Perhaps the most significant changes in the criminal law involves not the laws used to prosecute the husband, but those used to defend the wives who protect themselves by using retaliatory violence in response to physical or sexual assault. A recent Washington case[49] indicated that the so-called objective standard of "the reasonable man" in determining self-defense combined with jury instructions framed in the masculine gender, inherently precludes a jury from considering a woman's perspective of danger. In essence, the court in this case was stating that the reasonable person standard which was intended to be neutral, has in fact, a disparate impact on female defendants.[50]

This decision, holding that "all facts and circumstances known to the defendant" must be considered is particularly applicable in wife abuse cases. The defendant's attorney is now allowed to present to the jury all the circumstances of the abusive relationship between the woman and the husband. The attorney must convey the situation as perceived by the defendant, and the reasonableness of her fear by educating the judge and jury as to the battering syndrome and its debilitating effects on the victim.[51] This is particularly true if the woman has killed the abusive husband while he was unarmed or unsuspecting. The critical point is that the woman is "entitled to have the jury consider her actions in the light of *her* [emphasis added] own perceptions of the situation, including those perceptions which were the product of our nation's long and unfortunate history of sex discrimination,"[52] particularly with regard to application of the law between spouses.

When one examines the vastness of this country's criminal law system, these changes and understandings may appear almost microscopic. Certainly any improvement in the past system would be a blessing. The major point is that these laws are destroying the tip of an ever-diminishing iceburg of state and federal criminal statutes which are slowly being recognized as unfair and archaic. As public opinion and concern for this situation increases, legislatures will continue to change and improve the law, while the judiciary will exercise its not inconsiderable flexibility in ordering such approaches as pre-conviction probation, referral to treatment agencies, or dismissal after a period of supervised good behavior.[53]

Prosecutor's Response

The public's changing attitude toward the seriousness of wife abuse has caused many prosecutors to reassess their priorities in this regard and more vigorously prosecute these types of cases. New programs designed to aid and inform the battered spouse have been implemented in some of the larger metropolitan areas.[54]

The cornerstone of the criminal law is that the alleged act or omission is not an offense against any individual, but against society as a body.[55] As a consequence of this philosophy, it should not be left up to the battering victim, but instead the prosecutor, as to whether or not a case should be pursued. "By setting a policy that charges will not be dropped at the request of the victim, prosecutors prevent battered women from repeatedly testing their resolve to go to court."[56] Further, the battered woman is able to more completely recognize her role as a *witness* rather than the plaintiff.[57]

By putting the woman in this role, she is much less likely to be the target of intimidation by her mate, who would obviously like the charges dropped.

If she does, however, find herself a likely victim of harassment, prosecutors have the tools available to request that a husband's bail be conditioned on his staying away from the victim and on condition that he not threaten or otherwise intimidate her.[58] Such action should be, and sometimes is, taken routinely by the prosecutor.

Possibly the most beneficial change in policy is the effort now being made to inform and educate the battered woman in regard to the criminal process. As has been previously observed, many victims believe that a criminal conviction will necessarily result in a jail sentence, and therefore, cooperation is difficult to gain from one whose life would be affected by the incarceration almost as much as her assailant's. By educating the victim as to the flexibility possible in sentencing, a prosecutor gains cooperation and becomes able to plea bargain many cases by offering to recommend a sentence in keeping with the victim's objectives.[59]

These programs of information and assistance help prepare a woman for the inevitable problems and limitations of the criminal justice system. The expected hurdles of constant delays, the possibility of acquittal, and numerous court appearances will still be disturbing, but a realistic assessment of the system will better prepare her for the eventual outcome.

These somewhat enlightened programs are certainly a welcome sign for battered women, and a change in prosecutorial attitudes can only have a trickling-down effect throughout the criminal justice system. An improved priority for family violence cases will encourage more assertive police action and provide greater protection in a goal to reduce subsequent violence.[60]

THE NURSE IN THE LEGAL SYSTEM

An attorney views each case he or she handles in terms of its legal viability. That is, the availability of witnesses and the tangible evidence present.

A woman who is battered and seeks medical attention will undoubtedly come into contact with the nursing profession as one of the first neutral parties since the violent episode. Because of this, the nurse is in a unique position to aid the attorney if she takes special note of the injuries and conversations that occur in cases that appear to be a result of battering.

Rules of Evidence

To comprehend this statement fully, a more specific (if incomplete) explanation of the rules of evidence must be given. "Evidence" means testimony, writings, material objects, or other things *presented to the senses* that are offered to prove the existence or nonexistence of fact.[61] There are two fundamental types of evidence. They are direct evidence, sometimes termed "eyewitness" evidence, which proves a proposition directly rather than by inference; and circumstantial evidence which depends on inferences for its relationship to the material issue to be proven.

A witness's testimony based on his or her personal (direct) knowledge of the facts involved is generally admissable while testimony embracing his or her opinions, conclusions, or estimates often is not.

The reasoning for this is fairly simple. Because the jury system relies on nonexperts to decide cases, inexperienced jurors must be protected from improper and inappropriate influences.

A prime example of this protection is the rule against hearsay evidence. This type of evidence bears directly on a nurse's impact upon a case, since rarely does the nurse actually see the injury take place.

The definition of the rule against hearsay is simple enough to state in a general way: "Hearsay is oral testimony or documentary evidence as to somebody's (either the testifying witness's or someone else's) words or actions outside of court, where they are offered to prove the truth of the very matters they assert."[62] Although this definition at first glance may frighten many and appear to be a jumble of typical legal jargon, the reasoning behind it should be understood.

In order to encourage witnesses to put forth their best efforts and to expose inaccuracies which might be present, the Anglo-American legal system evolved three conditions under which witnesses ordinarily will be required to testify: oath, personal presence at the trial, and cross-examination.[63] The rule against hearsay is designed to insure compliance with these ideal conditions and when one of them is missing, the hearsay rule is operable.

Thus, when a statement is offered, and its value rests with the credibility of an out-of-court asserter (that is, someone who is testifying without the conditional safeguards), the inability to test this person's powers of memory, the accuracy of his reporting, or his tendency to lie, makes the testimony unreliable and therefore inadmissible in most cases.

There are, however, many exceptions to the hearsay rule which the nurse should be aware of and particularly alert for. Since credibility is the main issue in most hearsay problems, the court has made exceptions in instances where something in the statement's content or in the circumstances of its utterance serves to guarantee its *trustworthiness*.

One such exception is for a statement made while under the influence of a startling event. This so-called excited utterance [64] is important to the nurse because she is usually one of the first members of the "caring professions" to encounter the abused wife and therefore is present while the victim is still under the influence of the violent episode. Thus, the two requirements for an excited utterance are still present. First, the startling event and second, a statement made while still under stress and insufficient time for reflective thought.[65]

A second exception is present for statements made while in fear of impending death. This "dying declaration" is considered trustworthy since people do not wish to die with a "lie on their lips." Thus, if the victim/wife, in fear of impending death says "My husband beat me up," this is admissable. Conversely, if a husband shot by his wife were to state, "I've hit her for so many years and she never fought back before," a defense may be greatly aided.

Another important exception is the "regular course of business" doctrine. The gist of this doctrine is that business records should be admissable when the sources of information, and the method and time of preparation, indicate their trustworthiness.

Because the nurse has a duty to record certain facts in the patient's medical records, these records are characterized by standardization of the recorded facts and routinely used to make decisions upon which the health and life of the patient depend. Their trustworthiness seems assured. They must, however, reasonably relate to the diagnosis and treatment of the victim's condition. For example, entries in hospital records as to who hit her may be held unrelated to the woman's treatment. However, sometimes the *cause* of an injury is relevant to diagnosis and treatment.

The critical point in these exceptions is that the nurse take special note of what was actually said and record it as accurately as possible. The use of quotation marks for direct statements is considered a good tool in these instances, as the nurse will be able to use these records to refresh her memory should she be called upon to testify and she lacks sufficient memory to testify to the facts contained therein.[66]

Of course, the nurse may face the possibility of being called to testify to the circumstances that are peculiar to her knowledge and not hearsay. Such observations as the woman's physical condition (that is, scars, bruises) and her apparent relationship with her husband at the hospital are direct evidence.

Confidentiality

Although many state statutes expressly include nurses, they are not granted the "universal" privilege of confidentiality that physicians enjoy.[67] However, this is not to say that a conversation between an abused woman and the nurse will not be confidential, even in the areas that do not recognize the privilege.

Whenever the nurse is acting not as an independent person, but as an assistant or agent to a practicing physician, during a consultation with a "view toward curative treatment," the privilege of confidentiality exists.[68] Thus, a clinical record at a hospital kept by a nurse has been held privileged.[69] Indeed, the very fact that the nurse was working in a hospital made the communication confidential.[70]

The major belief would appear to be that nurses are within the physician-patient privilege when they are "necessary intermediaries for the physician," and only for such information as is "necessarily imparted to the nurse as an assistant to the physician."[71] It therefore appears that nurses in emergency room situations or those assisting private physicians would be covered by the privilege of the attending physician.

Because the privilege is limited to communications necessary to enable nurses to act in their professional capacity, they may be called to testify as to the conversations held or observations made which were related to professional activities. Thus, a nurse was able to testify that a person was mentally alert, or that their memory was good, because this information was such that any layperson could attest to it.[72]

In another case, a nurse was called to someone's home to attend in her professional capacity, and she was able to testify as to the person's physical and mental state, behavior, and also as to the condition of the apartment. The court expressed a view that the privilege did not extend to matters of description relating to or concerning the physical surroundings of the patient, to the patient's companions, to conversations between third persons and the patient, or to the reactions of the patient to the acts and conduct of third persons.[73]

Of course, these instances represent only a small portion of the vast array of reasons a nurse may be called to testify. Because of the complexity of the Evidence Codes, it is quite possible that in two seemingly exact cases, a nurse's testimony may be admissable in only one. However, the nurse, in her support of battered women, should strive to recall whatever information she can and offer that information to lawyers involved. The possibility of recalling a vital fact or incident should never be overlooked, and the lawyers can determine how best to present such information so that it is admissable in court.

Expert Testimony

Finally, if the nurse has sufficient skill, knowledge, or experience in the field of wife abuse as to make it appear that her opinion or inference will aid the judge or jury, she may be called to testify as an expert. Recent cases have indicated that such testimony is relevant, informative, and sufficiently reliable under scientific standards.[74]

The use of such expert testimony is helpful in overcoming attitudes which the judge and jury may have about battered women, such as the myth that any reasonable woman in fear of her husband would call the police or manage to escape. It will aid the lay observers in understanding that a battering relationship embodies psychological and societal problems and give them a realistic view of the peculiar interpersonal dynamics involved in this situation.[75]

Summary

All the areas of the law which are touched when a battering incident occurs are simply too numerous to mention. However, nurses who are aware of some of the law's complex functionings are capable of giving the attorney tremendous assistance.

The battered wife faces enormous difficulties if she seeks redress through the legal system. That this situation, and the discriminatory attitude of many lawmakers, still exists in this allegedly enlightened era is simply unacceptable.

Changes of attitudes and laws are being made, but until a condition of equality between the sexes exists in our society, such incidents will persist and require a combined effort to see that justice is done.

Chapter 14

1. Although this chapter will deal almost exclusively with married women, most of its information may be applied to violence between adults who are intimates, regardless of the living arrangements.
2. W. Prosser, *Handbook of the Law of Torts*, 4th ed. St. Paul, (Minn: West Publishing Co., 1971), p. 860.
3. W. Blackstone, *Commentaries*, Vol. 1, Sharswood Edition, (Philadelphia: J. B. Lippincott Co.) 1859.
4. E. Emerson Dobash and Russell Dobash, *Violence Against Wives* (New York: The Free Press, 1979), p. 63.
5. Poor v. Poor, 8 N.H. 307, 313 (1836).
6. Prosser, *Torts*, p. 861.
7. Ibid.
8. See, for example, New York Penal Law 120.
9. Maria L. Marcus, "Conjugal Violence: The Law of Force and the Force of Law," *California Law Review* 69 (1981): 16570.
10. Rollin M. Perkins, *Criminal Law* (New York: Foundation Press, 1969), p. 8.

11. S. Eisenberg and P. Micklow, "The Assaulted Wife: 'Catch 22' Revisited," 32 *Women's Rights Law Reporter* 3 (1977): 138, 147.
12. Prosser, *Torts*, p. 860.
13. Ibid., p. 861.
14. Ibid.
15. Ibid., p. 862.
16. Ibid. Ordinary negligent injury, for example, is nowhere a crime or a ground for divorce.
17. 61 N. C. 453 (1868).
18. Eisenberg and Micklow, "Assaulted Wife," p. 145.
19. Marcus, "Conjugal Violence," p. 1669.
20. See generally, Martin, *Battered Wives*.
21. Ibid., p. 14-15.
22. Cotner v. Henry, 393 U.S. 847 (1968).
23. Ravin v. State, 537 P.2d 494 (Alaska 1975).
24. Prince v. Massachusetts, 321 U.S. 158, 166 (1944).
25. Note, "Spousal Exemption to Rape," 65 *Marquette Law Review* (1981); 120, 123.
26. Model Penal Code, 213.1, Comment 8(c) (1980).
27. "Spousal Exemption," at 127.
28. Dobash and Dobash, *Violence Against Wives*, p. 51.
29. Ibid., p. 219.
30. Ibid., p. 218.
31. Lisa G. Lerman, "Criminal Prosecution of Wife Beaters," *Response* 4, no. 3 (1981): 2.
32. Martha H. Field and Henry F. Field, "Marital Violence and the Criminal Process: Neither Justice Nor Peace," *Social Service Review* 47, no. 2: 221–240. (1973).
33. Eisenberg and Micklow, "Assaulted Wife," p. 158.
34. Lerman, "Criminal Prosecution," p. 2.
35. Ibid.
36. Ibid., p. 4.
37. Ibid.
38. Lisa Lerman, "Protection of Battered Women: A Survey of State Legislation," *Women's Rights Law Reporter* 6 (Summer 1980): 271.
39. Dobash and Dobash, *Violence Against Wives*, p. 219.
40. Eisenberg and Micklow, "Assaulted Wives," p. 150.
41. Raymond I. Parmas, "Judicial Response to Intra-family Violence," 54 *Minnesota Law Review* (1970): 600.
42. Lerman, "Protection of Battered Women," p. 271.
43. It is a form of injunction, in which the court orders the defendant to do or not do specific acts.
44. Lerman, "Protection of Battered Women," p. 273.
45. Dobash and Dobash, *Violence Against Wives*, p. 61.
46. D. Martin, *Overview—Scope of the Problem*, U.S. Commission on Civil Rights, report "Battered Women: Issues of Public Policy," 9 (1978).
47. People v. Cameron, 126 Cal Rptr 44, 48 (5th Dist. 1975).

48. N.J. Stats. Ann. 2c:14-5 (Supp. 1981).
49. State v. Wanrow, 88 Wash. 2d 221, 559 P.2d 548 (1977).
50. Note, "The Use of Expert Testimony in the Defense of Battered Women," *University of Colorado Law Review* 52 (1981): 587, 591.
51. Ibid., p. 593.
52. State v. Wanrow, p. 232.
53. Marcus, "Conjugal Violence," p. 1670.
54. Most notably in Los Angeles; Seattle; Westchester County, New York; and Santa Barbara, California.
55. Perkins, *Criminal Law*, p. 6.
56. Lerman, "Criminal Prosecution," p. 6
57. Ibid.
58. Ibid.
59. Ibid., p. 8. Of course, a lighter sentence carries the danger of reinforcing the abusive behavior.
60. Ibid., p. 2.
61. Cal. Ev. C. 140. A more broad definition is sometimes found in other codes.
62. John Henry Wigmore, *Evidence*, Vol. 5, Section, 1364, (Boston: Little, Brown and Company, 1974) p. 21.
63. McCormick, *The Law of Evidence* (St. Paul, Minn.: West Publishing Co., 1972), p. 581.
64. McCormick, *Evidence*, at 704.
65. Ibid., p. 704.
66. Cal. Ev. Code 1237.
67. See, for example, the codes of New York, Arkansas, and New Mexico. A major exception to this physician-patient privilege involves nonaccidental injuries to children.
68. 10 Wigmore, *Evidence*, section 2382, p. 679.
69. Stalker v. Breeze, 114 N.E. 968, 1917.
70. Goodman v. Lang, 130 So. 50, 1930.
71. Meyer v. Russell, 214 N.W. 857, 1927.
72. Re Avery's Estate, 76 NYS2 d790 (1948).
73. In Re Schermerhorn (1950 Sup.) 98 NYS 2d361, 98 N.E. 2d475.
74. "Use of Expert Testimony," p. 593.
75. Ibid., p. 587.

The Nurse and the Legal System: Dealing with Abused Children

Joyce Underwood Munro

THE LEGAL CONCEPT OF CHILD ABUSE

Every case of child abuse and neglect encountered has legal ramifications for the nurse. The nature of nursing practice is such that entry into the lives of families is personal and frequent. Child abuse as a legal entity is a relatively new phenomenon that is historically based on laws against infanticide. This chapter begins with these historical roots and continues on to describe the legal concepts of corporal punishment, criminal procedure relative to child abuse, and modern child protection laws. Against this background, nursing responsibilities to the child and the community within the judicial system are delineated. The nurse's role in testifying regarding specific cases and potential as an expert witness are examined. The latter role is advocated as an important contribution which has not been previously utilized in the spectrum of nursing practice.

INFANTICIDE AND THE LAW

As long as there have been laws against murder, assault, and battery, there has been ambivalence as to whether they apply when a child is the victim. Infanticide was commonly practiced in ancient Thebes, even though it was a capital offense.[1] Figures in myth, history, and literature were "exposed," or abandoned as infants, including Egypt's Horus, the Jew's Moses, Sophocles's Oedipus, and Romulus and Remus. Throughout history, and no doubt before, children were killed for various reasons, either with the sanction of society or with society turning its head. Indeed, "anthropologically, infanticide refers to the killing of a newborn with the consent of the parent, family, or community."[2] This consent takes the form of decree by a group leader, as in Pharoah and Herod ordering the slaughter of the innocents, or by the group's tacit acceptance of individual acts. Such behavior is also found among primates. For example, after conquering a troop, the victorious male langur executes the infants in the defeated troop. The mothers of the dead infants, no longer nursing, quickly come into estrus again. The new infants conceived are fathered by the conquering male.[3]

Infanticide was also practiced and condoned as a form of population control, particularly in times of famine, war, and social stress. Sometimes unusual births or those resulting in deformed babies were followed by infanticide. Ancient Spartans were required to bring their infants for inspection by the elders; if an infant were deemed weak or defective, it was cast off a mountain.[4] Infanticide was the legally decreed fate of deformed children under the Roman Law of the Twelve Tables, and because he believed that mentally defective children were the instruments of the devil, Martin Luther ordered them drowned.[5] Only recently are the ethics of physicians and parents being questioned in cases of births of grossly defective children who are also born with a life-threatening condition easily corrected by surgery.

Illegitimate children were, and still are, more frequent targets of infanticide. Considering the social ostracism their mothers were often subjected to and the economic hardships of a single woman, these infants often paid the price of women's low status in society. Traditional recourse for mothers of illegitimate children included concealing the pregnancy and "overlaying" or exposing the infant; paying an unscrupulous midwife to arrange for the death of the child at birth; hiring herself out as a wet nurse, at the expense of her own child's food supply; and abandoning the infant on a doorstep, at a foundling home, or in the nearest sewer.

Concealing a pregnancy was unlawful in eighteenth-century Europe. Unmarried women were required to register their pregnancies, and if they did not have an infant to show at the end of term, they could be tried for infanticide. The penalties varied from high fines to a cruel execution. Interestingly enough, although many married women disposed of children they could not handle, only married women were ever acquitted of "overlaying."[6] In these two instances, there were different rules for prosecution of mothers committing infanticide. The married ones were treated much more leniently by the law.

Midwives were always available to do indirectly what an unwilling mother risked everything to do directly. In times when the medical profession left childbirth in the hands of midwives, midwives were called upon to establish and report the cause of death of infants and children. Thus it was possible for an unscrupulous midwife to do away with the unwanted infant, for a fee for her deed and silence.

The notion of foster care is ancient, and indeed is mentioned in the Code of Hammurabi and in the Bible.[7] It is only very recently that strict standards of supervision and care have been required of foster homes. There were too frequent instances of greedy foster parents doing away with their wards by starvation and ill-usage, while pocketing the fees received for their care.

The wet nurse system operated as another example of a legally condoned method of infanticide. During the nineteenth century in London, 80 percent of the illegitimate children put out to nurse died.[8] But in societies where putting children out to nurse was the norm for the well-to-do, as it was in the Italian Renaissance, the one who paid for the practice was the nurse's own infant, who generally starved or was in turn put out to nurse while his or her mother cared for the wealthy client's child.[9] The fate of the nurse's child was never discussed and was in fact repressed from the consciousness of a society that needed the nurse's services. Becoming a wet nurse, like becoming a prostitute, was one of the few sources of economic survival open to poor young women who found themselves with an illegitimate child. The interdependence of society on the wet nurse and of the nurse on her clients led to a striking situation: while infanticide was everywhere in Europe punishable by death, "it seems that infanticidal *mothers were punished by death. Wet nurses were not.*"[10] Thus the wet nurse was both a "professional feeder and a professional killer,"[11] and in accepting her commodity, society condoned the unfortunate consequences of the system.

The development of foundling hospitals represented a humane method of dealing with unwanted children. Although they were a good idea and gave women somewhere to place the children that they did not want or could not care for, the death rate of these institutionalized infants was alarming. Even at the best hospitals, only about one-third of the infants survived to become school age.[12] In addition to the problems of finding adequate wet nurses for all the young patients, no doubt many, if not most, of these infants suffered from failure to thrive and other ills of the institutionalized. When the hospitals were full, the surplus infants were put out to nurse, with its attendant hazards.

The use of child labor in the nineteenth century also led to deaths of children from starvation, overwork, injury, disease, and suicide. But the industrial revolution provided a market for these unwanted children. For years their hardships were ignored by industrializing societies which must have been aware of the exploitation of these children. Again, perhaps because society needed this cheap pool of labor at the time, society legally condoned this treatment of children.

CORPORAL PUNISHMENT

Corporal punishment of children has long been accepted in most Western societies as necessary in order to make the child obey and learn. The Bible intones, "He that spareth the rod hateth his son: but he that loveth him chasteneth him betimes."[13] Under the *Patria Protestas* of ancient Rome, the father had the power of life and death over his children, including the right to sell, discipline, abandon, or do whatever he pleased. Massachusetts in 1646 and Connecticut in 1651 imposed the death penalty on unruly children, although more often the punishment actually meted out was public whipping.[14] Harsh physical punishment was the usual form of discipline.

Beatings were also used to "drive out evil spirits" thought to be residing within children due to their "impish" playfulness or affliction with madness or epilepsy. Even today nurses in emergency rooms see badly beaten children of parents who firmly believe that God or the Bible told them that they had to beat their child for disobedience. Sometimes these parents do not stop until the child is dead. When tried for second-degree murder or for manslaughter, they steadfastly maintain that they had to beat the devil out of the child, and they seem somewhat incredulous that society does not agree. Some parents still threaten, much less seriously, "if you don't stop that, I'm going to beat the devil out of you."

Corporal punishment has been employed by parents, guardians, teachers, employers, and masters to whom a child was apprenticed. In the United States, parents and teachers in the public schools may legally administer corporal punishment to children. In 1977 the Supreme Court of the United States held that corporal punishment in the public schools was not cruel and unusual punishment under the Eighth

Amendment to the United States Constitution, nor was it a violation of a schoolchild's Fourteenth Amendment right to due process of law.[15] There still exists a common-law right for teachers (and parents) to punish children with physical force.

In addition to corporal punishment and the sometimes sanctioned practice of infanticide, children have been and continue to be mutilated by their caretakers. Footbinding, castration, headshaping, and other practices were considered acceptable in the societies in which they were practiced. Children were also mutilated to make them look more pathetic as street beggars. Countless child laborers were maimed and crippled in the machinery of the industrial revolution. Industrialists of the nineteenth century discovered, "that children, especially poor ones, constituted the world's most inexpensive and unprotected labor force, that they could be made to substitute for the machine."[16] As a measure of how acceptable child mutilation is even today, note that circumcisions are now routinely performed on infants whose parents have no religious mandate for doing so.

THE MODERN IDEA OF CHILD ABUSE

The law's historical ambiguity toward children continues today in some of the forms mentioned above. The criminal law provides that murder, manslaughter, assault and battery, mayhem, and other crimes apply no matter who the victim is. But the idea persists that somehow killing one's own child is different from other homicides. The common-law privilege to use corporal punishment makes it difficult to decide whether a child has been disciplined or is the victim of assault and battery. One commentator opens an article on criminal child abuse prosecutions with the statement, "Child abuse differs from other criminal assaults or homicides."[17] Some judges still occasionally dismiss cases of overdiscipline resulting in death or serious injury on the basis that a parent has a right to discipline his or her child, and the injuries were the result of an accident or of "things getting out of hand." At the other extreme, some parents are vigorously prosecuted for far less serious neglect or abuse, usually following intense media exposure of the case. These parents may be society's scapegoats. They are punished publicly for what the community is evidently powerless to prevent—child abuse.

In the nineteenth century, the law began to limit the power of parents over their children. Under the doctrine of *parens patriae*, that a general guardian of the community could intercede in family matters to protect children, courts began to remove cruelly treated children from their parents. By the end of the nineteenth century, England and France had enacted legislation for the protection of maltreated and abandoned children and children put out to nurse. At the same time, some cities in the United States were setting up homes for wayward (delinquent) children, which also took in abandoned and ill-treated children. The celebrated case of Mary Ellen in New York City in 1874 spurred the development of child protection legislation (see Chapter 5). Today all states have such legislation, which provides that the state can become the child's guardian or even remove the child from the parent's care if the child is subjected to cruelty, neglect, an unfit home, or abandonment.

By the late 1960s there was an explosion in medical knowledge about child abuse. The work of J. Caffey,[18] F.N. Silverman,[19] P.V. Wooley,[20] and C. Kempe et al.,[21] came to the attention of the medical profession and the "battered-child syndrome" became a medical diagnosis. In spite of the increased awareness of child abuse, many cases were nevertheless going unreported. In 1962 California enacted the first statute requiring physicians to report child abuse, and by 1966, forty-nine states had passed reporting statutes.[22] In response to the states' needs for funding to carry out their reporting and treatment programs, the Congress enacted the Child Abuse Prevention and Treatment Act, effective 31 January 1974, which set out criteria for state child abuse reporting statutes in order for the state to qualify for federal funds.[23] The states quickly amended their reporting laws in accord with the mandates of the federal legislation, and today all fifty states, Puerto Rico, Guam, and the Virgin Islands have reporting statutes modeled on the federal act.

The reporting laws do vary somewhat from state to state in their definitions of what should be reported. The categories of abuse and neglect which must be reported have been expanding, partly due to the impetus of the federal act, and partly due to increased public awareness of the various forms of exploitation that children suffer.

In order for the nurse to deal effectively with the child abuse issues that she might face, it is necessary to detail the various situations in which the nurse can come into contact with the legal system.

THE LAW AND VIOLENT FAMILIES

The Criminal Law and Child Abuse and Infanticide in the United States

The existing criminal laws against assault and battery, murder and manslaughter, and criminal sexual assault can be used to charge child abusers. In addition to these, there are special statutes on child torture and criminal child neglect. If the police are involved in an investigation of child abuse and neglect, they may attempt to have the responsible parent or guardian charged under the criminal law. The implications for the parent are serious. He or she can be jailed until the trial, if unable to post bond. The trial can be a humiliating experience, with the sordid details of the crime coming out in public. If the parent pleads guilty to the charge or to lesser charges, then he or she has a criminal record. This record is public, and the parent is obliged to reveal it to all prospective employers. The parent may be placed on probation and have his or her movements and habits controlled by the conditions of probation. The parent may be sentenced to prison if convicted of a more serious crime.

However, criminal prosecution of child abuse cases is not that common. Most commentators recommend the prosecution be used only in cases where the abuse results in serious injury or death.[24] The new thinking is that treatment, not punishment, should be the goal of the law. Punishment does not solve the problem of abuse, and when the parent returns home, he or she is likely to be embittered by the experience. This leaves the child at even greater risk from a hostile parent. Further, a parent who is afraid of the possibility of being sent to jail may be even more reluctant to seek necessary medical treatment for injuries he or she inflicts upon the child.

In addition, it is more difficult to prove child abuse in criminal court. The police must be able to establish which parent or other person in the household was the perpetrator, or no one can be charged. The prosecutor (known in some states as the state's attorney, district attorney, or public prosecutor) must present evidence that establishes the accused's guilt "beyond a reasonable doubt," sometimes a difficult burden of proof to meet. A jury may have difficulty believing that a parent would actually abuse his or her child. The only eyewitness may be the child victim. If the child is verbal, he or she may have to testify against the parent in order to obtain a conviction. This may be more damaging to the child and the family than dropping the prosecution.

When only a few child abuse cases are processed through the criminal justice system, there is a danger that this selective enforcement will fall more harshly on one segment of the population, notably the poor. Also, a parent whose case received extensive media coverage is more likely to be prosecuted than another parent who caused equally serious injury, but whose case does not come under the scrutiny of the press. Child health professionals and child protection workers often wonder what logic is behind police and prosecutors' decisions to prosecute. Media and political pressure can explain some of these discrepancies. Where a non-related adult member of the household is responsible for the abuse, the policy considerations are different. There is usually no rationale for reuniting a parent's boyfriend or girlfriend with the child. In fact, criminal prosecution may be the only effective way to remove the abuser from the family in instances where the parent is ambivalent and does not take steps to remove the offender.

The consensus that the criminal law should only be used in extreme cases of child abuse overlooks two factors. The first is that the criminal courts have a wide latitude in sentencing offenders. Although a prison term is unlikely to rehabilitate a child abuser, a creative probation order can set out a treatment plan. If substance abuse is a problem, the court can order attendance at inpatient or outpatient treatment centers. The court usually orders the probationer into some form of counseling or psychotherapy. It can order completion of parenting skills classes. It can also control the contact of the probationer with the child victim, either forbidding it completely or providing that it be under some appropriate supervision. The probation officer can refer the probationer for job training skills, budget counseling, and to other agencies which will aid in overcoming some of the pressures that may have contributed to the child abuse. While criminal prosecution may not be a good tool in dealing with some cases, "the *threat* of criminal prosecution may be necessary to induce some parents to have treatment."[25]

The second factor overlooked is that the policy of limiting criminal prosecution to cases of severe injury or death endorses the notion that child abuse *is* different from other forms of violence. Perhaps this is the result of the centuries-old common-law privilege of parents and teachers to use corporal punishment. The only other circumstances in which an individual is privileged to use force against another are in the case of self-defense, defense of others, and in limited circumstances, defense of property. There may come a time when our society decides that children do not have to be physically punished to make them obey and learn. Courts may get tired of deciding where to draw the line between discipline and assault and battery. If it were a crime for a parent to strike his or her child, as it is to strike another's child or an adult, some persons might be able to refrain from striking their children. This may not prevent child abuse, but it would be a clear policy statement that child abuse is no longer condoned by the criminal law and the way it is enforced.

Whether or not to prosecute is a policy decision, depending on the circumstances of a particular case. A sexual abuse case is a good example for demonstrating how social workers, the police, and the prosecutor work out the problem. There are two schools of thought on how to handle a sexual abuse case. One calls for criminal prosecution, figuring that the rape of one's child is as serious as rape of an adult stranger. The other adopts the treatment mode, reasoning that a parent in jail for criminal sexual assault is not going to be able to support or care for the family and is likely to be too hostile to benefit from therapy. There are critics of both views. Sometimes incarceration of the offender is the only way to protect the child and still keep the rest of the family intact. On the other hand, incarceration of the parent may lead the young victim to conclude that he or she put the parent in jail by reporting what had been going on between them. The remaining parent may indeed blame the child for the removal of the spouse. In some instances, the offending parent is amenable to treatment and the family can be kept intact while family therapy is pursued. A live-in partner of a parent may require different handling from that of a stepparent or biological parent.

Criminal courts are even beginning to consider child abuse syndrome as a factor mitigating guilt in criminal cases. In 1978 the Massachusetts Supreme Judicial Court relied on data concerning the child abuse syndrome to reduce the conviction of a surrogate father for first-degree murder in the beating death of a three year-old boy.[26] This case presents in some detail the criminal law's struggle to come to grips with child abuse. Should parents suffering from the "child abuse syndrome" be treated differently from other adult criminal defendants? If they are, does it devalue children as a class of victims?[27]

Modern Child Protection Laws and Procedure in Juvenile Court

State child welfare laws provide for judicial intervention by the juvenile or family court. Because the statutory scheme varies from state to state, it is important for the interested nurse to obtain a copy of her current state law. The laws are usually available in pamphlet form from the local department of social services or child welfare department. State legislatures change and update child welfare laws from time to time, and the changes may have a direct impact on the nurse's function in the system.

Generally speaking, state child welfare laws provide a mechanism for bringing cases to the attention of the court. Not all cases uncovered by means of the reporting laws will be brought to court. If parents agree to accept the services of a child protection worker and the risk to the child can be reduced so that the child may remain at home while the parents undergo treatment, there is no need for the court's intervention. If the case does warrant the attention of the court, then the protective services worker or some other authorized person files a petition with the court. Nurses need to check to see if they are authorized to bring petitions in their states.

The child welfare laws will also provide for a procedure for removal of a child from the home. In emergency situations, children in imminent danger of harm can be removed without a prior court hearing. In these instances, there is provision for a hearing on the removal within a very short period of time. In less threatening circumstances, the children may remain in the home pending the hearing on the petition.

The court procedure is usually divided into two stages: the adjudication (hearing on the petition, or trial), and the disposition (hearing on where the child should be placed). There may be a pretrial conference prior to the adjudication, where all the parties are gathered to determine whether some agreement can be reached without having to take the petition to trial. One or both of the parents may admit some or all of the allegations in the petition. If so, a hearing is usually unnecessary if the admissions are sufficient to constitute abuse or neglect under the statutory definitions.[28] If the problems in the home appear to be resolved and court intervention is no longer necessary or appropriate for the protection of the child, the parties may agree to dismiss the petition prior to adjudication. Then the court would no longer be involved, although the child's protective services worker may continue to work with the family on a voluntary basis.

If agreement cannot be reached at a pretrial conference, the hearing officer (called a referee or master in some states) or judge who is handling the trial would set a date for the hearing on the petition. The parties subpoena witnesses. On the date of the hearing, the witnesses, usually including the petitioner, testify and other matters may be admitted into evidence. In the early days of juvenile court, proceedings were informal, and the rules of evidence were not strictly followed. Frequently there were no attorneys representing the various parties. In recent years more careful attention has been paid to parents' and children's rights to counsel and due process in general. Proceedings are now more formal, and the rules of evidence are more strictly followed.

At the conclusion of the adjudication hearing, the hearing officer (or jury where the parents have a right to a jury trial in neglect and abuse cases) must give a decision on whether the allegations in the petition have been proved, usually "by a preponderance of the evidence." If not, the petition is dismissed for lack of sufficient evidence, and the court is no longer involved. However, if the petitioner has met this burden of proof, the court will find that the neglect or abuse has been proved. The children come under the wardship of the court, and some parental rights are thereby temporarily suspended.

The second stage of the proceedings is the dispositional hearing, to determine where the child should be placed and what treatment plan should be ordered for the family. If the hearing officer has enough information before him or her to make an informed disposition on the date of the trial, an order of disposition can be entered at that time. If further information is needed, then a separate dispositional hearing is scheduled. After testimony at the dispositional hearing, the hearing officer can make various orders. The child may be placed in the parental home under the court's supervision. The court can also place the child with a qualified relative, legal guardian, in a licensed foster home, or in a group home, depending on the particular circumstances of the case, the degree of risk to the child, and the available community resources.

In cases where the child remains under the supervision of the court, the court is usually directed by statute to review the parent's progress at prescribed intervals. If the problems leading to the abuse or neglect are basically resolved, the court can dismiss its intervention, returning the child if he or she had been placed outside the parents' home. If some progress has been made, and it is safe to return the child to the parents, the court can do so and still keep the child under its supervision.

There are a significant number of cases where the parents make little or no progress during the entire time that the child is out of their custody. Some parents disappear for long periods of time and cannot be located by the court or by the agency supervising the children for the court. In appropriate circumstances, after adequate legal notice, and upon proof by "clear and convincing evidence,"[29] the court can terminate the parents' rights to the child permanently. "Clear and convincing evidence" is more than a preponderance and less than beyond a reasonable doubt.

The various states have their own criteria for termination of parental rights, but it is usually done only in cases where the abuse or neglect is severe, repeated, and long-standing, and there is little likelihood the parents will become rehabilitated to the extent that the child can safely be returned to their custody. Termination of parental rights is also done in cases of long-term abandonment. Other criteria vary by state. Once the court terminates the parental rights and the applicable appeal period has passed, the child is legally free for adoption.

While the foregoing description of the procedures in juvenile court is general and somewhat oversimplified, it describes the basic flow of a case through the system. There is some variation between states and even within a state as to how some aspects of the process are handled. The juvenile courts also have jurisdiction over delinquency cases. Many of the delinquent children also came before the court years earlier as abused or neglected children.

INTRERACTION BETWEEN NURSING AND THE LEGAL SYSTEM

The Nurse's Responsibility: Reporting Child Abuse and Neglect

The early reporting laws only required physicians to report suspected child abuse or neglect. By 1974 the list of mandated reporters was extended to include nurses in twenty-one states.[30] Today all states require nurses to report, either under provisions specifically listing nurses or provisions requiring any person to report.[31]

What must be reported varies by state to some extent. It can also change as reporting laws are amended following a trend to expand the list of situations requiring a report. Generally speaking, a report is required in cases of physical abuse, emotional abuse,[32] some forms of neglect,[33] and sexual abuse.[34] Neglect can include such situations as abandonment; failure to provide food, clothing, shelter; and failure to provide adequate supervision and care (including failure to protect from obvious hazards and failure to seek necessary medical care or to send the child to school).

How certain does the reporter have to be before a report should be made? State laws vary, using terms such as "has cause to suspect," "has reasonable cause to believe," "probable cause to suspect," "reasonably suspects," and "has reason to believe or suspect." Words such as "probable cause," "reasonable," and "belief" are part of legal terminology. Practically speaking, what it means for the reporter is that she does not have to be positive that the child has suffered abuse or neglect; well-founded suspicion is enough. The reporter need not have to prove the abuse in order to make a report. Sometimes abuse and neglect will be obvious.

It is helpful to include reporting of suspected abuse and neglect because the reporter may not have access to all the pertinent data on the child. If, for example, a clinical nurse suspects abuse and makes a report to the appropriate authority, that agency will conduct an official investigation. That investigation can gather information unavailable to the reporting nurse in an inpatient setting, who probably would not be able to make home visits. Community health nurses, on the other hand, do have access to the home. Either investigation can help to confirm or rule out abuse. At this point, the parent may agree to accept services designed to reduce the risk to the child. If the parent fails to cooperate, court intervention may be necessary to save or protect the child's life or health. If reporters waited until they were *positive* the child was being abused or neglected, many children would slip through the protective net, sometimes with crippling or fatal results.

A report sometimes reveals that the case is already active with a protective services agency or the juvenile court. A report can also uncover patterns of hospital shopping, as the investigator checks the child's name against the central registry. It can also establish patterns of accidents to the child which show that the child is inadequately supervised. Furthermore, a reporter is usually not an eyewitness to abuse or neglect. So unless the parents admit it to the nurse, the child is able to talk about it, or the pattern of injury is obvious, the reporter will generally be somewhat less than certain that the child's problems are due to abuse or neglect.

Reporting statutes provide specific penalties for failure to make a mandated report. The penalty is either civil or criminal, or both. The criminal penalty is usually a misdemeanor, punishable by a fine or jail sentence or both. Some states have specifically legislated civil penalties. Thus, if a mandated reporter fails to report when she had reason to know or suspect abuse or neglect and the child is subsequently reinjured or killed, the negligent reporter can be sued for money damages. Even in states that do not provide a specific civil penalty for failure to report, there is common-law basis for such a lawsuit, for violation of statutory duty to report.[35]

Even though a specific statutory civil penalty may not be necessary to create the liability, having it spelled out can be a great help. It can make it easier to explain to parents why a report must be made.[36] It can be invaluable to nurses. "For example, nurses frequently relate how the mention of the potential liability for failure to report is the only argument that convinces reluctant hospital administrators to commence protective action."[37] Nurses sometimes run into conflict with supervising physicians. A nurse's opinion may be devalued and her experience ignored because she is not a medical doctor. Yet the particular nurse may actually have more skill than the physician in recognizing some cases of suspected abuse. If the physician refuses to report, or disagrees with the nurse's assessment, the nurse is in a delicate situation. Many hospitals and clinics have established in-house protocols under which only a physician or administrator can make the required report. If the nurse is unable to persuade the designated person to report, what can she do?

One commentator, a nurse, suggests that a nurse in this situation can sometimes remind the physician that the case may be referred to a child protection team physician, and/or she can, as a last resort, submit an anonymous report.[38] The best solution is to work out a procedure in advance which recognizes the nurse's professional status and skills and the fact that the nurse, too, is subject to penalties for failure to report.

The reporting laws give immunity from civil and criminal liability to reporters who make their reports in good faith. This immunity usually covers all acts required or permitted by the reporting law. In addition, the laws also provide that information received in a privileged communication, such as between patient and physician, between spouses, and between other classes of persons, can be divulged in reporting child abuse. Ordinarily the person in this confidential relationship who receives information is obliged to keep it to him or herself and may only tell another person or the court what the informant has given permission to disclose. This abrogation of privileges, and the grant of immunity from civil or criminal penalty for good faith report are both designed to encourage reporting. Although there is a good argument that these clauses abrogating the various privileges are legally unnecessary,[39] having them specifically spelled out helps calm fears a reporter may have about a lawsuit for disclosing confidential communications he may have heard in the physician-patient, spousal, or other listed relationship.

There are some special problems for the nurse in dealing with the reporting laws, in addition to disputes with physicians or administrators on whether to file a report. For instance, private physicians seem more reluctant to report the people who pay them, or they are reluctant to believe that parents would actually abuse their children. They may not understand the legal protections given to reporters. Thus a nurse who works with a private physician may have to do some subtle education, remembering that she, too, is liable for failure to report.

The visiting or public health nurse is probably in a position to make more reports than nurses with other assignments. In some communities a visiting nurse is assigned to do a follow-up home visit for all new births. At the home visit the nurse can assess the level of care given the new infant. If there are problems, she can educate the parents. If education fails to help, or if the infant is seriously neglected or is being abused, or if there are solid signs that the infant is at risk, but the parents will not accept intervention, then the nurse can make a report. If the parents never take the child for any routine clinic checkups, the visiting nurse may be the only mandated reporter who ever sees the child.

Another problem the nurse may encounter is lack of response from the agency assigned to investigate the report. Some protective services departments in large cities are monolithic bureaucracies. There may be inefficiency in some investigations, or the investigator may not appreciate the urgency of a situation in the same way the nurse does. In smaller towns and in rural areas, there may be a tendency away from reporting a neighbor, for fear of being branded an informer. The nurse, or her supervisor if necessary, can always contact the investigating worker's supervisor if there is a problem with the worker. Sometimes misunderstandings can be worked out this way.

The Role of the Nurse in The Legal System

Evidence

The nurse deals with evidence in two ways. First, she collects evidence for use in medical diagnosis of child abuse. Second, the nurse's testimony in a child abuse hearing is evidence that can be used to establish child abuse or neglect. How well the nurse collects and records data and observations affects how useful her testimony will be in court. And some understanding of the rules of evidence can make the nurse more aware of what data are important for proving child abuse or neglect.

Evidence can take two main forms: demonstrative evidence, which consists of things, and the assertions of witnesses about things. In child abuse cases, demonstrative evidence includes photographs of the child's injuries; x-rays; plotted growth charts; and skin injury maps which chart a pattern of bruises, burns, or other injuries. It includes presenting the child in court to demonstrate the injuries. The statements of witnesses about what they saw, heard, palpated, measured, were told, and in the case of expert witnesses, their opinions, are examples of the second type of evidence.

Evidence can also be characterized as direct or circumstantial. Direct evidence in child abuse cases includes the testimony of a witness who saw a parent beat the child, the child's testimony that the parent beat him or her, the parent's admission to the witness that he or she beat the child, and the parent's admission in court that he or she beat the child. Sometimes this kind of testimony is available in child abuse cases, but not often. It is usually necessary to resort to circumstantial evidence to prove the abuse or neglect. The court can infer that the child has been abused from testimony of witnesses who observed the injuries, from the testimony of witnesses to whom the parents gave inconsistent explanations of the injuries, from testimony of witnesses who observed the behavior of the child, and from various items of demonstrative evidence, such as photographs, x-rays, charts, and so forth.

Juvenile courts have also adopted the common-law tort theory of *res ipsa loquitur*, which essentially says that the child's condition speaks for itself, that any unexplained, nonaccidental injury to the child while in the parent's care can lead the court to conclude that the parent inflicted the injury or allowed it to be inflicted upon the child.[40] It should be noted that *res ipsa* is merely presumptive. It does, however, shift the burden of proof to the defendant.

A word about hearsay. When a party calls a witness to testify at a hearing, the other party has an opportunity to cross-examine that person. The purpose of cross-examination is to ask questions to test the witness's credibility. When a witness testifies in court about what another person (the "declarant") said, there is no opportunity to cross-examine the declarant to determine or assess credibility. Also, the declarant usually was not under oath when he made the statement. Because such secondhand testimony is deemed inherently unreliable, courts developed the hearsay rule. "Hearsay is a statement, other than one made by the declarant while testifying at the trial or hearing, offered in evidence to prove the truth of the matter asserted."[41] Because some hearsay statements were considered more reliable than others, a list of exceptions to the rule was developed. If the declarant's statement comes under one of the twenty-some exceptions, it can be admitted into evidence to prove the truth of what the declarant said.

The nurse will encounter admissible hearsay in a number of circumstances. Hospital, clinic, and agency records are admissible under the business record exception. To qualify, a business record must:

1. Be kept in the usual course of business;

2. The person who made the record or The person informing him or her must have firsthand knowledge of the matter, and both must have been acting in their usual business capacity;

3. The entries must be made at or near the time of the event being recorded; and

4. They must be original entries.

If these criteria are met, the business record is deemed reliable, since persons at the business, institution, or agency rely upon the accuracy of the entries made therein.

Not all parts of a business record are admissible into evidence and individual information can be challenged regarding accuracy. Statements which are diagnoses, either by a nurse or a physician, are usually not admitted to prove their truth, since the statement is the maker's opinion and the opposing party has a right to cross-examine him or her regarding how he or she formulated that opinion. If the portions of the medical record fall within another exception to the hearsay rule, then they can be admitted to prove the truth of the matter asserted.

A nurse's notes of her own observations can be read into the record if the nurse at the time of her testimony cannot remember the contents of the notes fully enough to give accurate and complete testimony.

Also, a child's excited utterances, "statements relating to a startling event or condition made while the declarant was under the stress of excitement caused by the event or condition,"[42] can be testified to by a nurse who hears them. For instance, if an injured and distraught child in the emergency room says to a nurse, "Daddy hurt me," the nurse can testify to what the child said, and it can be admitted as proof that the father abused the child. The nurse (or other person) who hears the child's statement should put it in the child's chart, with quotation marks around the exact words the child uttered, and identify all staff or others present who heard the child make the utterances. That way if the nurse who heard the statement leaves her job and goes to another state, another person who heard the utterances can be called to testify, and the evidence will not have been lost.

Statements made for purposes of medical treatment or a medical diagnosis in connection with treatment are admissible. For example, a child says to a nurse or physician who examines him or her at a clinic or emergency room, "It hurts where Mommy hit me," or "I got burned when Daddy held my hand on the stove." The person to whom these statements were made can testify to them. Some courts allow descriptions of past pain to be admitted, as well as present pain. And again, it is important to record the statement accurately.

A statement of a declarant's then-existing state of mind, emotion, sensation, or physical condition (including mental feeling, pain, and bodily health) is admissible. If a child says "I don't want to go home; I'm afraid of Daddy," the person who hears the statement can testify to it, and it can be admitted as proof that the child is afraid of the father.

Also admissible are statements made under belief of impending death, or so-called dying declarations. If the child makes such a verbalization, the nurse hearing it can testify regarding the statement. Or if a parent's boyfriend, on his deathbed, says to a nurse, "I beat my girlfriend's kid many times, and I'm sorry; I just couldn't seem to stop doing it," that is also admissible in a neglect case to show that the mother failed to protect the child from a known abuser.

A statement made against interest, where the statement tends to subject the declarant to civil or criminal liability, is also admissible. If the above boyfriend (in good health) says to the emergency room nurse, "I just couldn't seem to help myself; it got on my nerves when the baby cried. I just shook the baby and then the baby went limp, and she stopped crying." That statement is admissible as one made against interest, since the boyfriend can be sued or prosecuted for doing what he said.

Some out-of-court statements are *not* hearsay. If a party to a child abuse case (as opposed to the boyfriend, above, who is not a party if he is not legally related to the child) makes an admission that he or she hurt or neglected the child, that statement is admissible and is not considered hearsay at all. Parties in a child abuse case (besides the state and sometimes the child) are parents or legal guardians. If a nurse hears an admission it is important, as in all the above cases, to enter the exact words spoken by the parent, and to whom, into the child's chart. When the parents know that the state can prove that they admitted the abuse, the case generally will not go to trial, saving the court and witnesses time and money, and the parents the pain and humiliation of a contested trial they will almost surely lose.

A nurse may be subpoenaed to testify to a number of her observations. She may be needed to describe a child's physical condition, such as skin injuries, height, weight, and body hygiene. She may be needed to testify as to any parental admissions of abuse or neglect. She may be needed to testify as to statements she heard which fall within exceptions to the hearsay rule. The nurse may also be needed to testify as to her observations of the child's behavior (did the child flinch when the blood sample was taken, or behave stoically during painful procedures?), or of her observations of the interaction between parent and child. The floor nurse at a hospital has the time to make a number of important observations. Who visits the child? How do the visits go? How does the child react to the visits? How long do the visitors stay?

Nurses may in some instances be able to testify as expert witnesses. An expert, as opposed to a mere observer of events, can draw inferences from a set of facts and render an opinion about the facts. In order to be qualified in court to testify as an expert, the witness must have expertise in the field above and beyond what a layperson has, and the witness must have sufficient skill and expertise in her field that her opinion will aid the hearing officer, judge, or jury in its task of determining what happened. Physicians, particularly radiologists, are frequently called to give their opinions as to whether the injury is the result of nonaccidental means. There is no legal reason why, in appropriate cases, an experienced nurse could not be qualified as an expert witness and render her opinion. The only barriers to nurses with appropriate qualifications testifying as experts in certain situations are the reluctance of the courts to hear opinion testimony from other than the traditional medical expert, the physician, and the lack of imagination of tradition-bound attorneys who are overlooking a valuable resource. It should be noted that the nurse is asked to testify as an objective witness. She is to testify to the facts as she perceives them neither as an advocate or adversary. It is important that the nurse be nonjudgmental in the case. The nurse's role is to give the facts as she knows them, but not to judge those facts.

Testifying in Court

Familiarity with the conduct of a child abuse hearing can help reduce some of the witness's anxiety about testifying. There are generally three attorneys involved in a child abuse hearing, each one representing a different party. The nurse may be contacted by an attorney, usually the prosecutor or the child's attorney, to discuss what evidence may be offered. If no attorney contacts the nurse and she knows something important that is being overlooked, she can bring it to the attention of the hospital's medical social worker who is assigned to the case, or to her supervisor, or even contact the court for the names and telephone numbers of the prosecutor and child's attorney. Prosecutors often have huge case loads, and not all cases are thoroughly prepared. And attorneys, like all professionals, vary in their levels of expertise and competence.

No one can ignore a subpoena. But many times witnesses are called to testify, only to find that when they get to court, the case was settled without a hearing or the hearing was postponed. If the witness's workplace is relatively close to the court and there is a telephone number where they can be reached, they can ask the attorney who subpoenaed them to place them on call. Then they will only have to go to court if their testimony is needed.

The procedure for testifying is for the attorney who subpoenaed the nurse to call her to the witness stand. The witness will be asked to swear or affirm that she will tell the truth. The attorney who called the nurse will conduct what is called the direct examination, a series of questions designed to get the testimony on the court record. The other attorneys will cross-examine the witness. Their questions may try to confuse or upset the nurse or to get her to argue with them. They may try to point out inconsistencies in the testimony. In short, their job is to discredit testimony so the court will not believe what the nurse says. Most people asked to testify will probably be somewhat nervous. So the nurse should take the time she needs to answer a question. If she does not understand a question, the nurse should say so. Attorneys are not always articulate. She can ask to have a question rephrased or repeated. If the nurse answers "yes" or "no" to a question that she does not understand, she may inadvertently put an incorrect or opposite meaning to her testimony. If the nurse thinks an answer is beyond her expertise, she should say so. If she does not know the answer, she should also admit this.

In a well-prepared case, the nurse will have discussed her proposed testimony with one or more attorneys. She should not be afraid to say so if asked whether she discussed her testimony with anyone prior to coming to court. The attorneys she talked to were acting appropriately in preparing their case by discussing various issues pertaining to the case with the nurse.

If the nurse is asked a question, she should answer it even if she believes her answer will involve hearsay or other inadmissible evidence. As has been shown, hearsay is admissible under a number of circumstances. Even technically inadmissible evidence is admitted if no attorney objects to it. The parents' attorney may have a strategic reason to let that evidence come in. So the nurse should follow the direction of the hearing officer on whether to answer a question to which an attorney has made an objection.

The nurse should make notes from her records. A witness who can quickly recite the dates she made home visits is more effective than one who shuffles noisily through the chart or record, and consequently she will appear more believable. The nurse's credibility will rest on how she answers questions, as well as on the content of the answers. If she appears hesitant, unsure of herself, easily confused, or if she contradicts herself, her testimony will not carry much weight or authority. Preparation can prevent this from happening. If the nurse knows what to expect, she can take the time to be prepared for her testimony. The nurse's self-confidence and professionalism will show.

Follow-up

The nurse may be subpoenaed to testify at another stage in the proceedings. The court may order that a visiting nurse be allowed to check on the child regularly as a condition of keeping the child at home. The nurse may be subpoenaed to testify as to the child's (and parents') progress. In a child neglect case, she may be asked to monitor the child's progress in foster care. She may be assigned to monitor the child's siblings in the parents' home, or to file a report of suspected abuse when a new sibling is born to extremely dysfunctional parents in serious abuse cases.

Nurses could also be used more extensively by the court in treatment functions. Nurses can teach parenting classes, or teach individual parents informally in the home. They can offer support and counseling to parents who themselves were badly abused and neglected as children. Nurses can refer parents to various social agencies for services and treatment. Pediatric nurse practitioners can fill a number of specialized needs in the treatment of abusive families. Indeed, the juvenile court needs to be made more fully aware of all the resources available to the nursing profession.

Summary

The nurse is in an excellent position to assist the legal system in detecting, proving, and treating child abuse and neglect. The nurse in most states is required to report cases of suspected child abuse and neglect to the appropriate authority for investigation. In her record-keeping role, she can fully document and preserve the evidence of abuse or neglect for trial and treatment. Although courts traditionally have ignored the nurse's expertise as a witness, this will change as courts are made more aware of the education and experience nurses receive in the area of child abuse and neglect. Finally, nurses can also fill a number of educational and treatment functions to improve parenting skills in order to prevent child abuse and neglect or to reunite troubled families. A closer collaboration between the nursing profession and the legal system will aid both in their handling of child abuse and neglect cases.

Chapter 15

1. Samuel X. Radbill, "A History of Child Abuse and Infanticide," in *Battered Child*, ed. Ray E. Helfer and C. Henry Kempe (Chicago: The University of Chicago Press, 1974), p. 14.
2. Radbill, "History of Child Abuse," p. 6.
3. Maria W. Piers, *Infanticide: Past and Present* (New York: W. W. Norton & Company, 1978), p. 34.
4. Radbill, "History of Child Abuse," p. 8.
5. Ibid.
6. Piers, *Infanticide*, p. 68.
7. Radbill, "History of Child Abuse," p. 7.
8. Ibid.
9. See Piers, *Infanticide*, chapter 3, "About Wet Nurses," pp. 44-55, for a detailed analysis of the system.
10. Piers, *Infanticide*, p. 51.
11. Ibid., p. 52.
12. Ibid., p. 67.
13. Prov. 13:23.
14. Radbill, "History of Child Abuse," p. 4.
15. Ingraham v. Wright, 430 U.S. 651, 51 L. Ed2d 711, 97 S.Ct. 1401 (1977), where the U.S. Supreme Court upheld corporal punishment in the schools, saying "the State itself may impose such corporal punishment as is reasonably necessary for the proper education of the child and for the maintenance of group discipline," 430 U.S. 651, 662. See also James P. Stoneman II, "Corporal Punishment in the Schools: A Time for Change," *Journal of Juvenile Law* 4 (1980): 155.
16. Piers, *Infanticide*, p. 80.
17. Lloyd Leva Plaine, "Evidentiary Problems in Criminal Child Abuse Prosecutions," *Georgetown Law Journal* 63 (1974): 257.
18. J. Caffey, "Multiple Fractures," *American Journal of Roentgenology, Radium Therapy, and Nuclear Medicine* 56 (1946): 163-73.
19. F. N. Silverman, "The Roentgen Manifestations of Unrecognized Skeletal Trauma in Infants," *American Journal of Roentgenology, Radium Therapy and Nuclear Medicine* 69 (1953): 413-27.

20. P. V. Wooley, Jr. and W. A. Evans, Jr., "Significance of Skeletal Lesions in Infants Resembling Those of Traumatic Origin," *JAMA* 158 (1955): 539.

21. C. Kempe, T. Silverman, B. Steele, W. Droegemueller, and H. Silver, "Battered-Child Syndrome," *JAMA* 181 (1962): 17.

22. Marjorie R. Freiman, "Unequal Protection and Inadequate Protection Under the Law: State Child Abuse Statutes," *George Washington Law Review* 50 (1982): 242, 250.

23. Child Abuse Prevention and Treatment Act, 42 U.S.C. sections numbered 5101–5106 (1976 & Supp. LV 1980), Pub. L. No. 93-247, 88 Stat. 4 (1974).

24. Sandford N. Katz, Lillian Ambrosino, Melba McGrath and Kitt Sawitsky, "Legal Research on Child Abuse and Neglect: Past and Future," *Family Law Quarterly* 11 (1977): 151, 155; *Georgetown Law Review* 63 (1974): 258; and Monrad G. Paulsen, "The Law and Abused Children," in Kempe and Helfer, *Battered Child*, p. 154.

25. Katz et al., "Legal Research on Child Abuse," p. 156.

26. Commonwealth v. Cadwell, 374 Mass. 308, 372 N.E. 2d 246 (1978).

27. Comment, "Commonwealth v. Cadwell: Deliberate Premeditation, Extreme Atrocity and Cruelty, and the Battered-Child Syndrome—A New Look at Criminal Culpability in Massachusetts," *New England Law Review* 14 (1979): 812.

28. Or to designate the child a "minor in need of care" or "person in need of supervision," two of the newer terms being used in some states. It is important to repeat that child protection legislation is currently undergoing study and revision.

29. Santosky v. Kramer, 455 U.S. 745, 71 L.Ed.2d 599, 102 S.CT. 1388 (1982).

30. Paulsen, "Law and Abused Children," p. 161.

31. Marjorie R. Freiman, "Unequal Protection," p. 257.

32. Ibid., p. 254. As of late 1981, seven states (Georgia, Indiana, Iowa, Maryland, Minnesota, Oregon, and Wisconsin) do not require the reporting of emotional abuse.

33. Ibid. Only Idaho does not require the reporting of neglect, as of late 1981.

34. Ibid. New Mexico, South Dakota, Tennessee, and Texas do not require the reporting of sexual abuse.

35. Landeros v. Flood, 17 Cal. 3d 399, 551 P.2d 389, 131 Cal. Rptr. 69 (1976).

36. Douglas Besharov, "Legal Aspects of Reporting Known and Suspected Child Abuse and Neglect," *Villanova Law Review* 23(1978): 458, 482.

37. Ibid., p. 482.

38. Carole L. Bridges, "The Nurse's Evaluation," in *The Child Protection Team Handbook—A Multidisciplinary Approach to Managing Child Abuse and Neglect*, ed., Barton D. Schmitt (New York: Garland STPM Press, 1978): p. 71.

39. Douglas Besharov, "Legal Aspects," p. 477; Alan Sussman, "Reporting Child Abuse: A Review of the Literature," *Family Law Quarterly* 8 (1974): 245, 298.

40. See the opinion of the Hon. Harold A. Felix of the New York Family Court for a good discussion of the application of the doctrine of *res ipsa loquitur* in child abuse cases, In the Matter of S, 46 Misc. 2d 161, 162, 259 N.Y.S. 2d 164, 165 (1965).

41. *Federal Rules of Evidence*, Rule 801 (c).

42. *Michigan Rules of Evidence*, Rule 803 (2).

Implications for Nursing

Janice Humphreys

"So Many Faces Pass Through This House"

So many faces pass through this house
Younger, older, richer, poorer
Women with bruised marks
   surrounding their faces,
Babies with welt scars on
   unmentionable places.

     an excerpt from "So Many Faces Pass
     Through This House" by Barbee Finer

Reprinted from *Every Twelve Seconds*, compiled by Susan Venters (Hillsboro, Oregon: Shelter, 1981) by permission of the author.

The case for violence in families as a health problem of concern to nursing has been made, and the issue now becomes what are the future implications for nursing? Once nursing as a profession acknowledges that family violence can and does happen, what direction does it take? If nursing theory is the direction, what empirical validation through nursing research exists? What principles of nursing practice are followed and how does nursing education respond to this new demand? The purpose of this chapter is to examine the implications of family violence for nursing. The discussion will particularly focus on the issues of nursing theory, research, and practice as they relate to violence in the family.

NURSING CONCEPTUAL MODEL OF FAMILY VIOLENCE

A nursing theory of family violence currently does not exist. If the definition of a nursing theory given by Jacqueline Fawcett is accepted, that is "a set of propositions consisting of defined and interrelated units which presents a systematic view of person, the environment, health, and nursing by specifying relations among relevant variables,"[1] it should be clear that much work remains to be done before such theoretical specificity can be achieved. It would, however, seem possible to make certain statements about the four key concepts—environment, person, health, and nursing.

Margaret Newman defines a conceptual model as "a matrix of concepts which together describe the focus of inquiry."[2] She goes on to say that although a conceptual framework or model is not testable, it does provide direction to the development of research questions and subsequent theories. It is suggested that this book conceptualizes a nursing framework that addresses each of the four key concepts. What follows is a delineation of these concepts as they appear throughout the text. It is further proposed that these concepts require attention toward describing the nature of the relationships between each.

Environment

The environment in which family violence occurs must of necessity condone, either implicitly or explicitly, aggression against family members. The phenomenon cannot exist in a culture that does not allow it. The factors within a society that provide this approval of violence are not altogether clear. The mode of transmission of violence and its cultural tolerance, al-

Implications for Nursing

though tied to the family by some investigators, also exists in the larger sphere of culture.

Environment which condones violence in families has also been shown to selectively allow its commission only against certain members. Clearly gender and age biases play a major role in support of violence. Violence is not experienced equally by all members of the family. The nature of the role that gender and age play, however, is not completely clear and as has been discussed, is not even accepted by some investigators. In the presence of repeated evidence to the contrary, some theorists consistently fail to acknowledge that family violence is usually physical aggression directed at women, children, and the elderly by men. Is it possible that the factors of the environment that support gender and age-biased violence also perpetuate the myths of its nonexistence? These factors need clarification.

Person (Family)

Throughout this text the focus has been on the family. Family has been referred to as the basic unit of nursing. Although the nurse may care for an individual she does so only within the context of the larger unit, the family. It has been repeatedly stated that an enormous number of families are violent, committing numerous and varied aggressive acts against their members. Although child abuse, battering of women, and abuse of the elderly are examined separately, they are really only manifestations of violence in families. Clinicians, especially those in the community, clearly practice nursing with families.

The theorist and researcher, however, somehow have difficulty placing the family in so central a role. Even the four key concepts of any nursing model refer only to person, not family. To address the family from a theoretical or research standpoint is fraught with problems. Ann Whall, who strongly advocates the family as the basic unit of nursing, has described that problems occur when in an effort to have any kind of family theory, nursing accepts as is theories from other disciplines.[3] She goes on to propose how nursing theories might be applied to families.

Family is further complicated by the mere fact that theorists and researchers have difficulty defining what they mean by family, or they fail to define it at all. Families experiencing violence, as have been shown, are often experiencing general alteration in their functioning. Certainly any definition of family must be broad and flexible enough to include all the relevant members.

Susan Meister's conceptualization of the family and family well-being and her attention to the individual's perception of who they consider to be their family contain intriguing ideas (see Chapter 3). Application of these concepts to violent families could provide tremendous insight and advancement of nursing knowledge of families.

Health

After wrestling with the problems of securing a definition for family, the issue of what is health arises. Certain victims of family violence are clearly experiencing physical alterations. The physical damage inflicted upon abused family members is the most obvious evidence of impediments to health. However, the impact of violence upon even nonabused members has been shown to be enormous. In looking at health the nurse must not only attend to the present physical damage, but also the long-term psychological, emotional, and spiritual harm. Judith Smith in a philosophical inquiry into the idea of health describes a model which would seem to address the aspects of health that a nursing definition must consider.[4] The eudaimonistic model presents an ideal of health that is much more than the absence of disease. Included in the suggested model are "views of human nature that extend the idea of health to general well-being and self-realization."[5] Illness would therefore be any condition that impedes self-actualization. By this definition, the nurse is not only concerned with the bleeding wound, but also the potential or actual alteration in self-concept of the victim. In viewing violence, such a definition is a necessity and once the nature of family is described, easily adapted to the larger unit.

Nursing

Through this text, attention has been paid to preventing family violence and addressing the strengths of individuals and families experiencing the same. These ideas are believed essential to any nursing framework and may even seem too obvious to state. Much of the literature on family violence, however, attends only as an afterthought to prevention and generally not at all to individual or family strengths. It is much easier to find theories and articles about family violence and its attendant pathology than it is to locate descriptions of family strengths. Clinical practice with families experiencing violence has revealed that both individuals and the family as a unit possess great stamina, creativity, and resiliency. Yet the literature on family violence does not describe these findings.

It is also fair to say that nursing has not made the contributions that it must to family violence literature. As part of its contributions it is hoped that nursing will consider family strengths and violence prevention in its conceptualizations.

The four key concepts—environment, person, health, and nursing—can be tied to the problem of family violence. A nursing framework that addresses family violence must consider the socio-cultural condoning of gender- and age-biased violence, the person as a member of the larger basic unit of family, health as a concept that is an integration of strength of body and self-realization, and nursing as a discipline that promotes strengths and prevents violence. This nursing framework is described as a starting point for the further description and clarification that remains to be done.

NURSING THEORY AND FAMILY VIOLENCE

There has been no research on family violence to date using nursing theory as a basis. The nursing literature that suggests appropriate nursing interventions does so on the basis of theory from other disciplines. The problem with such interventions are twofold: first, the theory is generally poorly tested or untested; and second, the nurse must try to create nursing actions from another discipline's model. Georgia Kemm Millor has developed a theoretical framework for nursing research in child abuse and neglect (see Chapter 5).[6] Empirical research by Millor to test her assumptions is near completion. Numerous other research projects could select other aspects of Millor's framework for nursing study. Systematic testing of this nursing framework could do much to advance the knowledge base of child abuse and neglect in nursing.

Nursing interventions that have been described in the literature suffer from the same problems previously identified in research in child abuse and neglect. The literature on nursing interventions with victims of family violence tend to be presented in a case study or discussion format. The interventions are based upon generally accepted principles of nursing and yet the reader has only the experience and the opinion of the author to support the interventions. In all fairness, the same could be said of many of the suggested nursing actions described in the current text. Nursing as a profession must approach the development of client care in a more sophisticated fashion. Nursing research based upon nursing theory is required, and empirical study testing the effectiveness of interventions is necessary. Rising health care costs and accountability of nursing as a profession mandate that interventions be developed and aimed at maximum effectiveness.

Application of Nursing Theory

The following discussion will illustrate how nursing theory may be applied to the problem of family violence. In addition, beginning research questions are identified. The nursing conceptual model developed by Dorothea E. Orem will be used as a basis for suggested nursing research into the area of adolescent abuse.

The general theory of nursing set forth by Orem is particularly suited to nursing research into family violence. Orem's model revolves around the concept of self-care. As such, victims of violence who seek assistance can be viewed as demonstrating both the ability to identify the need for action and the ability to take action to promote life, health, and well-being. The strengths of individuals from violent families are easy to identify in light of self-care. Finally, Orem's model lends itself to client nurse problem solving to increase client abilities and decrease, as Orem defines it, the therapeutic self-care demand.

Orem describes self-care as "the practice of activities that individuals initiate and perform on their own behalf in maintaining life, health and well-being."[7]

According to Orem, the requirement for nursing exists when a client is unable to meet his or her own needs for the basics of life. Nursing interventions must accomplish self-care or assist the individual in the development or regulation of self-care.

Self-care has been described by Orem primarily in terms of the competent adult. Children and dependent adults are viewed as having some self-care abilities; however, these are not seen as developing and are not clearly described. Recently, other researchers[8] have expanded upon Orem's model by applying theories of development to self-care.

Mary J. Denyes has developed and tested an instrument to measure self-care capabilities in adolescents. The findings of her research indicate that adolescents possess interest in their health and self-care.[9] A study by this author using Denyes's instrument to describe self-care capabilities of low-income, urban, female adolescent parents and nonparents has been recently completed.[10]

From initial data on self-care capabilities in adolescence, six components have been identified:

1. Ego strength and health decision-making capability,
2. Relative valuing of health,
3. Health knowledge and decision-making experience,
4. Physical energy levels,
5. Feelings,
6. Attention to health.[11]

Adolescence is a time of life when various patterns of living are explored and accepted or rejected by the individual. Self-care capabilities need particular attention during the adolescent phase of rapid development and identity establishment. The opportunity to promote self-care practices is particularly pertinent to the self-care conscious adolescent. Despite recent nursing interest in self-care as a basis for nursing intervention, no research has been conducted regarding the self-care capabilities of the abused adolescent.

Clinical experience with violent families has provided the author with many opportunities to assess abused adolescents. Observations from experience reveal that adolescents have great interest in their bodies and their health, yet professionals frequently express frustration and mistrust of adolescents as clients. Adolescents who run away from home are frequently maltreated, females often sexually abused. The act of "running away from home" rather than being a delinquent action is an excellent example of self-care. While in the home, the abused adolescent cannot get necessary professional assistance and is a likely subject of repeated parent attacks. By running away, the adolescent immediately puts a stop to the abuse and becomes eligible for multidisciplinary assistance. Professionals who work with adolescents who flee their abusive homes often fail to see the strength and resourcefulness of the youth's action and instead treat a child as a juvenile delinquent. Nursing research into abused adolescent self-care capabilities will add to the refinement of the phenomenon. The nurse who works with abused adolescents will be better able to identify and encourage client self-care practices. Knowledge of the abused adolescent's self-care strengths may aid decision making on the part of the professionals who must suggest placement or recommend emancipation.

Appropriate research questions might then be:

1. How do abused adolescents perceive their self-care capabilities?
2. What differences exist in the degree of perceived self-care capability between abused adolescents and non-abused adolescents?
3. What differences exist in the degree of perceived self-care capability between abused male adolescents and abused female adolescents?
4. What differences exist in the degree of perceived self-care capability between sexually abused adolescents and non-sexually abused adolescents?

Other nursing theories may be used as a basis for nursing research into family violence. Orem's model has merely been used as an example. The point to be made is that nursing research based upon nursing theory is necessary for advancing the knowledge base of nursing in family violence.

NURSING RESEARCH AND FAMILY VIOLENCE

The need for nursing research in the area of family violence is tremendous. Nurses are in an ideal position to make a major contribution to the knowledge base of family violence and yet, with a few exceptions, only occasional nursing research studies have been reported. Nursing is not alone in its need to conduct systematic inquiries into family violence. Although other disciplines have carried out research studies and reported in the literature, the progress to date in understanding and preventing family violence has been small.

Child abuse, as the most widely known and studied form of family violence, provides an excellent example of the problems associated with much of the research. In a content analysis of 2,698 abstracts in the National Center on Child Abuse and Neglect series, *Child Abuse and Neglect Research: Projects and Publications,* from 1976 to 1979, F. G. Bolton, Jr., Roy H. Laner, Dorothy S. Gai, and Sandra P. Kane identify the great lack of research that can "survive rigorous scientific scrutiny."[12] Child abuse reports tend to be more of the discussion than empirical type. Sample sizes are often small, nonrepresentative, convenience based, and usually lack controls. There is almost a total absence of longitudinal or trend analysis.

In particular is the problem of excessive use of official records for child abuse and neglect research rather than direct subject contact. Only 17.2 percent of the research did not rely upon official records. "An added concern is the fact that 84.4 percent of the official records utilized were in a form completed by an official in the organization under study."[13] Over one-half (53 percent) of the authors did not even have contact with their subjects and drew all their conclusions based upon official records.[14]

When the child abuse and neglect works were broken down, 77.2 percent were found to be on "general maltreatment" rather than dealing with one specific area. Of those reports that did identify one aspect of child abuse and neglect, only 1.8 percent dealt with neglect and 0.05 percent dealt with emotional maltreatment. The greatest number of studies from one discipline was 39.7 percent from the "Medical/Biological/Physiological" field.

Bolton and his colleagues found that much of the early work on child abuse and neglect focused upon the search for definitions. Although the number of reports dealing with definitions has decreased, only 10.4 percent address prevention and treatment.[15] The most serious outcome of such inadequate study is the impact on child welfare funding.

> "The funneling of money into programs built upon a less than secure base, largely as a result of the lack of solid empirical knowledge, is truly wasted and may even border upon damaging due to its false promises."[16]

Fortunately, some nursing investigations have overcome these limitations. In an unpublished study, Wendy G. Goldberg, a nurse researcher and clinician, and Michael C. Tomlanovich, obtained some interesting results in a survey of emergency room patients.[17] Out of 492 emergency department patients systematically surveyed over a two-month period, 107 were found to be victims of domestic violence on a self-report survey. Patients included in the study were males and females at least sixteen years old. Domestic violence victims were found to be willing to reveal themselves on a survey, but even with the incentive of participating in the study, they were reluctant to directly ask for help.

Domestic violence victims tended to describe their abusive relationships in a devalued, understated style. Their reports may reflect the general social unacceptability of being a victim of family violence. In contrast, those victims who used emergency departments at all tended to use them repeatedly. In this case, their devalued descriptions may reflect past experience with health care providers and the lack of assistance, or a combination of this and a sense of the general unacceptability of family violence victim status.

The domestic violence victim's chief complaints, triage assessments, and diagnoses were most often categorized as medical rather than traumatic or psychiatric. Further, victims often requested pain medication from the emergency room staff and complained of "pain" (on the survey form), but were seldom given such medication either in the emergency department or at discharge from the emergency room. Therefore, domestic violence victim's expressions of pain may reflect a more global painful existence rather than a localized organic problem.

The Goldberg and Tomlanovich study identitified that the factors most closely associated with requests for counseling were if one were injured by weapons, if one had a negative view of the overall relationship, and if one's children had been hurt by the abusive partner. The study results clearly reinforce the importance of adequate assessment of every client for the existence or potential for abuse.

An example of generally accepted clinical practices and assumptions being refuted with empirical data is a study by Eleanor J. Bullerdick Corey, Carol L. Miller, and Frederick W. Widlak. The study attempted to examine the validity of previous demographic findings as characteristics of abused children.[18]

> Demographic characteristics and medical history items suggested by some investigators as factors that influence child abuse were shown in the study to be of doubtful value in discriminating between hospitalized battered children and their non-battered counterparts.[19]

The characteristics associated with abuse in children may merely be those associated with hospitalization. In addition, Corey reports that the siblings of abused children tended to be abused as well. Therefore nurses cannot rest once they are certain of the safety of one abused child in the family; siblings are likely to be abused as well and even if not, require appropriate nursing interventions (see Chapter 11).

Richard J. Gelles, in a review of research done in the seventies on family violence, identifies several areas of need. Research must move beyond mere descriptive efforts toward "a systematic program of research to empirically test theories and also to use available data to build new theories of family violence."[20] Research should test theories unlike much of the current theoretical knowledge which is based upon post hoc explanations of data. Gelles suggests that longitudinal designs be employed to provide greater in-

Implications for Nursing

sight concerning time, order, and causal relationships in family violence research. The use of more nonclinical samples would help "to overcome the confusion which arises out of confounding factors which lead to public identification of family violence with those factors causally related to violent behavior in the home."[21] Finally, Gelles recommends that data collection and measurement techniques increase in number and diversity. Researchers no longer need to fear that subjects can not or will not disclose violence in their family.

Nursing research into family violence is needed in many areas. Several of these topic areas are:

1. Intrafamilial sexual abuse
2. Threats to victim body image from violence
3. Relationship between violent family functioning and individual well-being
4. Incidence and description of elderly abuse
5. Wife abuse and pregnancy
6. Abuse and the grieving response
7. Abuse, victim stress, and its manifestations
8. Relationship between suicide and abuse
9. Relationship between substance abuse and violence against family members
10. Resolution of personal and professional feelings about family violence
11. Nursing interventions with individual victims of family violence
12. Nursing interventions that assist violent families in achieving well-being

NURSING PRACTICE

The professional nurse in clinical practice—whether it be in a hospital, in the community, or in private practice—has contact with potential or actual family violence. The practicing nurse may not initially be aware that clients are perpetrating and/or experiencing abuse. Victims of family violence are by no means always obvious even to a critical eye. The first step toward identifying family violence is for the nurse to be aware of the problem. Increased awareness on the part of the nurse can prevent the potential for violence from becoming a fact.

The mere fact that the practicing nurse is aware of family violence, its forms, and magnitude will increase the number of clients that are identified as "at risk." The author's clinical experience as a pediatric clinical nurse specialist, with a constant clinic population, demonstrated that as awareness and knowledge of family violence increased so did the number of clients experiencing the problem. It is unlikely that the client population changed all at once, rather it was an understanding of the indicators of violence that increased in the practitioner. Awareness of the problem of family violence should therefore make the nurse more sensitive to certain assessment findings. Another consequence, however, should be that the nurse includes assessments about family violence as part of the nursing care given to every client. Just as the nurse always asks the client's age, marital status, and so on, so should inquiries be made into family and individual stresses, family conflict resolution, and childrearing patterns. Clients do not question such nursing assessments and are often pleased to know that a health care provider is interested in more than just their physical health. The nurse is also setting the framework for future client interactions. Routine assessment of family functioning lets the client know that such topics are appropriate in client-nurse discussion.

Effective nursing care, as always, begins with the client or family's concerns. Actual or potential violence in the family may be a problem; however, it may not be the reason for seeking out nursing care. Primary attention given to the client's concerns indicates to the client that the nurse acknowledges their importance, initiates the process of establishing a trusting relationship, and increases the likelihood of the joint development of an effective plan of care. The collaborative role of the nurse indicates her respect for the clients and their freedom to make their own decisions regarding the kind of nursing care they need. Such nursing care, therefore, logically builds upon the strengths of individuals and families. Nursing in this manner can effectively be provided in any setting. The successful development of such nursing in a nontraditional setting was carried out by the major authors and is described as an example of its appropriateness for other nurses.

The initial contact took place between Jacquelyn Campbell and the director at the battered women's shelter. At first the staff could identify only the need for occasional first aid, development of emergency protocols, blood pressure screening, and health appraisal form completion as appropriate nursing functions. The agency had only minimal contact with nursing or its services.

The role the nurse played within the agency gradually began to evolve. A sign-up list was established whereby any resident of the shelter could request to see the nurse during her weekly visits. Additional clients might just appear at the time of the nurse's established hours. Eventually, some clients began to be referred by the agency staff. Again, initially only those clients with established medical problems were referred by staff to the nurse. There was a wide range of reasons given by the residents for wanting to see the nurse. One nine-year-old girl with severe atopic dermatitis referred herself as she wanted to go swimming with the other children. The shelter's staff was fearful that she was "contagious." Another shelter resident, this one a woman hit in the head with a hammer, sought out the nurse because she needed her stitches removed. Many other visits to the nurse were for reasons that can be found in any setting: diarrhea, colds, weight reduction, stress control, pregnancy, infant feeding, sore throats, headaches. The nurse is really called upon to be a generalist.

Later on, Janice Humphreys joined as the second nurse volunteer. Nursing visits were now alternated between the two with a written record of clients seen, assessment, intervention, and needed follow-up established both in the "nurse's log" and in the individual client's agency record. Additional consultation between the nurses frequently occurred by phone.

Through the sharing of experiences at the shelter with the faculty at the College of Nursing, Wayne State University, and the offer of graduate student placement, a master's student in nursing was assigned to the shelter for a clinical learning experience. The student became so intrigued with the opportunities for nursing in such a setting that she continued her involvement even after her course work was completed. The outcome of the student's experience was a master's thesis that investigates the role of play therapy with the children of battered women. The following year, another master's student was placed at the shelter. She too became interested in the women and children and is now a volunteer and engaged in conducting an ethnography into the lives of the battered women and their children in the shelter.

Both authors continue to practice at battered women's shelters. The involvement that began as volunteer work in a shelter has expanded considerably. Both were elected to board of director positions with shelters and other domestic violence groups. Participation also routinely includes speaking engagements on behalf of battered women's shelters, generally on the topic of family violence. Education of other health care professionals has also become a regular activity.

The purpose of this discussion has been to suggest that in addition to nursing practice with violent families in traditional settings, there is a wealth of opportunity and need for nurses to investigate and expand practice in innovative areas. What began with one nurse's offer to volunteer at a battered women's shelter has grown into a relationship between agency (staff and residents) and nursing that strengthens both.

NURSING EDUCATION AND FAMILY VIOLENCE

The nurse who is practicing in a truly holistic sense must be prepared to deal with family violence whatever the type or location of practice. Nursing education has for the most part acknowledged its inability to expose students to every possible health problem or concern. Appropriately, the baccalaureate nursing student is instructed in the basis of all nursing care, the nursing process, and is then familiarized with certain theories or principles. The student is assisted to develop a flexible and inquiring mind so that whatever client alteration is identified, even though previously unencountered, she will be able to systematically assess, plan, implement, and evaluate to the client's greatest benefit. In the case of physical alterations experienced by a client, the nursing student is often admirably prepared to tackle any circumstance. Appropriate nursing interventions where a client impairment is experienced related to diabetes mellitus, renal failure, or cardiac insufficiency are usually thoroughly familiar to the nursing student. Nursing interventions where family violence has occurred, however, probably go almost unmentioned in many nursing programs and likely receive nursing educational time equal to their incidence in the general population in no present program. The example of wifebeating occurring more often than diabetes during pregnancy is an excellent case in point. Many nursing students spend large amounts of time both reading and listening to the many problems related to diabetes during pregnancy. The same cannot be said for the study of abuse of women which occurs even more often prenatally.

The reasons for the lack of nursing education directed at family violence are as complex as the problem itself. Nursing as a profession exists in the United States within the larger field of health care. Both are in turn subject to the values and culture of the dominant group, white middle-class males. Nursing as a profession, composed in majority by females, exists as an atypical group within the larger patriarchal culture. Nurses (women) outnumber all other health care providers (men) and yet in many ways have been subject to oppression and control by the male minority. This situation is repeated for women in general in the United States.

Nursing continues to strive for its autonomy and yet as predominately female professionals nurses must attempt to meet the health needs of their clients all the while overcoming obstacles other providers have never experienced. For nursing to have neglected family violence as an issue for nursing education is not too surprising. Like the battered woman who is continually told she is worthless, stupid, and incapable of having her own ideas or making her own decisions, nursing has not been regarded as possessing knowledge that is valuable and worthy of respect given to other professionals. Achieving and maintaining feelings of self-worth was and is an arduous task for both the battered woman and nursing. Until the time that adequate self confidence in nurses could be achieved, nursing could not acknowledge the health care implications of male domination. Male oppression of women persists as an experience common to both nursing as a profession and most of its practitioners as individuals. It might be said that the discipline of nursing is disturbingly familiar with the discriminating forces affecting battered women. The reality of prevention of third-party reimbursement for nursing services by physicians, male-controlled insurance companies, and male legislators is very much like the reality of the abusive husband who controls every cent received by his battered wife, only on a larger scale. Until nursing recognized its own oppression, it was difficult to acknowledge the oppression of battered women and was therefore easier to neglect the problem.

It should be further noted that many battered women have been so mentally debilitated that they spend large amounts of time trying to determine if something "they did" was wrong and fear that they are the "only battered women in town." Nursing may have been just too close to the problem for a long time to have been able to see it clearly. Because of the nature of nursing and due to its largely female constituents, nurses are in an excellent position to be advocates and providers for the dependent female victims of family violence.

Other factors that may have contributed to the general lack of attention given to family violence by nursing have to do with the characteristics of violence. As was discussed in Chapter 5, violence in the family is associated with poverty. Poor American populations have typically been underserved in respect to problems associated with their low socioeconomic class. In addition, there is often a tendency for society to "blame the poor" for its difficulties. As a member of the larger society, nursing deserves equal responsibility for its neglect of family violence.

It has also been discussed at length in earlier chapters that the causes of violence in the family are multifaceted and complex. As such, the tendency is sometimes to focus on the physical injury and not on the reasons why. Understanding the nature of family violence, although essential to all levels of prevention, does not come easily. Treatment of impairment or injury caused by neglect or abuse on the other hand often does achieve immediate results.

The implication of this discussion is *not* to suggest that client physical alterations are not important and should not receive so much attention in nursing education. Indeed physical impairments are of great concern to nurses and clients alike. Clinical experience has revealed that battered women and children often seek out nursing care for what they perceive to be a physical problem and because the nurse is known to be knowledgeable in that area. The nurse was approached in the first place because nursing education is well grounded in anatomy, physiology, and physical care. The point to be made is that violence in families must also be a concern to professional nurses. The first step in increasing the nursing assessments of family violence is to raise the awareness of the profession to the problem. An ideal method of familiarizing nurses with family violence as a health problem is to include the topic in basic and advanced nursing education. One method of including family violence within nursing education is the incorporation of a special course into the curriculum.

COURSE DESCRIPTION

Out of the concern of the major authors of the text, a course was developed to prepare senior-level undergraduate students in a midwestern baccalaureate program to provide nursing care to victims of family violence.

Objectives of the Course

The formalized cognitive course objectives were as follows:

a. Analyzes theoretical approaches to the problem of violence in the family

b. Analyzes the applicability of nursing care measures and community resources designed to assist dysfunctional families for nursing care of violent families

c. Analyzes the influence of culture and community on the problems of violence

d. Formulates appropriate nursing interventions for the problem of violence in the family on the primary, secondary, and tertiary prevention levels

e. Utilizes the nursing process to provide nursing care to selected families experiencing violence

The purpose of the course was to provide students with the opportunity to integrate previous learning about families, adaptation, nursing care of children, communication skills, health assessment, and nursing process with new concepts of violence and alteration in fit between family resources and demands in order to provide holistic and comprehensive nursing care to families experiencing violence. The course was a four-credit-hour elective that combined both formal classroom lecture/discussion (three hours per week) and individualized student clinical experiences (three hours per week). The course focused on the causes and extent of violence in the family; the influence of culture and community on violence in the family; and nursing interventions for the problem at the primary, secondary, and tertiary prevention levels. Areas of violence in the family examined included child abuse, wife abuse, sexual abuse, violence involving adolescent family members, abuse of elderly family members, and homicide.

In addition to providing educational opportunities in the cognitive and psychomotor domains, the course addressed the affective domain of providing nursing care to victims of family violence. The decision to include learning experiences in the affective domain was based upon the theoretical framework presented by Dorthy E.

Reilly in her book *Teaching and Evaluating the Affective Domain in Nursing Programs.*[22]

Briefly, Reilly describes and supports the notion that nurses as health care providers have a responsibility to deal with all of the needs of clients within the guidelines of the standards of practice and according to the Code for Nurses. Nursing education in turn has an obligation to prepare students to meet this responsibility. Nursing students have been provided with assistance in the areas of cognitive and psychomotor learning. The affective domain, however, remains essentially untouched in nursing education. The general thinking on this subject is that students will learn about this area as they focus on theory and skills. "Events in our society are now convincing educators that the affective domain of learning is not only a crucial component of any program planning which prepares health providers but it demands the same pedagogical considerations as the other domains."[23]

In order for the learning of values to take place, two criteria must be met in teaching—experience and critical thinking. Teaching strategies suggested by Reilly that provide both experience and critical thinking include group discussion based upon student experiences, multimedia presentations, "exposure to varied value related patterns of behavior and lifestyles," and clinical practice with a group and with one family in particular.[24] Each of these strategies was incorporated into the senior-level course described. "The primary goal of this educational endeavor [including the affective domain] is in assisting the learners in the development of values that support a self-identity that is compatible with the responsibilities inherent in the role of a health care provider in a complex ever-changing pluralistic society."[25] In view of the factors suggested earlier as possibly contributing to the lack of nursing attention to family violence, nursing education is particularly in need of learning opportunities in the affective domain.

In an effort to crudely measure student nurses' attitudes and experience with family violence a presurvey and a postsurvey were conducted. Fifteen demographic variables were also included. The small number (N = 15) of students and the short-term nature of the course preclude generalizability. Some interesting results, however, were noted.

The majority of the students were aware of their own values and were generally nonjudgmental in their attitudes about victims of family violence. Little to no change was noted in the students' values surveyed from before and after the course. This may have been mainly due to the students' supportive attitude upon entering the course.

Of particular note was the finding that almost all the nursing students reported some kind of close personal contact with violence. The majority of students reported that either they had experienced physical abuse as a child or as an adult or that a close friend had experienced some kind of physical violence. It must be remembered that the course offered was an elective and chosen by the nursing students themselves. However, self-selected or not, experience with personal violence is common and likely to have been experienced by a large number of nursing students in any class. The need for nursing education focused upon family violence and including learning opportunities in the affective domain becomes even greater.

Two additional studies with working nurses and undergraduate student nurses

Implications for Nursing

bring to light information about nurses' attitudes toward female victims of violence. In an investigation of staff nurses' reactions toward rape victims versus nonsexual beating victims, Cheryl S. Alexander found no significant difference in the nurses' perception of victim blame for either group. The practicing nurses did not attribute a significant degree of responsibility for the crime to either type of victim.[26] In a different study, Shirley Petchel Damrosch found that graduating baccalaureate nursing students were significantly more likely to attach responsibility for rape to the victim if the woman committed a perceived act of carelessness (failed to lock her car door). When the nursing students were told the study results, their reaction was one of surprise, that they, as a group, had discriminated against the careless victim. As Damrosch points out, the key difference between her study sample and that of Alexander's may be the subjects' exposure to victims of violence.[27] The need for nursing students to have experience with victims of violence as part of their basic education assumes even greater importance.

Summary

The current text attempts to bring together the three major areas, theory, research, and practice that give direction to the nursing care of victims of family violence. The book approaches violence from a nursing perspective and examines the problem as it affects individuals and the family as a unit.

The implications of family violence for nursing are great. The nurse in clinical practice is called upon to have awareness of the problem and the needs of those victims of family violence. The demands upon both nursing and families increase as economic cutbacks require that social agency resources decrease. Nursing can meet the demands placed upon it in the care of victims of family violence. To better prepare future nurses, educational content on family violence should be included in every nursing program. Nursing research, particularly that based upon nursing theory, is still needed to increase the knowledge base of nursing in the care of victims of family violence. Violence only exists as we as a society and a profession allow it. The existence of violence is never acceptable, especially when it is inflicted with our most basic unit, the family. Nursing as a discipline is challenged to provide leadership in developing theory, research, and effective practice.

Chapter 16

1. Jacqueline Fawcett, "The What of Theory Development," in *Theory Development: What, Why, How?* (New York: National League for Nursing, 1978), p. 25.
2. Margaret Newman, *Theory Development in Nursing* (Philadelphia: F. A. Davis Co., 1979), p. 6.
3. Ann Whall, "Congruence between Existing Theories of Family Functioning and Nursing Theories," *Advances in Nursing Science* 3, no. 1 (October 1980): 59–67.
4. Judith Smith, "The Idea of Health: A Philosophical Inquiry," *Advances in Nursing Science* 3, no. 3 (April 1981): 43–50.

5. Ibid., p. 44.

6. Georgia Kemm Millor, "Theoretical Framework for Nursing Research in Child Abuse and Neglect," *Nursing Research* 30, no. 2 (March-April 1981), pp. 78-83.

7. Dorothea E. Orem, *Nursing: Concepts of Practice*, 2nd ed. (New York: McGraw Hill, 1980) p. 35.

8. Mary J. Denyes, "Development of an Instrument to Measure Self-Care Agency in Adolescents" (unpublished doctoral diss., University of Michigan, 1980); K. M. Eichelberger, D. H. Kaufman, M. E. Rundahl, and N. E. Schwartz, "Self-Care Nursing Plan: Helping Children to Help Themselves," *Pediatric Nursing* 6, no. 3 (1980): 9-13.

9. Denyes, "Development of an Instrument."

10. Janice Humphreys, "Self-Care Capabilities of Low Income, Urban, Female Adolescent Parents and Non-Parents" (paper presented at the Michigan Nurses Association Annual Convention, Saginaw, Michigan, 26 October 1982).

11. Denyes, "Development of an Instrument."

12. F. G. Bolton et al., "Study of Child Maltreatment When is Research . . . Research?" *Journal of Family Issues* 2, no. 4 (December 1981), pp. 531-39.

13. Ibid., p. 537.

14. Ibid.

15. Ibid., p. 535.

16. Ibid., p. 538.

17. Wendy G. Goldberg, personal communication to J. Campbell, 26 October 1982.

18. Eleanor J. Bullerdick Corey, Carol L. Miller, and Frederick W. Widlak, "Factors Contributing to Child Abuse," *Nursing Research* 24 (July/August 1975): 293-95."

19. Ibid, p. 294.

20. Richard J. Gelles, "Violence in the Family: A Review of Research in the Seventies," *Journal of Marriage and the Family* 42 (November 1980): 873-85. p. 882.

21. Ibid., p. 883.

22. Dorothy E. Reilly, ed. *Teaching and Evaluating the Affective Domain in Nursing Programs* (Charles B. Slack, 1978).

23. Reilly, p. 34.

24. Ibid., pp. 43-47.

25. Ibid., p. 35.

26. Cheryl S. Alexander, "The Responsible Victim: Nurses' Perceptions of Victims of Rape," *Journal of Health and Social Behavior* 21 (March 1980): 22-23.

27. Shirley Petchel Damrasch, "How Nursing Students' Reactions to Rape Victims Are Affected by a Perceived Act of Carelessness," *Nursing Research* 30, no. 3 (May-June 1981): 168-70.

Selected References

THEORIES OF VIOLENCE AND AGGRESSION

Abel, Ernest L. "The Relationship between Cannabis and Violence: A Review." *Psychological Bulletin* 84 (March 1977): 193-211.

Abrahamsen, David. *Our Violent Society.* New York: Funk & Wagnalls, 1970.

———. *The Psychology of Crime.* New York: Columbia University Press, 1960.

Alland, Alexander. *The Human Imperative.* New York: Columbia University Press, 1972.

Allen, Martin. "A Cross-Cultural Study of Aggression and Crime." *Journal of Cross-Cultural Psychology* 3 (September 1972): 259-71.

Allen, Richard, Daniel Safer, and Lino Covi. "Effects of Psychostimulants on Aggression." *Journal of Nervous and Mental Disease* 160 (February 1975): 138-43.

Andison, F. Scott. "TV Violence and Viewer Aggression: A Cumulation of Study Results, 1956-1976." *Public Opinion Quarterly* 41 (Fall 1977): 314-31.

Archer, Dane, et al. "Cities and Homicide: A New Look at an Old Paradox." *Comparative Studies in Sociology* 1 (1978): 73-95.

Ardrey, Robert. *The Territorial Imperative.* New York: Atheneum, 1976.

Bach-Y-Rita, George. "Episodic Dyscontrol: A Study of 130 Violent Patients." *American Journal of Psychiatry* 127 (May 1971): 1473-78.

Bach-Y-Rita, George, and Arther Veno. "Habitual Violence: A Profile of Sixty-Two Men." *American Journal of Psychiatry* 131 (September 1974): 1015-17.

Balkwell, Carolyn, et al. "On Black and White Family Patterns in America: Their Impact on the Expressive Aspect of Sex-Role Socialization." *Journal of Marriage and the Family* (November 1978): 743-48.

Bailey, William C. "Some Further Evidence on Homicide and a Regional Culture of Violence." *Omega* 7 (1976): 145-70.

Bandura, Albert. *Aggression: A Social Learning Analysis.* Englewood Cliffs, N.J.: Prentice-Hall, 1973.

———. "Influence of Models' Reinforcement Contingencies on the Acquisition of Imitative Responses." *Journal of Personality and Social Psychology* 1 (June 1965): 589–95.

Bellak, Leopold, and Maxine Antell. "An Intercultural Study of Aggressive Behavior on Children's Playgrounds." *American Journal of Orthopsychiatry* 44 (July 1974): 503–511.

Bergen, Bernard, and Stanley Rosenberg. "Culture as Violence." *Humanitas* 12 (May 1976): 195–205.

Berkowitz, Leonard. "Experimental Investigations of Hostility Catharsis." *Journal of Consulting and Clinincal Psychology* 35 (February 1970): 1–7.

Berkowitz, Leonard, and Joseph Alioto. "The Meaning of an Observed Event as a Determinant of Its Aggressive Consequences." *Journal of Personality and Social Psychology* 28 (November 1973): 206–217.

Berkowitz, Leonard and Anthony LePage. "Weapons as Aggression Eliciting Stimuli." *Journal of Personality and Social Psychology* 7 (1967): 202–207.

Blumenthal, Monica, et al. *Justifying Violence.* Ann Arbor, Mich.: Braun-Brumfeld, 1972.

Blumer, Dietrich, and Claude Migeon. "Hormones and Hormonal Agents in the Treatment of Aggression." *Journal of Nervous and Mental Disease* 160 (January 1975): 127–37.

Braziller, George. *Violent Crime.* U.S. Commission on the Causes and Prevention of Violence, 1969.

Brennan, John J. "Mentally Ill Aggressiveness—Popular Delusion or Reality." *American Journal of Psychiatry* 120 (June 1964): 1181–84.

Briggs, Jean L. *Never in Anger.* Cambridge: Harvard University Press, 1970.

Buss, Arnold. *The Psychology of Aggression.* New York: John Wiley & Sons, 1961.

Carthy, J. D., and F. J. Ebling, eds. *The Natural History of Aggression.* London: Academic Press, 1964.

Cloward, Marshall, and Lloyd Ohlin. *Delinquency and Opportunity.* Glencoe, Ill.: Free Press, 1960.

Cocozza, Joseph J., and Henry Steadman. "Some Refinements in the Measurement and Prediction of Dangerous Behavior." *American Journal of Psychiatry* 131 (September 1974): 1012–15.

Coleman, Lee S. "Perspectives on the Medical Research of Violence." *American Journal of Orthopsychiatry* 44 (October 1974): 675–87.

Coles, Robert. "Violence in Ghetto Children." *Children* 14 (May-June 1967): 101–104.

Curtis, Lynn A. *Criminal Violence.* Lexington, Mass.: D. C. Heath & Co., 1974.

———. *Violence, Race, and Culture.* Lexington, Mass.: D. C. Heath & Co., 1975.

Delgado, Josi M. R. "The Neurological Basis of Violence." *International Social Science Journal* 33 (1971): 27-35.

Diener, Edward. "Effects of Altered Responsibility, Cognitive Set, and Modeling on Physical Aggression and Deindividuation." *Journal of Personality and Social Psychology* 31 (1975): 328-37.

Divale, William Tulio, and Marvin Harris. "Population, Warfare, and the Male Supremacist Complex." *American Anthropologist* 78 (September 1976): 521-38.

Doerner, William. "A Regional Analysis of Homicide Rates in the United States." *Criminology* 13 (May 1975): 90-101.

Eckhardt, William. "Anthropological Correlates of Primitive Militarism." *Peace Research* 5 (1 February 73): 5-10.

Elkin, A. P. *The Australian Aborigines.* Natural History Library Edition 1964. Garden City, N.Y.: Doubleday Co., 1938.

Elliott, Frank. "The Neurology of Explosive Rage." *Practitioner* 217 (July 1976): 51-59.

Ember, Melvin. "Warfare, Sex Ratio, and Polygyny." *Ethnology* 13 (April 1974): 197-206.

Erlanger, Howard S. "The Empirical Status of the Subculture of Violence Thesis." *Social Problems* 22 (December 1974): 280-92.

———. "Is There a 'Subculture of Violence' in the South?" *Journal of Criminal Law and Criminology* 66 (December 1975): 483-90.

Eron, Leonard. "Prescription for Reduction of Aggression." *American Psychologist* 35 (March 1980): 244-52.

Eysenck, H. J. *Crime and Personality.* 3rd ed. London: Routledge & Kegan Paul, 1977.

Fawcett, Jan, ed. *Dynamics of Violence.* Chicago: American Medical Association, 1971.

Fenigston, Allen. "Does Aggression Cause a Preference for Viewing Media Violence?" *Journal of Personality and Social Psychology* 37 (December 1979): 2307-17.

Frazier, Shervert H., ed. *Aggression.* Baltimore: Williams & Wilkins Press, 1974.

Fromm, Erich. *The Anatomy of Human Destruction.* New York: Fawcett Crest Books, 1973.

Galle, Omer R., Walter R. Gove, and J. Miller McPherson. "Population Density and Pathology: What are the Relations for Man?" *Science* 176 (7 April, 1972): 23-30.

Gastil, Raymond. "Homicide and a Regional Culture of Violence." *American Sociological Review* 36 (June 1971): 412-27.

Gerbner, George. "The Demonstration of Power: Violence Profile No. 10." *Journal of Communications* 29 (Summer 1979): 177-96.

Gerbner, George, et al. "Cultural Indicators: Violence Profile No. 9." *Journal of Communications* 28 (Summer 1978): 196-207.

Gerson, Lowell W., and Donald A. Preston. "Alcohol Consumption and the Incidence of Violent Crime." *Journal of Studies on Alcohol* 40 (March 1979): 307–312.

Gillies, Hunter. "Homicide in the West of Scotland." *British Journal of Psychology* 28 (February 1976): 126–32.

Goldstein, Jeffrey. *Aggression and Crimes of Violence.* New York: Oxford University Press, 1975.

Goldstein, Murray. "Brain Research and Violent Behavior." *Archives of Neurology* 30 (January 1974): 1–35.

Golin, Sanford, and Michael A. Romanowski. "Verbal Aggression as a Function of Sex of Subject and Sex of Target." *Journal of Psychology* 97 (September 1977): 141–49.

Goodwin, Donald W. "Alcohol in Suicide and Homicide." *Quarterly Journal of Studies on Alcohol* 34 (March 1973): 144–56.

Graham, Kathryn. "Theories of Intoxicated Aggression." *Canadian Journal of Behavioral Science* 12 (April 1980): 141–58.

Halloran, J. D. "The Mass Media and Violence." *Forensic Science* 5 (June 1975): 209–217.

Hamburg, David A. "Recent Research on Hormonal Factors Relevant to Human Aggressiveness." *International Social Science Journal* 23 (1971): 36–47.

Hepburn, John. "Subcultures, Violence, and the Subculture of Violence: An Old Rut or a New Road." *Criminology* 9 (May 1971): 87–98.

Herjanic, M., and D. Meyer. "Notes on Epidemiology of Homicide in an Urban Area." *Forensic Science* 8 (November-December 1976): 235–45.

Hosken, Fran P. "Female Circumcision in Africa." *Victimology* 2 (1977–78): 487–98.

Kaplan, Howard B. *Self-Attitudes and Deviant Behavior.* Pacific Palisades, Calif.: Goodyear Publishing Co., 1975.

Kaplan, Howard B., and Robert D. Singer. "Television Violence and Viewer Aggression: A Reexamination of the Evidence." *Journal of Social Issues* 32 (Fall 1976): 35–70.

Kutash, Irwin L. and others, ed. *Violence: Perspectives on Murder and Aggression.* San Francisco: Jossey-Bass Publishers, 1978.

Laborit, Henri. "The Biological and Sociological Mechanisms of Aggression." *International Social Science Journal* 30 (1978): 727–49.

Leavitt, Ruby. *Peaceable Primates and Gentle People: Anthropological Approaches to Women's Studies.* New York: Harper & Row, 1975.

Liston, Robert. *Violence in America.* New York: Julian Messner, 1974.

Lorenz, Konrad. *On Aggression.* New York: Bantam Books, 1966.

Lunde, Donald T. *Murder and Madness.* San Francisco: San Francisco Book Co., 1976.

Lundsgaarde, Henry P. *Murder in Space City*. New York: Oxford University Press, 1977.

McCarthy, Elizabeth D., et al. "Violence and Behavior Disorders." *Journal of Communications* 25 (Autumn 1975): 71-84.

McConahay, Shirley A., and John B. McConahay. "Sexual Permissiveness, Sex Role Rigidity, and Violence across Cultures." *Journal of Social Issues* 33 (1977): 134-43.

Madden, Denis J., and John R. Lion, eds. *Rage, Assault, and Other Forms of Violence*. New York: Spectrum Publications, 1976.

Maletzky, Barry M. "The Episodic Dyscontrol Syndrome." *Diseases of the Nervous System* 34 (March 1973): 178-85.

Maple, Terry, and Douglas R. Matheson, eds. *Aggression, Hostility, and Violence*. New York: Holt, Rinehart & Winston, 1973.

May, Rollo. *Power and Innocence*. New York: W. W. Norton, 1972.

Megargee, Edwin I., and Jack E. Hokanson, eds. *The Dynamics of Aggression*. New York: Harper & Row, 1970.

Megargee, Edwin I. "Undercontrolled and Overcontrolled Personality Types in Extreme Antisocial Aggression." *Psychological Monographs* 80 (1966): 3-20.

Mesnikoff, Alvin M., and Carl G. Lauterbach. "The Association of Violent Dangerous Behavior with Psychiatric Disorders: A Review of the Literature." *Journal of Psychiatry and the Law* 3 (Winter 1975): 415-45.

Monroe, Russell R. "Anticonvulsants in the Treatment of Aggression." *Journal of Nervous and Mental Disease* 160 (January 1975): 119-26.

Monroe, Russell. *Brain Dysfunction in Aggressive Criminals*. Lexington, Mass.: D. C. Heath & Co., 1976.

Montagu, Ashley, ed. *Learning Non-Aggression*. New York: Oxford University Press, 1978.

———. *The Nature of Human Aggression*. New York: Oxford University Press, 1976.

Morrison, James R., and Kenneth Minkoff. "Explosive Personality as a Sequel to the Hyperactive-Child Syndrome." *Comprehensive Psychiatry* 16 (July/August 1975): 343-48.

Moyer, K. E. *The Psychobiology of Aggression*. New York: Harper & Row, 1976.

Mulvihill, Donald J., and Melvin M. Tumin. *Crimes of Violence*. Vol. 12. *A Staff Report Submitted to the National Commission on the Causes and Prevention of Violence*. Washington, D.C.: U.S. Government Printing Office, 1966.

Neopolitan, Jerry. "Parental Influence on Aggressive Behavior: A Social Learning Approach." *Adolescence* 16 (Winter 1981): 831-40.

Newcombe, Alan. "Some Contributions of the Behavioral Sciences to the Study of Violence." *International Social Sciences Journal* 30 (1978): 750-68.

O'Connor, James, and Alan Lizotte. "The Southern Subculture of Violence: Thesis and Patterns of Gun Ownership." *Social Problems* 25 (April 1978): 420-429.

Owen, David. "The 47, XYY Male." *Psychological Bulletin* 78 (September 1972): 209-233.

Owens, David. "The Social Structure of Violence in Childhood and Approval of Violence as an Adult." *Aggressive Behavior* 1 (1975): 193-211.

Paddock, John. "Studies on Antiviolent and 'Normal' Communities." *Aggressive Behavior* 1 (1975): 217-33.

———. "Values in an Antiviolent Community." *Humanitas* 12 (May 1976): 183-94.

Page, Monte, and Rick Scheidt. "The Elusive Weapons Effect." *Journal of Personality and Social Psychology* 20 (December 1971): 304-318.

Palmer, Stuart. *The Violent Society*. New Haven. College and University Press, 1970.

Parker, Robert Nash, and M. Dwayne Smith. "Deterrence, Poverty, and Type of Homicide." *American Journal of Sociology* 85 (November 1979): 614-23.

Persky, H., K. D. Smith, and G. K. Basu. "Relationship of Psychologic Measures of Aggression and Hostility to Testosterone Production in Men." *Psychosomatic Medicine* 33 (1971): 265-77.

Prescott, James W. "Body Pleasure and the Origins of Violence." *The Futurist* 9 (April 1975): 64-74.

Rochlin, Gregory. *Man's Aggression*. Boston: Gambit, 1973.

Rose, Harold M., ed. *Lethal Aspects of Urban Violence*. Lexington, Mass.: Lexington Books, 1979.

Russell, Claire, and W. M. J. Russell. "The Natural History of Violence." *Journal of Medical Ethics* 5 (1979): 108-117.

Saul, Leon. "A Psychoanalytic View of Hostility: Its Genesis, Treatment, and Implications," *Humanitas* 12 (May 1976): 171-82.

Schmutte, Gregory, Kenneth Leonard, and Stuart Taylor. "Alcohol and Expectations of Attack." *Psychological Reports* 45 (August 1979): 163-67.

Scott, John Paul. "Agnostic Behavior: Function and Dysfunction in Social Conflict." *Journal of Social Issues* 33 (Winter 1977): 9-21.

Sebastian, R. J. "Immediate and Delayed Effects of Victim Suffering on the Attacker's Aggression." *Journal of Research in Personality* 12 (September 1978): 312-28.

Singer, Jerome, ed. *The Control of Aggression and Violence*. New York: Academic Press, 1971.

Spellacy, Frank. "Neuropsychological Discrimination between Violent and Nonviolent Men." *Journal of Clinical Psychology* 34 (January 1978): 49-52.

Storr, Anthony. *Human Destructiveness*. New York: Basic Books, 1972.

Toch, Hans, ed. *Psychology of Crime and Criminal Justice*. New York: Holt, Rinehart & Winston, 1979.

Toch, Hans. *Violent Men.* Chicago: Aldine Publishing Co., 1969.

Valzelli, Luigi. *Psychobiology of Aggression and Violence.* New York: Raven Press, 1981.

Walen, John, ed. *The Neuropsychology of Aggression.* New York: Plenum Press, 1974.

West, D. J. "The Response to Violence." *Journal of Medical Ethics* 5 (1979): 128-31.

Whiting, Beatrice B. "Sex Identity Conflict and Physical Violence: A Comparative Study." *American Anthropologist* 67 (December 1965): 123-40.

Witkin, Herman A., et al. "Criminality in XYY and XXY Men." *Science* 193 (13 August 1976): 547-55.

Wolfgang, Marvin. "A Preface to Violence." *Annals of the American Academy of Political and Social Science* 364 (March 1966): 1-7.

Wolfgang, Marvin, and Franco Ferracuti. *The Subculture of Violence.* London: Tavistock Publications, 1967.

Yelsma, Paul, and Julie Yelsma. "Self-Esteem of Prisoners Committing Directly Versus Indirectly Destructive Crimes." *Perceptual and Motor Skills* 44 (April 1977): 375-80.

ABUSE OF FEMALE PARTNERS

Appleton, William. "The Battered Woman Syndrome." *Annals of Emergency Medicine* 9 (February 1980): 84-91.

Bard, Morton, and Joseph Zacker. "Assaultiveness and Alcohol Use in Family Disputes." *Criminology* 12 (November 1974): 281-92.

Borland, Marie, ed. *Violence in the Family.* Atlantic Highlands, N.J.: Humanities Press, 1976.

Byles, John A. "Violence, Alcohol Problems, and Other Problems in Disintegrating Families." *Journal of Studies on Alcohol* 39 (March 1978): 551-53.

Campbell, Jacquelyn. "Misogyny and Homicide of Women." *Advances in Nursing Science* 3 (January 1981): 67-85.

Carlson, Bonnie. "Battered Women and Their Assailants." *Social Work* 22 (November 1977): 455-65.

Carroll, Joseph C. "The Intergenerational Transmission of Family Violence." *Aggressive Behavior* 3, no. 3 (1977): 289-99.

Cate, Rodney, et al. "Premarital Abuse." *Journal of Family Issues* 3 (March 1982): 79-90.

Chapman, Jane Roberts, and Margaret Gates, eds. *The Victimization of Women.* Beverly Hills, Calif: Sage Publications, 1978.

Chester, Robert, and Jane Streather. "Cruelty in English Divorce: Some Empirical Findings." *Journal of Marriage and the Family* 34 (November 1972): 706-710.

Daly, Mary. *Gyn/Ecology. The Metaethics of Radical Feminism.* Boston: Beacon Press, 1978.

Davidson, Terry. *Conjugal Crime: Understanding and Changing the Wifebeating Problem.* New York: Hawthorn Books, 1978.

DeBliek, Doreen J. "Prevalence of Domestic Violence Reported by Female Psychiatric Inpatients." Unpublished field study, Wayne State University, 1981.

DeLorto, D. O., and A. D. LaViolette. "Spouse Abuse." *Occupational Health Nursing* 28 (August 1980): 17-19.

Dibble, Ursula, and Murray Straus. "Some Social Structure Determinants of Inconsistency between Attitudes and Behavior: The Case of Family Violence." *Journal of Marriage and the Family* 42 (February 1980): 71-80.

Dobash, R. Emerson, and Russell Dobash. *Violence against Wives.* New York: Free Press, 1979.

———. "Social Science and Social Action: The Case of Wife Beating." *Journal of Family Issues* 2 (December 1981): 439-70.

Drake, Virginia Koch. "Battered Women: A Health Care Problem in Disguise." *Image* 14 (June 1982): 40-47.

Eekelaar, John M., and Sanford Katz, eds. *Family Violence.* Toronto: Butterworth & Co., 1978.

Elbow, Margaret. "Theoretical Considerations of Violent Marriages." *Social Casework* 58 (November 1977): 515-26.

Faulk, M. "Men Who Assault Their Wives." *Medicine, Science, and the Law* 14 (July 1974): 180-83.

Fasteau, Marc. *The Male Machine.* New York: McGraw-Hill, 1974.

Fauman, Beverly J. "Psychiatric Intervention with Victims of Violence." *Topics in Emergency Medicine* 3 (March-April, 1982): 85-93.

Ferrarro, Kathleen. "Processing Battered Women." *Journal of Family Issues* 2 (December 1981): 415-38.

Finkelhor, David, Richard J. Gelles, Gerald T. Hotaling, and Murray A. Straus, eds. *The Dark Side of Families.* Beverly Hills, Calif. Sage Publications, 1983.

Finley, B. "Nursing Process with the Battered Woman." *Nurse Practitioner* 6 (July/August 1981): 11-13.

Fleming, Jennifer Baker. *Stopping Wife Abuse.* Garden City, N.Y.: Doubleday, Anchor Books, 1979.

Flynn, Janice, and Janice Whitcomb. "Unresolved Grief in Battered Women." *Journal of Emergency Nursing* 7 (November/December 1981): 250-54.

Flynn, John. "Recent Findings Related to Wife Abuse." *Social Casework* 63 (January 1977): 13-20.

Gaquin, Deirdre. "Spouse Abuse: Data from the National Crime Survey." *Victimology* 2 (Fall-Winter, 1977-78): 623-43.

Selected References

Gayford, J. J. "The Aetiology of Repeated Serious Physical Assaults by Husbands on Wives." *Medicine, Science, and the Law* 19 (January 1979): 19–24.

Gelles, Richard. "Power, Sex, and Violence: The Case of Marital Rape." *Family Coordinator* 26 (April 1977): 339–47.

———. "Violence and Pregnancy: A Note on the Extent of the Problem and Needed Services." *Family Coordinator* 24 (January 1975): 81–86.

———. "Violence in the Family: A Review of Research in the Seventies." *Journal of Marriage and the Family* 42 (November 1980): 873–85.

———. *The Violent Home*. Beverly Hills, Calif.: Sage Publications, 1972.

Goldberg, Wendy, and Anne Carey. "Domestic Violence Victims in the Emergency Setting." *Topics in Emergency Medicine* 3 (January 1982): 65–75.

Goode, William. "Force and Violence in the Family." *Journal of Marriage and the Family* 33 (November 1971): 624–36.

Green, Maurice R., ed. *Violence and the Family*. Boulder, Col.: Westview Press, 1980.

Gullattee, Alyce C. "Spousal Abuse." *Journal of the National Medical Association* 71, no. 4 (1981): 335–40.

Hanks, Susan E., and C. Peter Rosenbaum. "Battered Women: A Study of Women Who Live with Violent Alcohol-Abusing Men." *American Journal of Orthopsychiatry* 47 (April 1977): 291–306.

Heffner, Sarah. "Wife Abuse in West Germany." *Victimology* 2 (Fall-Winter, January 1977–78): 472–76.

Hendrix, Melva Jo. "Home is Where the Hell Is." *Family and Community Health* 4 (August 1981): 53–59.

Hendrix, Melva Jo, Gretchen E. LaGodna, and Cynthia A. Boben. "The Battered Wife." *American Journal of Nursing* 78 (April 1978): 648–53.

Heyman, Steven. "Dogmatism, Hostility, Aggression, and Gender Roles." *Journal of Clinical Psychology* 33 (July 1977): 694–98.

Hilberman, Elaine. "Overview: The 'Wife-beater's Wife' Reconsidered," *American Journal of Psychiatry* 137, no. 11 (1980): 1336–47.

Hilberman, Elaine, and Kit Munson. "Sixty Battered Women." *Victimology* 2 (Fall-Winter 1977–78): 460–470.

Hornung, Carlton A., B. Claire McCullough, and Taichi Sugimoto. "Status Relationships in Marriage: Risk Factors in Spouse Abuse." *Journal of Marriage and the Family* 43 (August 1981): 675–92.

Hosken, Fran P. "Female Circumcision in Africa." *Victimology* 2 (Fall-Winter, 1977–78): 487–98.

Houghton, B. D. "Domestic Violence Training: Treatment of Adult Victims of Family Violence." *Journal of the New York State Nurses Association* 12 (December 1981): 25–33.

Iyer, Patricia W. "The Battered Wife." *Nursing* 10 (September 1980): 52–55.

Janosik, Ellen Hastings, and Lenore Bolling Phipps. *Life Cycle Group Work in Nursing.* Monterey, Calif.: Wadsworth Health Sciences Division, 1982.

Janssen-Jurreit, Marielouise. *Sexism: The Male Monopoly on History and Thought,* trans. Verne Moberg. New York: Farrar, Straus & Giroux, 1982.

Kalmuss, Debra S., and Murray A. Straus. "Wife's Marital Dependency and Wife Abuse." *Journal of Marriage and the Family* 44, no. 2 (1982): 277-86.

Labell, Linda S. "Wife Abuse: A Sociological Study of Battered Women and Their Mates." *Victimology* 4 (1979): 258-67.

Landon, Julia. "Images of Violence Against Women." *Victimology* 2 (Fall-Winter, 1978): 510-24.

Langley, Roger, and Richard Levy. *Wife Beating: The Silent Crisis.* New York: E. P. Dutton, 1977.

Lester, David. "A Cross-Culture Study of Wife Abuse." *Aggressive Behavior* 6 (1980): 361-64.

Levinger, George. "Sources of Marital Dissatisfaction among Applicants for Divorce." *American Journal of Orthopsychiatry* 36 (October 1966): 803-807.

Lichtenstein, Violet R. "The Battered Woman: Guideline for Effective Nursing Intervention." *Issues in Mental Health Nursing* 3 (July-September 1981): 237-50.

Lieberknecht, K. "Helping the Battered Wife." *American Journal of Nursing* 78 (April 1978): 654-56.

Lystaad, Mary Hanemann. "Violence at Home: A Review of the Literature." *American Journal of Orthopsychiatry* 45 (April 1975): 328-45.

Mahon, Lisa. "Common Characteristics of Abused Women." *Issues in Mental Health Nursing* 3 (January-June 1981): 137-57.

Makepiece, James M. "Courtship Violence among College Students." *Family Relations* 30, no. 1 (1981): 97-102.

Martin, Del. *Battered Wives.* San Francisco: Glide Publications, 1976.

Martin, J. P., ed. *Violence and the Family.* Chichester: John Wiley & Sons, 1978.

Masumura, Wilfred T. "Wife Abuse and Other Forms of Aggression." *Victimology* 4 (1979): 46-59.

Moore, Donna, ed. *Battered Women.* Beverly Hills, Calif: Sage Publications, 1979.

NiCarthy, Ginny. *Getting Free.* Seattle: Seal Press, 1982.

O'Brien, John E. "Violence in Divorce Prone Families." *Journal of Marriage and the Family* 33 (November 1971): 692-98.

Pagelow, Mildred Daley. *Woman-Battering.* Beverly Hills, Calif.: Sage Publications, 1981.

———. "Factors Affecting Women's Decisions to Leave Violent Relationships." *Journal of Family Issues* 2 (December 1981): 391-414.

Peterson, Roger. "Social Class, Social Learning, and Wife Abuse." *Social Service Review* 54 (September 1980): 390-406.

Selected References

Pleck, Joseph H., and Jack Sawyer, eds. *Men and Masculinity.* Englewood Cliffs, N.J.: Prentice-Hall, 1974.

Renvoize, Jean. *Web of Violence.* London: Routledge & Kegan Paul, 1978.

Rounsaville, Bruce J. "Battered Wives: Barriers to Identification and Treatment." *American Journal of Orthopsychiatry* 48, no. 3 (1978): 487–99.

_____. "Theories in Marital Violence: Evidence from a Study of Battered Women." *Victimology* 3 (1978): 11–31.

Roy, Maria, ed. *Battered Women.* New York: Van Nostrand, 1977.

Sammons, Lucy N. "Battered and Pregnant." *Maternal Child Nursing* 6 (July-August 1981): 246–50.

Sandelowski, Margarete. *Women, Health, and Choice,* Englewood Cliffs, N.J.: Prentice-Hall, 1980.

Scott, P. D. "Battered Wives." *British Journal of Psychiatry* 125 (November 1974): 433–41.

Shainess, Natalie. "Vulnerability to Violence: Masochism as Process." *American Journal of Psychotherapy* 33 (April 1979): 174–89.

Shipley, S. B., and D. C. Sylvester. "Professionals' Attitudes toward Violence in Close Relationships." *Journal of Emergency Nursing* 8 (March-April 1982): 88–91.

Silverman, Phyllis R. *Helping Women Cope with Grief.* Beverly Hills, Calif.: Sage Publications, 1981.

Snell, John et al. "The Wifebeater's Wife." *Archives of General Psychiatry* 11, no. 2 (1964): 107–112.

Stark, Evan, Anne Flitcraft, and William Frazier. "Medicine and Patriarchal Violence: The Social Construction of a 'Private' Event." *International Journal of Health Services* 9 (1979): 461–93.

Star, Barbara. "Comparing Battered and Non-battered Women." *Victimology* 3, nos. 1–2 (1978): 32–44.

_____. "Patterns in Family Violence." *Social Casework: The Journal of Contemporary Social Work* 61 (June 1980): 339–47.

Steinmetz, Suzanne K. *The Cycle of Violence: Assertive, Aggressive and Abusive Family Interaction.* New York: Praeger Publishers, 1977.

_____. "Women and Violence: Victims and Perpetrators." *American Journal of Psychotherapy* 34, no. 3 (1980): 334–49.

Steinmetz, Suzanne K., and Murray A. Straus, eds. *Violence in the Family.* New York: Harper & Row, 1974.

Straus, Murray A., Richard J. Gelles, and Suzanne K. Steinmetz. *Behind Closed Doors: Violence in American Families.* New York: Doubleday, 1980.

Straus, Murray K., and Gerald T. Hotaling, eds. *Social Causes of Husband-Wife Violence.* Minneapolis: University of Minnesota Press, 1980.

Symonds, Alexandra. "Violence against Women—The Myth of Masochism." *American Journal of Psychotherapy* 33 (April 1979): 161–73.

Taylor, Stuart P., and Ian Smith. "Aggression as a Function of Sex of Victim and Male's Attitudes Toward Females." *Psychologial Reports* 35 (December 1974): 1095–98.

Toby, Jackson. "Violence and the Masculine Ideal: Some Qualitative Data." *Annals of the American Academy of Political and Social Sciences* 364 (March 1966): 19–28.

Tolson, Andrew. *The Limits of Masculinity*. New York: Harper & Row, 1977.

Ulbrich, Patricia, and Joan Huber. "Observing Parental Violence: Distribution and Effects." *Journal of Marriage and the Family* 43 (August 1981): 623–31.

Walker, Lenore. *The Battered Woman*. New York: Harper & Row, 1979.

———. "Battered Women: Sex Roles and Clinical Issues." *Professional Psychology* 12, no. 1)1981): 81–91.

Watts, Deborah L., and Christine A. Courtois. "Trends in the Treatment of Men Who Commit Violence Against Women." *Personnel and Guidance Journal* 60 (December 1981): 245–49.

Weinfourt, Rita. "Battered Women: The Grieving Process." *Journal of Psychiatric Nursing and Mental Health Services* 17 (April 1979): 40–47.

CHILD ABUSE

Berger, Audrey. "The Child Abusing Family: I. Methodological Issues and Parent-Related Characteristics of Abusing Families."*American Journal of Family Therapy* 8, no. 3 (Fall 1980): 53–66.

———. "The Child Abusing Family: II. Child and Child-Rearing Variables, Environmental Factors and Typologies of Abusing Families." *The American Journal of Family Therapy* 8, no. 4 (Winter 1980): 52–68.

Blum, Robert William, and Carol Runyan. "Adolescent Abuse: The Dimensions of the Problem." *Journal of Adolescent Health* 1, no. 2 (December 1980): 121–26.

Bolton, F. G., Jr., Roy H. Laner, and Sandra P. Kane. "Child Maltreatment Risk among Adolescent Mothers: A Study of Reported Cases." *American Journal of Orthopsychiatry* 50, no. 3 (July 1980): 489–504.

Bolton, F. G., Jr., Roy H. Laner, Dorothy S. Gai, and Sandra P. Kane. "The 'Study' of Child Maltreatment: When is Research . . . Research?" *Journal of Family Issues* 2, no. 4 (December 1981): 531–39.

Bremner, Robert H., ed. *Children and Youth in America: A Documentary History*, Vol. 1, 1600–1865. Cambridge: Harvard University Press, 1970.

———. *Children and Youth in America: A Documentary History*, Vol. 2, 1866-1932. Cambridge: Harvard University Press, 1970.

Selected References

Bush, Malcolm. "Institutions for Dependent and Neglected Children: Therapeutic Option of Choice or Last Resort?" *American Journal of Orthopsychiatry* 50 no. 2 (April 1980): 239-55.

Bybee, Rodger W., ed. "Violence Toward Youth in Families." *Journal of Social Issues* 35, no. 2 (1979).

Caffey, John. "Multiple Fractures in the Long Bones of Infants Suffering from Chronic Subdural Hematoma." *American Journal of Roentgenology, Radium Therapy, and Nuclear Medicine* 56 (1946): 163-73.

Carter, Bryan D., Ruth Reed, and Ceil J. Reh. "Mental Health Nursing Intervention with Child Abusing and Neglectful Mothers." *Journal of Psychiatric Nursing and Mental Health Services* 13, no. 5 (September/October 1975): 11-15.

Caulfield, Coleen, Mildred A. Disbrow, and Michelle Smith, "Determining Indicators of Potential for Child Abuse and Neglect: Analytical Problems in Methodological Research." In *Communicating Nursing Research.* Vol. 10, *Optimizing Environments for Health: Nursing's Unique Perspective,* edited by Marjorie V. Batey. Boulder: Western Interstate Commission for Higher Education, 1977, 141-62.

"Child Abuse and Neglect." *Victimology: An International Journal* 2, no. 2 (Summer 1977): 175-414.

Cook, Joanne Vliant, and Roy Tyler Bowles, eds. *Child Abuse: Commission and Omission.* Toronto: Butterworth & Co., 1980.

Corey, Eleanor J. Bullerdick, Carol L. Miller, and Frederick W. Widlak. "Factors Contributing to Child Abuse." *Nursing Research* 24, no. 4 (July-August 1975): 293-95.

Derdyn, Andre P. "A Case for Permanent Foster Placement of Dependent, Neglected, and Abused Children." *American Journal of Orthopsychiatry* 47 no. 4 (October 1977): 604-614.

Disbrow, M. A., H. Doerr, and C. Caulfield. "Measuring the Components of Parents' Potential for Child Abuse and Neglect." *Child Abuse and Neglect: The International Journal* 1 (1977): 279-96.

Elmer, Elizabeth. "A Follow-up Study of Traumatized Children." *Pediatrics* 59, no. 2 (February 1977): 273-79.

Finkelhor, David, Richard J. Gelles, Gerald T. Hotaling, and Murray A. Straus, eds. *The Dark Side of Families: Current Family Violence Research.* Beverly Hills: Sage Publications, 1983.

Garbarino, James. "The Human Ecology of Child Maltreatment: A Conceptual Model for Research." *Journal of Marriage and the Family* 39 no. 4 (November 1977): 721-35.

Garbarino, James, and Gwen Gilliam. *Understanding Abusive Families.* Lexington, Mass.: D.C. Heath & Company, Lexington Books, 1980.

Gelles, Richard J. "Violence toward Children in the United States." *American Journal of Orthopsychiatry* 48 no. 4 (October 1978): 580-592.

———. "Violence in the Family: A Review of Research in the Seventies." *Journal of Marriage and the Family* 42, no. 4 (November 1980): 873–85.

Gelles, Richard J. and Murray Straus. "Determinants of Violence in the Family: Toward a Theoretical Integration," In *Contemporary Theories About the Family*, Vol. 1, ed. Wesley R. Burr, Reuben Hill, F. Ivan Nye, and Ira Reiss. New York: Free Press, 1979.

Gil, David G. "Primary Prevention of Child Abuse: A Philosophical and Political Issue." *Psychiatric Opinion* 13, no. 2, (April 1976): 30–3.

———. "Violence Against Children." *Journal of Marriage and the Family* 32, no. 11 (November 1971): 637–48.

Giovannono, J., and A. Billingsley. "Child Neglect Among the Poor: A Study of Parental Inadequacy in Families of Three Ethnic Groups." *Child Welfare* 49 (1970): 196–204.

Heindl, M. Catherine, ed. *The Nursing Clinics of North America*. Philadelphia: W. B. Saunders Co., 1981, 16, no. 1.

Helfer, Ray E., and C. Henry Kempe, eds. *Child Abuse and Neglect: The Family and the Community*. Cambridge, Mass.: Harper & Row Publishers, Ballinger Publishing Co., 1976.

Helfer, Ray E., James K. Hoffmeister, and Carol Schneider. *MSPP: Michigan Screening Profile of Parenting*. Boulder: Test Analysis and Development Corp., 1978.

Helfer, Ray E. "The Etiology of Child Abuse." *Pediatrics* 51, no. 4 (April 1973): 777–79.

Kempe, C. Henry, Frederic Silverman, Brandt Steele, William Droegemueller, and Henry Silver. "The Battered Child Syndrome." *JAMA* 181, no. 1 (1962): 17–24.

Kempe, C. Henry, and Ray E. Helfer, eds. *The Battered Child*. 3d ed. Chicago: University of Chicago Press, 1980.

Korbin, Jill E., ed. *Child Abuse and Neglect: Cross-Cultural Perspectives*. Berkeley: University of California Press, 1981.

Leader's Manual: A Curriculum on Child Abuse and Neglect. Department of Health, Education, and Welfare, publication no. (OHDS) 79-30220, September 1979.

Martin, J. P. ed. *Violence and the Family*. Chichester: John Wiley & Sons, 1978.

Millor, Georgia Kemm. "A Theoretical Framework for Nursing Research in Child Abuse and Neglect." *Nursing Research* 30, no. 2 (March-April 1981): 78–83.

Morse, Abraham E., James N. Hyde, Eli H. Newberger, and Robert B. Reed. "Environmental Correlates of Pediatric Social Illness: Preventive Implications of an Advocacy Approach.", *American Journal of Public Health* 67, no. 7 (July 1977): 612–15.

National Analysis of Official Child Abuse and Neglect Reporting: 1977, Department of Health, Education, and Welfare, publication no. (OHDS) 79-30232, 1979.

O'Connor, Susan, Peter M. Vietze, Kathryn B. Sherrad, Howard M. Sandler, and William A. Altermeier III. "Reduced Incidence of Parenting Inadequacy Following Rooming-in." *Pediatrics* 66, no. 2 (August 1980): 176–82.

Selected References

Pelton, Leroy H. "Child Abuse and Neglect: The Myth of Classlessness." *American Journal of Orthopsychiatry* 48, no. 4 (October 1978): 608–17.

Richardson, Susan. "Abusive Parents and Their Nonabusive Partners." *Communicating Nursing Research*, Vol. 13, *Directions for the 1980s*. Boulder: Western Interstate Commission for Higher Education, 1980, p. 43.

Scharer, Kathleen. "Nursing Therapy with Abusive and Neglectful Families." *Journal of Psychiatric Nursing and Mental Health Services* 17, no. 8 (September 1979): 12–21.

Seaberg, James R. "Predictors of Injury Severity in Physical Child Abuse." *Journal of Social Service Research* 1, no. 1 (Fall 1977): 63–76.

Straus, Murray A., Richard J. Gelles, and Suzanne K. Steinmetz, *Behind Closed Doors: Violence in the American Family*. Garden City, N.Y.: Doubleday, 1980.

Walker, Wendy Fontaine. "Child-Rearing Experiences, Support Systems and Couple Cohesiveness as Antecedent Factors in Parent-Child Interaction in Child Abuse." *Communicating Nursing Research*. Vol. 12, *Credibility in Nursing Science*. Boulder: Western Interstate Commission for Higher Education, 1979, p. 29.

SEXUAL ABUSE

Armstrong, Louise. *Kiss Daddy Goodnight: A Speakout on Incest*. New York: Hawthorn Books, 1978.

Browning, Diane H., and Bonny Boatman. "Incest: Children at Risk." *American Journal of Psychiatry* 134 (1977): 69–72.

Burgess, Ann W., and Lynda L. Holmstrom. *Rape: Crisis and Recovery*. Bowie, Md.: Robert J. Brady, Co., 1979.

Burgess, Ann W., and Lynda L. Holmstrom. "Rape Trauma Syndrome." *American Journal of Psychiatry* 131 (1974): 981–86.

Burgess, Ann W., and Lynda L. Holmstrom. "Sexual Trauma of Children and Adolescents." *Nursing Clinics of North America* 10 (September 1975): 551–63.

Burgess, Ann W., Lynda L. Holmstrom, and Maureen P. McCausland. "Child Sexual Assault by a Family Member: Decisions Following Disclosure." *Victimology* 2 (1977): 236–50.

Burgess, Ann W., Nicholas A. Groth, Lynda L. Holmstrom, and Suzanne M. Sgroi. *Sexual Assault of Children and Adolescents*. Lexington, Mass.: D. C. Heath & Co., 1978.

DeMott, Benjamin. "Criminal Intimacies." *Psychology Today* 16, no. 8 (1977): 72–74.

Finkelhor, David. *Sexually Victimized Children*. New York: Free Press, 1979.

———. "What's Wrong with Sex between Adults and Children?" *American Journal of Orthopsychiatry* 49, no. 4 (1979): 692–97.

Finkelhor, David, and Kristi Yllo. "Forced Sex in Marriage." *Crime and Delinquency* 28, no. 3 (July 1982): 459-78.

Geis, Gilbert. "Rape in Marriage: Law and Law Reform in England, the United States, and Sweden." *Adelaide Law Review* (June 1978): 284-302.

Groth, A. Nicholas, Ann W. Burgess, and Lynda L. Holmstrom. "Power, Anger, and Sexuality." *American Journal of Psychiatry* 134 (1977): 1239-43.

Herman, Judith, and Lisa Hirschman. "Families at Risk for Father-Daughter Incest." *American Journal of Psychiatry* 138, no. 7 (July 1981): 967-70.

Lukianowicz, Nancy. "Incest I: Paternal Incest." *International Journal of Psychiatry* 120 (1972): 301-318.

Molnar, G., and P. Cameron. "Incest Syndromes: Observations in a General Hospital Psychiatric Unit." *Canadian Psychiatric Association Journal* 20 (1975): 373-77.

Peters, Joseph. "Child Rape: Defusing a Psychological Time Bomb." *Hospital Physician* 9, no. 46 (1973).

———. "Children Who Are Victims of Sexual Assault and the Psychology of Offenders." *American Journal of Psychotherapy* 30, no. 3 (1976): 398-421.

Russell, Diana R. *Rape in Marriage*. New York: MacMillan, 1982.

Schulman, J. "Expansion of the Marital Rape Exemption." *National Center on Women and Family Law Newsletter* (July 1980): 3-4.

Schultz, L. G., ed. *The Sexual Victimology of Youth*. Springfield, Ill.: Charles C. Thomas, 1979.

Sgroi, Suzanne M. "Sexual Molestation of Children: The Last Frontier in Child Abuse." *Children Today* 4, no. 44 (1975): 18-21.

Summit, Roland. "Recognition and Treatment of Child Sexual Abuse." In *Providing for the Emotional Health of the Pediatric Patient*, ed. C. E. Hollingsworth. New York: Spectrum, 1981.

Vaden, K. Amanda. *Betrayal*. Montgomery, Ala.: Preferred Healthstyles, 1982.

ELDERLY ABUSE

Block, Marilyn, and Jan D. Sinnott. *The Battered Elder Syndrome: An Exploratory Study*. College Park, Md.: Center on Aging, 1979.

Douglass, Richard, and Tom Hickey. "Domestic Abuse of the Elderly: Research Findings and a Systems Perspective for Service Delivery Planning." In *Abuse and Maltreatment of the Elderly: Causes and Intervention*, edited by Jordon Kosberg. Boston: John Wright, 1983.

Lau, Elizabeth, and Jordon Kosberg. "Abuse of the Elderly by Informal Care Providers." *Aging* (September/October, 1979): 10-15.

Selected References

Pedrick-Cornell, Claire, and Richard J. Gelles. "Elder Abuse: The Status of Current Knowledge." *Family Relations* 31 (1982): 457–65.

O'Malley, H. "Elder Abuse: A Review of the Literature." Boston: Legal Research and Services for the Elderly, 1979.

Rathbone-McCuan, E. "Elderly Victims of Family Violence and Neglect." *Social Casework* 61, no. 4 (1980): 296–304.

Steuer, J. and E. Austin. "Family Abuse of the Elderly." *Journal of the American Geriatrics Society* (August 1980): 372–76.

U. S. Department of Health and Human Services. *Elder Abuse.* Washington, D.C.: Administration on Aging, 1980.

Sengstock, Mary C., and Jersey Liang. *Identifying and Characterizing Elder Abuse.* Detroit: Institute of Gerontology, 1981.

Sengstock, Mary C., and Jersey Liang. "Domestic Abuse of the Aged: Assessing Some Dimensions of the Problem." In *Interdisciplinary Topics in Gerontology: Social Gerontology,* ed. Michael Kleiman. (New York: Karger, in press.)

Index

A

Abuse of female partners
  Advocacy, 272–273
  Alcohol, 86, 99
  Approaching battered women, 247–249
  Assessment, 249–257
  At risk indicators, 253–255, 256
  Batterer, 272; see also Machismo
  Child abuse, 88, 100, 219–220, 251, 252; see also Child abuse
  Control, 100–101
  Courts, 104, 273; see also Legal system
  Cultural attitudes, 91, 95, 97, 98
  Cycle of violence, 106
  Dating situations, 94, 101
  Definition, 75
  Denial, 107, 248, 264
  Depression, 105–106, 265
  Drug abuse, 86
  Emergency rooms, 75, 80, 354–355
  Emotional/psychological responses, 76, 250–251, 255, 264–265
  Evaluation of nursing care, 273–274
  Grieving, 263–265, 270
  Guns, 251; see also Guns
  Historical perspective, 81–84
  Health problem, 75–76
  History taking, 249–252, 253–255

Abuse of female partners (Contd.)
  Homicide, 78–80
  Housing, 273
  Incidence, 3, 80, 341–343
  Interventions, 258–273
    Assertiveness training, 261
    Groups, 268, 271
    Marriage counseling, 266
    Mental health, 260, 262, 264–265, 270–272
  Jealousy, 102–103, 261
  Laws, see Legal system
  Law enforcement, 341–358
  Learned helplessness, 105–106
  Machismo, see Machismo
  Marital Rape, 252
  Masochism, see Masochism
  Media, 259
  Myths, 104–105
    Masochism; see Masochism
  Nursing diagnosis, 255–257
  Physical exam, 252, 255, 256, 269
  Physical injuries, 75–76
    Care of, 269–70
    Documentation, 255, 354–355
  Physicians, 103
  Planning, 257
  Police, 104
  Poverty, 89

Index

Abuse of female partners (*Contd.*)
  Pregnancy, 81, 102, 262
  Prescribed medication, 81
  Prevention
    Primary, 258–261
    Secondary, 261–267
    Tertiary, 267–273
  Psychiatric
    Theories, 84–85
    Treatment, 81
  Psychological responses, 106–107
  Research issues, 84
  Sample nursing process, 275–278
  Self awareness, 249, 274
  Self-defense, 78
  Self esteem; *see* Self esteem
  Shelters, 104
    Nursing role in, 267–271, 412–413; *see also* Children of battered women
  Social isolation, 90
  Social learning theory, 87–88, 99
  Socialization, 342–343
  Societal response to victims, 103–104
  Socio-economic status, 89
  Strengths of battered women, 255–256, 269
  Stress, 88–90, 99
    Related symptoms, 76, 257, 266
  Television influence, 87
  Theories of causation, 84–94
  Unemployment, 89
Adolescence, 408
Adolescent abuse, 234
Adolescents
  Rape, 201
  Runaways, 192, 238, 319
Advocacy, 172–173, 230–231, 272–273; *see also* Elder abuse
Aggression
  Animals, 17–19
  Concept analysis, 14–15
  Definitions, 14–17, 29
  Frustration, 25, 33–34

Aggression (*Contd.*)
  Theoretical frameworks; *see also* Violence, theoretical frameworks
  Anthropology, 38–40; *see also* Culture
Assertiveness, 15, 261
Assessment, *see* Nursing Care
Attachment, 59

B

Bandura, A., 24, 29, 30, 31, 32
Bannon, J., 7, 104
Battered child syndrome, 123–124; *see also* Child abuse and neglect
Battered women, *see* Abuse of female partners
Blaming the victim, 414
Bowlby, J., 59
Burgess, A., 59, 93

C

Campbell, J., 79, 102, 412
Child Abuse; *see also* Child Abuse and Neglect
  Age, 121, 123
  Assessment, 121, 283–291
  At risk populations, 121
  Child characteristics, 121, 123, 131, 132, 136
  Corporal punishment, 125, 126, 130, 132, 136; *see also* Corporal punishment
  Culture, 127–128, 131, 136
  Definitions, 123–125
    Legal, 361
  Development, 133
  Evaluation, 305
  Gender differences, 121, 123
  History, 125–129, 283–289
  Incidence of, 3, 120
  Intervention, 292–305
  Laws, *see* Legal system

Child Abuse (*Contd.*)
  Medical perspective, 124, 129–130
  Nursing care, 382–313; *see also* Child abuse, Theoretical frameworks, Nursing frameworks
  Parent characteristics, 136–138
  Patterns of behavior, 136–138
  Physical examination, 290–291
  Plan, 291–292
  Prevention
    Primary, 293–298
    Secondary, 298–303
    Tertiary, 303–305
  Reporting mandate, 381–382
  Research, 120–121; *see also* Nursing research
  Sample nursing process, 306–313
  Socioeconomic status, 121, 122, 131
  Stress, 122, 123, 130–131, 132
  Theoretical frameworks
    Environmental-stress model, 130–131
    Human ecological model, 133–134
    Mental illness model, 129–130
    Nursing framework, 134–136
    Social learning models, 132–133
    Social-psychological models, 131–132
  Types, 123–125
  Wife abuse, connection with, 219–220
Child maltreatment, *see* Child abuse
Child neglect, *see* Child abuse
Children of battered women, *see also* Children of violent families
  Characteristics from research, 317–318
  Shelters, 317, 318, 327, 334
Children of violent families
  Adolescents, 238, 319, 322, 323
  Aggression, 317, 319
  Assessment, 321–327
  Assessment through play, 325–327
  Characteristics, 318–320
  Development, 318, 324, 325, 328, 332
  Developmental assessment, 324
  Developmental stimulation, 328–329
  Evaluation, 335–336
  History, 321–323

Children of violent families (*Contd.*)
  Identification, 318
  Infant temperament, 323
  Interaction with parents, 320
  Interventions, 328–335
    Behavioral, 334–335, 337–338
    Group, 332–334
    Play, 329–332
  Nursing diagnosis, 327
  Observation, 321–322, 327
  Physical
    Assessment, 324–325
    Symptoms, 319
  Plan/Goals, 328
  Role modeling, 320
  Role reversal, 319, 321
  Sample nursing process, 337–338
  Self esteem, 318, 324–327
  Speech, 325
  Social learning theory, 316–317, 324
  Stress, 317
  Trust establishment, 321–323
Childrearing
  Father involvement, 39
Confidentiality, *see* Legal system
Communication, 101, 266
Community health nursing, 81, 248, 263
Compulsive masculinity, *see* Machismo
Corporal punishment, 39–41, 218–219, 221, 232
  Legal concepts, 387–388, 391
Courts, *see* Legal system
Criminal Justice System, *see* Legal system and Law enforcement
Crisis Intervention, 234
Culture
  Abuse of female partners, 90–92, 97
  Nonviolent, 15–17, 24, 38–40, 95, 231
  Violence, 33, 36
Curtis, L., 34–35, 37–38, 98

D

Davidson, T., 82, 100
Denyes, M. J., 407

Index

Depression
  Battered women, 250-251
Dobash, R. E. & Dobash, R., 4, 8, 75, 77, 78, 81, 82, 83, 99, 101, 104, 105, 106
Domestic Violence, *see* Abuse of Female Partners, Child abuse, Elder Abuse, Family Violence
Drake, V., 75, 78, 80, 81, 106, 248, 261

E

Elder abuse
  Abuser characteristics, 153-156
  Agency services, 171
  Assessment, 174-180
  Demographic characteristics, 151-156
  Direct physical abuse, 147
  Emotional neglect, 147
  Evaluation, 182-183
  Family development, 163-167
  Financial abuse, 147
  Frequency, 147-151
  Gender, 151
  History, 177
  Identification, 168-171
  Intervention, 180-184
  Nursing care, 173-183
  Physical examination, 176
  Physical neglect, 147
  Prevention, 231
  Psychological/Emotional abuse, 147
  Race, 151
  Research, 173; *see also* Nursing research
  Socio-economic status, 151
  Theoretical frameworks
    Psychopathological, 157-158
    Situational stress, 158-160
    Social learning, 160-163
    Violation of rights, 147
Emergency room, 75, 80, 248, 262, 409-410
Emotional abuse, *see* Child abuse, Elder Abuse, Abuse of Female Partners

Erikson, E., 60
Evaluation, *see* Nursing care
Evidence, *see* Legal system
Expert Testimony, *see* Legal system

F

Failure to thrive, 286, 289
Family
  At risk, 192
  Communication, 222, 227
  Conflict resolution, 219, 221, 222, 227, 232
  Convoy, 56-60
  Definition, 405
  Development, 54, 56, 58, 59, 60, 163-167, 223
  Fit
    Person-environment, 65-68
    Resources and demands, 56
  Functioning, 8, 9, 54, 60, 61
  Functions, 226
  Genogram, 222, 226
  Help-seeking, 63-65
  Interaction, 54
  Myths, 146
  Networks, 56-58, 62-66
  Resources and demands, 56, 65-66
  Roles, 54, 59, 222, 227
  Strengths, 220
  Stress, 58, 63
  Structure, 54, 222
  Support systems, *see* support systems
  Systems framework, 54
  Unit of focus for nursing, 405
  Violent, 217-44; *see also* Violent family
Family therapy, 236-237
Family Violence
  Alcohol, 138
  Child abuse, 133; *see also* Child abuse
  Development, 133, 136-137
  Conceptual Model, 404-406
  Economy, impact of, 5-6
  Health problem, 3-4

Family Violence (*Contd.*)
  Law enforcement, 7–8; *see also* Law enforcement
  Medical model, 7–8
  Multidimensional problem, 6–7
  Nursing research, *see* Nursing Research
  Nursing, relevance to, 1, 4–7
  Prevention, 9
  Stress, 5
  Social work, 7–8
  Theoretical frameworks, 8
  Types, 1
Family well-being, 54–70, 224, 405
  Definition, 65–67
  Dimensions, 55, 65–67
  Violence, and, 55, 56, 67–69
Feetham, S., 61, 226
Feminism, 92, 348
Freud, S., 24, 85, 196–8; *see also* Psychoanalytic theory
Fromm, E., 27, 38

G

Gender differences, *see* Machismo, Violence, Gender differences
Gelles, R., 3, 21, 76, 77, 80, 86, 88, 101, 120, 122, 124, 130, 132, 148, 161, 168, 218, 219, 252, 266, 410, 411
Gil, D., 33, 123, 125, 297, 298
Goode, W., 99–100, 101
Group Therapy, *see* Nursing care, Abused Children, Battered Women, Rape Victims, Children of Battered Women
Guns, 37, 96, 225, 230

H

Health
  Definition, 405–406
Helfer, R., 121, 124, 131, 132

Homicide, 33, 35–38, 40, 77–80, 96–97, 148, 230, 347–348
  Female partners, 79
  Incidence, 14
  Self defense plea, 347–348, 377
Humphreys, J., 412

I

Intervention, *see* Nursing Care

K

Kempe, C., 121, 123–124, 129, 131–132
Kinlein, M., 250

L

Laws; *see* Legal system
Law Enforcement
  Abused women, 341–358
    Arrest of Abuser, 344, 350, 351
    Culture, 343
    Dispatch, 344, 346
    Dropping charges, 346, 348
    History, 343–354
    Homicide, 347
    Injuries to police, 342
    Involvement, 341–343
    Legislation, 353
    Nursing, interface with, 354–357
    "Peace Bond", 346, 375
    Police Training, 350, 351–352
    Policy and procedure, 344, 348, 349, 351
    Police as mediators, 349–351
    Prosecution, 344
    Reporting to police, 354–355, 356
    Self defense, 347–348
    Socio-economic status, 342
    Traditional police response, 343–347
    Weapons, 346–347

Index

Law Enforcement (*Contd.*)
  Child abuse, 360-369
    Arrest, 368
    Detection, 367-368
    Evidence, 367-368
    Nursing, interface with, 366-367
    Police entry into homes, 363
    Police investigation, 362, 363-365
    Police officer role, 363
    Reporting mandate, 361-362
    Search warrant, 363
    Sexual abuse, 365-366
Legal System
  Abuse of Female Partners, 344, 371-381
    Attrition of cases, 374
    Civil proceedings, 372, 375
    Confidentiality, 380
    Criminal Law, 372-374, 376-377
    Evidence, 378-379
      Preservation, 356-357
    Expert testimony, 381
    Filing charges, 374
    Hearsay, 378-379
    Historical precedents, 373
    Homicide, 377
    Inequities in laws, 371, 373, 374, 376
    Laws, 372-374, 375, 376
    Legal concept of wife abuse, 371
    Marital rape, 376
    Marriage contract, 373
    Medical record, 379-380
    Nursing, interface with, 378-381
    "Peace bonds", 346, 375
    Prosecution, 374-375, 377-378
    Protection order, 375
    Testimony, Nursing
  Child abuse, 385-401
    Adjucation hearing, 392
    Child welfare laws, 391-392
    Corporal punishment, 387-388, 391
    Court interventions, 392
    Criminal law, 389-391
    Cross examination, 399-400

Legal System (*Contd.*)
    Custody, 383
    Dispositional hearing, 392-393
    Evidence, 393, 396-399
    Expert testimony, 400-401
    Foster care, 386-393
    Hearsay, 397
    Historical precedent, 385-387
    Illegitimacy, 386
    Infanticide, 385-386
    Juvenile court, 382-383, 396
    Legal concept of child abuse, 385
    Medical record, 397-398
    Nursing, interface with, 393-400
    Nursing responsibility to report, 393-396
    Poverty, 390
    Probation, 390-391
    Prosecution, 389-391
    Protective services, 393-394
    Reporting laws, 389, 393-394, 395
    Subpoena, 399
    Testimony, nursing, 398-400

M

Machismo, 38, 40, 41, 85, 88, 90, 91, 94-103, 105, 196, 260, 343
  Abuse of female partners, 99-100
  Characteristics, 96
  Culture, 95, 98-99
  Definition, 96
  Guns, 96
  Homicide, 97
  Jealousy, 102
  Powerlessness, 99-100
  Socialization, for, 95-96
Martin, D., 79
Media
  Abuse of female partners, 87, 99
  Violent family, 133, 230
Medical record as legal document; *see* Legal system
Megargee, E., 26

Meister, S., 61, 66, 405
Millor, G., 134-136
Moyer, K., 15, 18, 19, 25

N

Newberger, E., 6, 124, 284, 299
Nursing
    Autonomy, 414
    Conceptual model of family violence, 404-406
    Community health, 394, 395
    Family as unit of focus, 405
    Female profession, 414
    Maternal-child health, 81
    Battered women, 247-274; *see also* Abuse of female partners, Assessment, Nursing diagnosis, Interventions, Planning, Evaluation
        Emergency room, *see* Emergency room
Nursing care
    Abuse of female partners, 258-278; *see also* Abuse of female partners; assessment, intervention, evaluation
    Child abuse, 282-313; *see also* Child abuse; assessment, intervention, evaluation
    Community health, 226, 231
    Elder abuse, 173-183; *see also* Elder abuse; assessment, intervention, evaluation
    Group Interventions, 205-211
    Sexual abuse, 205-211
    Violent Family, 220-244; *see also* Family, violent; assessment, nursing diagnosis, intervention, evaluation
Nursing education
    Affective domain, 413-414
    Course in family violence, 414-417
    Family violence, 413-417
Nursing perspective, 7
Nursing practice, 411-413
Nursing research, 408-411
    Family violence, 409-411

Nursing research (*Contd.*)
    Need for, 7-8; *see also* Family violence; Nursing research
    Research questions, 411
Nursing theory
    Application, 407
    Family violence, 406-407

O

Order of protection, *see* Legal system
Orem, D., 407

P

Pagelow, M., 88, 107, 108, 194
Patriarchy, *see* Women, status
Pelton, L., 122
Police, *see* Law enforcement
Pornography, 98, 193, 259
Poverty, 414
    Abuse of female partners, 89
    Violence, 34-36
Pregnancy
    Battering during, 81
Prevention, *see* Abuse of female partners, Child abuse, Elder abuse, Sexual abuse, Violent family
Protection order, *see* Legal system
Protective services, 235, 362, 364, 393, 394
Psychological abuse, *see* Child abuse, Abuse of female partners, Elder abuse
Psychoanalytic theory
    Sexual abuse, 196, 198, 199, 203
    Violence, 25-28
Psychoanalytic viewpoints
    Abuse of female partners, 85
Psychosomatic disorders, *see* Stress, related symptoms

R

Rape, *see also* sexual abuse
    Conjugal, 103

Index

Rape (*Contd.*)
    Marital, 252, 376
    Nursing attitude toward victims, 416–417
Research
    Family violence, 409–411
Roles
    Family, 54, 59, 222
Russell, D., 190, 194

S

Sandelowski, M., 92
Self-awareness, 220, 227, 282–283
Self-care, 407
Self esteem
    Battered women, 106–107, 255
    Children of violent families, 318, 324–325, 326–327
    Incest victim, 205–207
    Theories of violence, 28
Sengstock, M., 146
Sex roles, 40
Sexual abuse, 190–211; *see also* Child abuse, Abuse of Female Partners
    Adolescents, 234
    Attitudes about, 192, 203
    Children (non-incestual), 193, 200–201
    Emotional response, 202–204
    History, 195
    Incest, 191–192, 197–201, 225
        Definition, 192
        Incidence, 192
    Myths, 195–197
    Nursing care, 205–211
    Physiological response, 202
    Power dynamics, 190, 193, 199, 200, 201
    Rape, 193, 194–197, 199–200, 201–202
    Rape of spouse, 194
    Rape trauma syndrome, 201–202
    Self esteem, 202, 205, 207, 209
    Theoretical frameworks, 194–201
    Victim response, 201–205
Shelter, *see* Abuse of female partners

Siblings of abused children, *see* children of violent families
Social learning theory, *see* Abuse of female partners, child abuse, children of violent families, elder abuse
Social networks, 57–58; *see also* Family; network
Social support
    Family, 61–63, 66, 90, 223, 233; *see also* Family
Socio-economic status
    Violence, 35, 38
    Family, 68
Spouse abuse, *see* Abuse of female partners
Support systems, 234
Stark, E., 4, 75, 103
Steinmetz, S., 3, 14, 76–77, 80, 87, 90, 99, 130, 132, 146, 148, 161, 219, 224, 252
Straus, M., 2, 14, 76, 80, 90, 91, 99, 124, 129, 130, 132, 146, 148, 161, 218, 219, 225, 252
Stress
    Family, 223, 233
    Related symptoms, 202
Suicide, 202, 224
    Battered women, 107, 255

T

Television, *see* Media
Toch, H., 28

U

Unemployment, 35, 89

V

Victim
    Blame, 37, 105, 202
    Definition, 2

Victim (*Contd.*)
  Incest, response to, 203–205
  Rape, response to, 201–203
Violence
  Attitudes, 15, 16, 30, 33, 218
  Alcohol, 20–22
  Anthropology, 16; *see also* Culture
  Brain disorders, 22–23
  Concept analysis, 15–16
  Definition, 1, 15
  Episodic dyscontrol, 23–24
  Family, *see* Family violence
  Gender differences, 24, 37
  Heredity, 22
  History, 16
  Hormones, 19, 20, 21, 23
  Incidence, 2–4
  Inter-generational transmission, 132, 133, 136
  Limbic system, 19, 22
  Machismo, 96–98; *see also* Machismo
  Media, 30–31; *see also* Media
  Poverty, *see* Poverty
  Race, 34–37
  Roles, 38
  Socio-economic status, *see* socio-economic status
  Subculture, 36–38, 97
  Theoretical frameworks, 17–41
    Instinctivist, 17, 18
    Neurophysiological, 18–24
    Psychological, 24–29; *see also* Psychoanalytic theory
    Social learning, 23, 29–32
    Sociological, 32–38
  Unemployment; *see* Unemployment
Violence against women, 92–94
  Genital mutilation, 93
  Historical forms, 92
Violent Family
  Assessment, 220–228
  At risk characteristics, 221, 222–224, 232

Violent Family (*Contd.*)
  Children, *see* Children of violent families
  Communication, 222, 227, 233
  Conflict resolution, 219, 221, 222, 227, 232
  Crisis intervention, 234
  Definition, 217
  Evaluation, 238–239
  History, 221–225
  Intergenerational transmission, 153, 161, 218–219
  Interventions, 229–238
    Courts, 237
  Nursing diagnosis, 228
  Physical assessment, 226–227
  Plan/goal, 228–229
  Prevention
    Primary, 229–231
    Secondary, 233–237
    Tertiary, 237–239
  Referrals, 235, 238
  Roles, 222, 227
  Sample nursing process, 239–243
  Sibling fighting, 224–225
  Social learning theory, 218–219
  Stress; *see* Stress
  Wife abuse and child abuse connection, 219–220

W

Walker, L., 77, 78, 79, 85, 86, 88, 101, 102–107, 263
Well-being, *see* Family, Well-being
Wife abuse, *see* Abuse of female partners
Wolfgang, M., 16, 33, 36, 78, 148
Women
  Identity formation, 206, 208
  Status, 39–40, 41, 92, 95, 203
  Violence against, 39–41; *see also* Abuse of female partners, Sexual abuse